BASICS IN ADOLESCENT MEDICINE

A Practical Manual of Signs, Symptoms and Solutions

BASICS IN ADOLESCENT MEDICINE

A Practical Manual of Signs, Symptoms and Solutions

Tomas J. Silber
Children's National Medical Center

Harshita J. Saxena
Walter Reed National Military Medical Center

editors

World Scientific

NEW JERSEY • LONDON • SINGAPORE • BEIJING • SHANGHAI • HONG KONG • TAIPEI • CHENNAI

Published by

World Scientific Publishing Co. Pte. Ltd.
5 Toh Tuck Link, Singapore 596224
USA office: 27 Warren Street, Suite 401-402, Hackensack, NJ 07601
UK office: 57 Shelton Street, Covent Garden, London WC2H 9HE

Library of Congress Cataloging-in-Publication Data
Basics in adolescent medicine : a practical manual of signs, symptoms, and solutions / edited by Tomas Silber, Harshita Saxena.
p. ; cm.
Includes bibliographical references.
ISBN 978-9814329538 (hardcover : alk. paper)
I. Silber, Tomas J. II. Saxena, Harshita.
[DNLM: 1. Adolescent Medicine--methods. 2. Signs and Symptoms. WS 460]

616.00835--dc23

2012046459

British Library Cataloguing-in-Publication Data
A catalogue record for this book is available from the British Library.

Typeset by Stallion Press
Email: enquiries@stallionpress.com

Printed in Singapore by World Scientific Printers.

To Rosita, for her love, companionship and half a century of patience, the family that sprung from us and the teenagers we were.

— Tomas J. Silber

To my mom — always on my mind, forever in my heart.

— Harshita J. Saxena

CONTENTS

AUTHOR CONTRIBUTORS

Anisha Abraham, MD, MPH
Honorary Associate Professor
Department of Pediatrics
Prince of Wales Hospital
Clinical Consultant
J.C. School of Public Health and Primary Care
Chinese University of Hong Kong
Shatin, N.T., Hong Kong

Anthony P. Acquavella, MS, MD, MPH, FAAP, FSAHM
Associate Professor
The University of the Sciences
Medical Director
Graduate Physician Assistant Program
Philadelphia, PA

Stephanie Addison, MD
Assistant Professor of Pediatrics
Pediatrics and Adolescent Medicine
Emory University
Atlanta, GA

Promise Ahlstrom, MD
Pediatrics and Adolescent Medicine
Chevy Chase Pediatrics
Washington, DC

William M. Barnes, PhD, MBA
Executive Director of Community Support Services
Children's National Medical Center
Washington, DC

Karen Bernstein, MD, MPH
Director, Division of Adolescent Medicine
Advocate Children's Hospital
Park Ridge, IL

Brooke Bokor, MD, MPH
Assistant Professor of Pediatrics
The George Washington University School of Medicine & Health Sciences
Associate Director
Adolescent Medicine Fellowship Program
Children's National Medical Center
Washington, DC

Jose J. Casas-Rivero, MD, PhD
Adolescent Medicine
Hospital Universitario La Paz
Madrid, Spain

Elizabeth G. Cius, MD
Clinical Associate
Division of Adolescent Medicine
Children's National Medical Center
Washington, DC

Liana R. Clark, MD, MSCE
Medical Director Adolescent Vaccines
Global Medical Affairs and Policy
Health Engagement & Customer Value
Merck Vaccines
West Point, PA

Nailah Coleman, MD, FAAP, FACSM
Attending
Goldberg Center for Community Pediatric Health
Children's National Medical Center
Washington, DC

Lawrence J. D'Angelo, MD, MPH
Professor, Pediatrics, Medicine, Epidemiology and Prevention and Community Health
The George Washington University School of Medicine & Health Sciences
Chief, Division of Adolescent and Young Adult Medicine
Children's National Medical Center
Washington, DC

Daniel N. Davidow, MD
Associate Clinical Professor
Medical College of Virginia-Virginia Commonwealth University
Medical Director
Cumberland Hospital for Children and Adolescents
New Kent, VA

Sadhana Dharmapuri, MD
Assistant Professor
Division of Adolescent Medicine
Medical College of Wisconsin
Milwaukee, WI

Evelyn Simpkins Evans, MD, FAAP
Director of Adolescent Medicine Clinic
Selma Pediatrics
Selma, AL

Jonathan Fanburg, MD, MPH
Pediatrics and Adolescent Medicine
Maine Medical Partners — Pediatrics
MaineHealth
Portland, ME

Isabel Goldenberg, MD
Medical Director
Student Health Service
The George Washington University
Washington, DC

Rita Hagler, BSN, MSN, CPNP
Division of Adolescent Medicine
Children's National Medical Center
Washington, DC

Kirsten B. Hawkins, MD, MPH, FAAP
Assistant Professor of Clinical Pediatrics
Georgetown University School of Medicine
Chief, Section Adolescent Medicine
MedStar Georgetown University Hospital
Washington, DC

Leslie A. Hayes, MD, FAAP
Director of Adolescent Medicine Services
Department of Pediatrics
Brooklyn Hospital
Brooklyn, NY

Nneka A. Holder, MD, MPH
Assistant Professor
Northeast Ohio Medical University
Attending Physician
Adolescent Medicine
Akron Children's Hospital
Akron, OH

Avril Melissa Houston, MD, MPH, FAAP
Chief Medical Officer
Rockville, MD

Mariana Kastrinakis, MD, MPH
The George Washington University School of Medicine & Health Sciences

Amy E. Klamberg, NP, CPNP-PC
Division of Adolescent Medicine
Children's National Medical Center
Washington, DC

Daniel E. Korin, MD
Pediatric Attending
Pediatrics 2000
New York, NY

Dana Kornfeld, MD, FAAP
Clinical Associate Professor
The George Washington University School of Medicine & Health Sciences
Physician, Pediatric and Adolescent Care Center
Bethesda, MD

Michael A. Lee, MD
Assistant Clinical Professor
Yale University
Director Concussion Center
CCMC, Fairfield Connecticut Branch
Southport, CT

Maureen E. Lyon, PhD, ABPP
Associate Research Professor in Pediatrics
The George Washington University School of Medicine & Health Sciences
Clinical Health Psychologist
Children's National Medical Center
Washington, DC

Jennifer Maehr, MD, FAAP
Medical Director
Maryland Department of Juvenile Services
Baltimore, MD

Donna Marschall, PhD
Assistant Professor of Psychiatry and Behavioral Sciences & Pediatrics
The George Washington University School of Medicine & Health Sciences
Director, HIV Services Mental Health Program
Children's National Medical Center
Washington, DC

Tiffany L. Meyer, MD, MPH
Medical Director
Nova Pediatrics
Springfield, VA

Robyn Miller
Senior Fellow
Division of Adolescent Medicine
Children's National Medical Center
Washington, DC

Gregg Joseph Montalto, MD, FAAP
Assistant Professor of Pediatrics
Uniformed Services of the Health Sciences

Alan Morrison, DO, FACP
Assistant Clinical Professor of Medicine
The George Washington University School of Medicine and Health Sciences
Internal Medicine for Adults and Adolescents
Washington, DC

Rosina Pellerano, MD
Medical Management of Eating Disorders
Miami, FL

Noel V. Pesce, MD, FAAP
Pediatrics and Adolescent Medicine
Pediatric Associates of Montgomery County
Wheaton, MD

Rick Place, MD
Associate Clinical Professor of Emergency Medicine
The George Washington University School of Medicine and Health Sciences
Pediatric Medical Director
Department of Emergency Medicine
Inova Fairfax Hospital for Children
Falls Church, VA

David S. Reitman, MD, MBA
Assistant Professor and Attending in Adolescent Medicine
Georgetown University Hospital
Washington, DC

Karen Rosewater, MD, MPH
Clinical Instructor of Pediatrics
Mount Sinai Medical Center
Adolescent-Young Adult Medicine (AYAM) of NYC
New York, NY

Harshita J. Saxena, MD
Department of Pediatrics
Division of Adolescent Medicine
Walter Reed National Military Medical Center
Bethesda, MD

Natwarlal Shah, MD, FAAP
Pediatrics and Adolescent Medicine

Tomas Silber, MD, MASS
Professor of Pediatrics
The George Washington University School of Medicine & Health Sciences
Director, Adolescent Medicine Fellowship
Children's National Medical Center
Washington, DC

Karen E. Simpson, MD, FAAP
Pediatrics and Adolescent Medicine
Baton Rouge, LA

Barbara K. Snyder, MD
Chief, Adolescent Medicine
Department of Pediatrics
Rutgers Robert Wood Johnson Medical School
New Brunswick, NJ

Karen Soren, MD
Associate Professor of Pediatrics and Population and Family Health
Columbia University Medical Center
Director, Adolescent Medicine
New York-Presbyterian Morgan Stanley Children's Hospital
New York, NY

Oscar Taube, MD
Assistant Professor of Pediatrics
University of Maryland School Of Medicine
Coordinator, Adolescent Medicine
The Herman and Walter Samuelson Children's Hospital at Sinai
Sinai Hospital
Baltimore, MD

Carleen Townsend-Akpan, NP, CPNP-PC
Division of Adolescent and Young Adult Medicine
Children's National Medical Center
Washington, DC

Maria Trent, MD, MPH, FAAP, FSAHM
Associate Professor of Pediatrics
Director, Adolescent Medicine Fellowship Program
Johns Hopkins School of Medicine
Baltimore, MD

Amy L. Weiss, MD, MPH
Assistant Professor of Pediatrics and Adolescent Medicine
Division of Adolescent Medicine
University of South Florida
Tampa, FL

Krishna White, MD, MPH
Clinical Assistant Professor
Thomas Jefferson University
Director, Adolescent Medicine Program
Nemours/A.I. duPont Hospital for Children
Wilmington, DE
Philadelphia, PA

Michele D. Wilson, MD
Clinical Associate Professor of Pediatrics
University of Pennsylvania School of Medicine
Attending Physician
Children's Hospital of Philadelphia Cobbs Creek Care Network
Philadelphia, PA

Erin Wolf-Barnett, MS, RD, LD
Registered Dietitian
CenteRD Nutrition, LLC
Rockville, MD

Kathy Woodward, MD
Director of In-Patient and Community Health Services
Division of Adolescent and Young Adult Medicine
Children's National Medical Center
Washington, DC

FOREWORD

As a pediatric clinician-educator with a long time investment in medical education, I always look for what is evidence-based or best practice when I review curricula or scholarly works. So, when the co-editors asked me to provide a foreword to introduce their book, I approached the task by seeking the answer to 3 questions:

1) Why another book on Adolescent Medicine?
2) What adult learning principles are imbedded in the text?
3) What is the credibility of the co-editors and contributors?

Why another book on Adolescent Medicine?

Excellent texts have been published: what is different about this one? I will enumerate what makes this book so unique and why it would be an important addition in anyone's library, personal or hospital/medical school.

- It is aimed at a targeted audience of practicing generalists, physician extenders and trainees at the undergraduate and graduate levels who interact with adolescent patients in the ambulatory and inpatient settings. This book is therefore directed to adult learners who expect to quickly access chunks of critical information around the common problems they will be seeing.
- The goal is to facilitate discerning diagnoses and treatment plans in an expedited manner without having to leaf through extended texts or many computer pages. Hence the format is ideal for primary care physicians, physician extenders, residents and students who seek succinct approaches to a variety of adolescent problems at the point of care setting; i.e., those who provide care in the office setting will especially benefit by the problem oriented structure of this handbook.

- The editors have organized chapters the way physicians think; i.e., they are problem-based (e.g., menstrual disorders). Each chapter begins with a "Test your knowledge question" that allows the reader to gauge what they may know about the subject matter, followed by a short clinical scenario, thereby activating readers to be thinking about what is to follow.
- The co-editors selected a format that eschews providing extensive overviews of every single topic in adolescent medicine, as most texts do that very well, but instead chose to highlight the basic assessment, diagnostic, and treatment principles of common adolescent problems. A caregiver can rapidly access information (the average reading time for each section is 2 to 4 minutes) while the patient waits for that individual to relate the diagnosis and plan.

How does the book encourage adult learning and higher level thinking?

- By all authors systematically highlighting those key aspects germane to the presenting problem, like what questions to ask, what to look for on the physical examination and which are the appropriate lab tests and imaging studies, they are motivating learners by encouraging them to think about the problem and treatment plan proactively. This differs from just reading text in a passive manner.
- Another technique is creating chapters that contain summarizing tables, allowing for easy and succinct visualization of problems. This models the way physicians think; i.e., at higher cognitive levels and not just through memorizing knowledge.
- Asking "What is different in adolescence" is probably the most valuable component in every chapter, calling attention to how clinical manifestations and management may be different for teenagers than what is seen in other age groups. Again, this encourages the learner to compare their previous knowledge and experiences with what they have to know about adolescents.
- The editors have encouraged readers to be reflective and to self-assess by placing at the end of each chapter the detailed answers to the multiple choice questions that tested the readers knowledge. This is also a good exercise for those that want to prepare themselves for the various Board Examinations, as the latter increasingly contain questions pertaining to the medical care of adolescents.

- To promote continual professional development, the editors have not included exhaustive references as comprehensive texts do, but have provided link web references and resources with each chapter. This approach is more compatible with how adult learners in general and *millennials* in particular, access information.

What is the credibility of the educators?

- The editors of this volume, Drs. Tomas J. Silber and Harshita J. Saxena, have created a point-of-care handbook that offers an approach other than what currently available texts do. This is no coincidence as this idea emanated from years of educating future caregivers in adolescent medicine. The Division of Adolescent Medicine at Children's National Medical Center (CNMC), among the first programs of its kind in the United States, is celebrating its 50th anniversary this year and has a long history of excellence in the field.
- Quite unique about the handbook is that the contributing authors are either former or current faculty, former or current fellows in adolescent medicine at CNMC and/or former pediatric residents who rotated through the adolescent service and went on to specialize in Adolescent Medicine. They all show a professional culture.
- Having former trainees as contributing authors is a testimony to the outstanding training these fellows and residents received at CNMC and to their ongoing commitment to the healthcare of adolescent patients all over the country and world. The breadth and depth of former trainee experiences and leadership abilities in the field brings further credibility regarding author expertise.
- As the senior editor, Dr. Silber is internationally known, having been awarded both the recognition award for outstanding achievement in adolescent health by the Society for Adolescent Health and Medicine as well as the Adele Hoffman Award by the Section on Adolescent Health of the American Academy of Pediatrics. In his decade as director of the Adolescent Medicine Fellowship Program at Children's National, he has been a devoted clinician-educator, advocate, mentor, teacher and researcher. It was his vision that was the impetus for the handbook.
- Dr. Saxena is a second generation graduate of the Adolescent Medicine Program at Children's National, her mother having completed the same fellowship with Dr Silber before her. She has demonstrated in this handbook

not only her professional standing, but also a special gift for organization and writing, enabling this multiple-authored text to coalesce and at the same time convey its contemporary electronic media feel. Moreover, having been in charge of the Adolescent Medicine medical student and resident rotations at Children's National, she has brought to the organization of these pages her thought and caring teaching expertise, collaborating with Dr Silber in the ongoing and insightful feedback that unified all contributions.

In summary, this book makes a significant and unique contribution to the adolescent literature because:

1) It offers content and resources not as rapidly and readily accessible in other works on adolescent medicine, and
2) Does this without sacrificing science and evidence-based knowledge.
3) Adult learners will enjoy how the handbook content melds with adolescent patients they see each day.

Larrie Greenberg, M.D.
Internal consultant, Faculty Development
Clinical Professor, Pediatrics
The George Washington University School of Medicine
Washington, DC
mcalwg@gwumc.edu

PREFACE

For whom is Basics in Adolescent Medicine written?

- For those interested in rapidly accessible, practical and updated information to successfully approach the medical care of teens.
- The handbook is ideal for the busy clinician who likes to have "at hand" a symptom based review that provides quick access to the knowledge they need in real time with tips to update their skills.
- The handbook format can also serve as a stimulating and reassuring introduction for medical students and residents on their first Adolescent Medicine rotation, allowing them to rapidly orient to the medical needs of adolescents, their most common illnesses and their unexpected emergencies.

What is the Content of Basics in Adolescent Medicine?

The handbook is divided into five sections:

- Section 1 develops an approach to the adolescent "**well visit**," covering topics ranging from routine screening, vaccinations and anticipatory guidance.
- Section 2 instructs on how to manage **common patient concerns**, ranging from the predictable teen visit for acne and gynecomastia to the more worrisome patients with multiple somatic complaints and eating disorders.
- Section 3 addresses the **reproductive health care of teens**, from the management of sexually transmitted infections to preventive services such as contraceptive counseling.
- Section 4 focuses on **urgent and emergency situations** with which teenagers can unexpectedly arrive at the office, ranging from testicular torsion to a slipped capital femoral epiphysis.
- Section 5 expands on **special circumstances** ranging from the management of the chronically ill adolescent to the use of psychopharmacology.

How is Basics in Adolescent Medicine organized:

- This volume is practitioner centered, focusing on the symptoms that bring the teen to the clinician. It provides this information through 69 concise chapters, with over 100 tables and figures to focus the reader on most salient points. Rather than a rapidly aging bibliography, BAM provides a wide array of responsible web references and resources for quick access to information.
- Each chapter highlights the approach to the presenting symptom (differential diagnosis), how to investigate it (history, physical, laboratory and imaging), how to treat and when to refer (disposition). A unique feature of each chapter includes a section on what is *unique to adolescents* as opposed to adults or children seen for similar complaints.
- Knowledge is tested at the start of each chapter with over 100 multiple choice questions, with detailed answers included at the end of each chapter.

Who has written Basics in Adolescent Medicine?

- This is the work of a team of experts, Adolescent Medicine Teaching Faculty and Subspecialists, who have either taught or trained at the Division of Adolescent and Young Adult Medicine at Children's National Medical Center. This textbook is being published on the occasion of celebrating half a century of educating and training in the medical care of adolescents at Children's National Medical Center.
- The editors of BAM are the Director of the Children's National Adolescent Medicine Fellowship Program (TJS) and the Former Director of Education for Residents and Medical Students (HS).

Enjoy taking care of adolescents and get ahead with BAM!

Tomas J. Silber, MD, MASS and Harshita J. Saxena, MD

ACKNOWLEDGEMENTS

Children's National Medical Center opened the first Adolescent Inpatient Unit in 1959, using for that purpose the former Polio Ward which was mercifully no longer needed. Not long thereafter, the patients seen in follow up and newcomers were taken care of in an "Adolescent Clinic." By 1964 an Adolescent Medicine Fellowship Program was established and has since graduated many leaders in the field nationally and internationally.

The physician contributors to this volume have either completed their Pediatrics residency training at Children's National, are graduates from the Fellowship Program in Adolescent Medicine, or faculty in the Division of Adolescent and Young Adult Medicine (and some have done all three). All have participated in a culture of intense clinical work with teens, self-propelled learning and devotion to teaching. Moreover the multidisciplinary contributors have all worked under the leadership of a Children's National alumni and hence partaken of that spirit. While it takes a village to raise a child it takes a mission to pass the adolescent medicine torch to successive generations of practitioners. This mission has been nourished by Children's National and that is why this place of encouragement and academic pursuit is so prominent in our collective acknowledgement.

This volume has been a response to the many students, rotating residents from pediatrics, internal medicine and family medicine and the occasional practitioner who wanted to "refresh" their adolescent medicine knowledge. As we provided them with information and articles, we found the resources to guide them through a medical problem to be limited. The editors are grateful for their questions and desire to learn in a practical way. This stimulated us to think about the format of this book and led to multiple exchanges with all our contributors, whom we would have liked to acknowledge individually but that would take another book. Instead we thank them here: for putting up with innumerable calls and e-mails as we streamlined chapters and developed the multiple choice questions. The merits of this book are due to their work.

There is a special place in our heart for the thousands of adolescents we have treated. We have seen teenagers becoming young men and women and have been saddened by their tragedies and awed by their resiliency. This volume is a thank you for the privilege of practicing Adolescent Medicine.

Throughout the years that it took to put all this together, Joy Quek, our managing publisher was indeed a joy to work with, as she has distinguished herself in her diligence and her dedication to comply with all our requests, especially the tables so essential to this text.

Last, but not least, we need to acknowledge our loved ones, without whose steady support anything worthwhile would not have been possible.

TJS would like to acknowledge his wife, who has accompanied him for more than half a century through the adventures of life, the struggles of immigration and the hardship of time alone during the long hours of medical work and writing. "*I am very grateful to her and to my three grown children, whom I love so dearly, for allowing me to pursue my dreams. We are now in the process of returning this 'time debt' to our six lovely grandchildren.*"

HJS would like to acknowledge her mother, Dr. Sunita B. Saxena who passed on her love of Adolescent Medicine with tales of teen resiliency. "*A brilliant physician with a most generous and loving spirit, she remains an ever present positive force in my life. I would also like to acknowledge my encouraging father, sister and dear family and friends for being constant cheerleaders — I am so grateful for your love and support. To Tomas J. Silber for extending an invitation to work with him on this project — we have forged a great partnership and I have learned so much from you. Finally, to my dear husband and the beautiful family we are growing — a very special thanks for patiently enduring the countless hours that have gone into this project. Aarohi, Avani and Akshay, you are the light of my life and coming home to you will always be the most favorite part of my day.*"

SECTION I

WELL ADOLESCENT CARE

1

THE ANNUAL PHYSICAL

Krishna White and Rita Hagler

TEST YOUR KNOWLEDGE

1. It is recommended that a 17 year old patient presenting for an annual physical exam be offered all the following screening tests EXCEPT:

   A. Vision screen
   B. HIV antibody test
   C. Urinalysis
   D. Fasting lipoprotein panel
   E. Chlamydia nucleic amplification test

2. A 16 year old female has come for her annual physical exam. Her BMI is 76% and she has a normal blood pressure. Menarche was at age 12, is regular and lasts 8 days. She is uncertain about her last menstrual period. Since her last physical, she has become sexually active with 2 partners and she uses condoms intermittently. Her family medical history is negative for cardiac disease, hypertension, diabetes and hypercholesterolemia. What would be the *BEST* set of laboratory tests to order at this visit?

   A. Hemoglobin and hematocrit, Papanicalaou smear, and screening for sexually transmitted infections.
   B. Fasting lipoprotein profile, hemoglobin and hematocrit, and screening for sexually transmitted infections.

Refer to end of chapter for answer on page 9.

C. Fasting lipoprotein profile, Papinicolaou smear and screening for sexually transmitted infections.
D. Hemoglobin and hematocrit, and screening for sexually transmitted infections.
E. No screening tests are required.

A 17 year old male presents for a physical exam appointment and states: "I just need this form completed so I can get my driver's license."

BACKGROUND

- There are many reasons that adolescents present for physical exams: school or college entry requirements, sports participation clearance, immunizations and entry into the juvenile justice or foster care system. Sometimes an adolescent may present for a "physical" but really have a hidden agenda (i.e. worries about being pregnant or having a sexually transmitted infection).
- The American Academy of Pediatrics (AAP)/Bright Futures recommends annual physical exams for adolescents 11–21 years old. These visits are grouped into early (11–14), middle (15–17), & late (18–21) adolescent visits.
- Despite this recommendation, the majority of adolescents do not have annual preventive visits. Of those seen, only a small percentage receive adequate preventive counseling, health promotion or screening.

ASSESSMENT

HISTORY

- Consider pre-visit paper or electronic questionnaires to help with time constraints.
- Ascertain adolescent and parent/guardian concerns and address the goals of the visit.
- Give a brief summary of the visit structure (e.g. that the parent and teen will be seen separately as well as together during the assessment).
- Obtain the history of present illness, past medical history, medicines, allergies, immunizations, and family history from the adolescent *and* their parent/guardian if possible, as adolescents often skip or minimize complaints.
- Use **HEEADSSS** (Table 1) for a developmentally appropriate psychosocial history.

- **H**ome, **E**ducation/Employment, **E**xercise/Eating, **D**rugs, **S**uicidality/Depression, **S**exuality, **S**afety and **S**pirituality.
- HEEADSSS was developed to progress from less to more intrusive questions.
- Questions should be asked without a parent in the room unless the patient specifically requests otherwise. Document who was in the room when the history was taken.
- You may want to confirm some details such as grades, eating habits and mood symptoms with the parent/guardian.
- Ask adolescents who are capable of answering, screening questions with follow up questions as appropriate. This also applies to developmentally delayed and chronically ill adolescents whose sexual lives are often overlooked.
- Avoid the temptation to counsel on risky behaviors before obtaining a complete history to assure that patient continues to answer questions open and honestly.

PHYSICAL

- Measure vitals and plot blood pressure on appropriate sex/age reference charts.
- Assess height and weight and calculate BMI. Plot changes over time on a growth curve with the aid of old records.
- Annual Snellen eye chart & audiometry screening are no longer recommended.
  - Complete Snellen vision screen once in early, middle, & late adolescence. At other visits do risk assessment, & screen only if positive.
  - Complete hearing risk assessments at each visit, with audiometry follow up if positive.
- Examine patients *unclothed and draped* in a gown.
- If a parent/guardian is not in the room, *strongly consider a chaperone* during the examination.
- Perform a comprehensive physical exam. Pay special attention to cardiac and musculoskeletal exams for sports physicals.
- Document Tanner stages of sexual maturity rating (Table 2).

STUDIES

- Laboratory screening of the adolescent is driven by the history and physical and includes universal screening performed at every visit, or selective screening dictated by positive findings on risk assessment (Table 3).
- Screening tests provide an objective assessment of risk and the opportunity to counsel and educate adolescents.
- The Affordable Care Act requires most health insurance plans to cover preventive health services recommended by Bright Futures and the United States Preventive Task Force (USPTF), such as screenings, vaccinations, and counseling without copayment, co-insurance, or deductibles.

ROUTINE TESTS (Tables 3 and 4)

Universal

Tests should be done for *all* adolescents:

- Vision: Snellen eye chart assessment in early, middle and late adolescence.
- Dyslipidemia: Fasting lipoprotein profile between 9–11 years and again at 17–21 years.
- HIV: The Centers for Disease Control and Prevention (CDC) recommends all adolescents >13 years have at least one HIV test.
  - The USPTF does not recommend for or against routine HIV screening in adolescents.
  - The AAP recently released guidelines stating that routine HIV screening should be offered to all adolescents at least once by 16–18 years of age in health care settings when the prevalence of HIV in the patient population is more than 0.1.

Selective Screening

Screening tests are limited to those with positive risk assessments and may include:

- Vision
- Hearing
- Anemia
- Dyslipidemia
- Sexually transmitted infections (STIs)

- Pregnancy
- Alcohol/Drug Use
- Cervical Dysplasia

Tuberculosis Screening. Should be done for adolescents with the following positive risk factors:

- Travel outside the United States in the past 5 years to high risk areas.
- History of incarceration.
- Family member or contact with Tuberculosis.
- Family member with a positive Tuberculin skin test.
- Immunosuppressed.

DISPOSITION

- If confidential information was obtained, ask your patient what can and cannot be disclosed to their parent/guardian.
- Praise your patient for positive healthy behaviors before counseling them about risky or unhealthy behaviors.
- Complete a standard physical exam form even if not requested at the time of the visit. A copy of this should be kept on file if the patient requests proof of an exam before their next visit.
- Review contact information to ensure you can contact the patient with pending test results. If reporting confidential test results (i.e. STI screening results), establish a way to contact the patient directly (i.e. their cell phone).
- Arrange for follow up in a year, or earlier if your patient is chronically ill or high risk.
- Anticipatory guidance should be provided to patients at all visits.
- Summarize your findings or recommendations with the adolescent and their parent/guardian at the end of the visit, maintaining confidentiality if appropriate.

What is unique about the annual physical exam in adolescents?

- Adolescents are among those least likely to have access to health care and they have the lowest rate of primary care use of any age group in the United States.

- Adolescents should be interviewed both with and without their parents/guardians.
- Though adolescents and young adults are generally healthy, it is important to focus on risky behaviors at each annual visit because most mortality (e.g. accidents, homicide and suicide) and morbidity (e.g. STIs, depression, and unintended pregnancy) come from risky behaviors.
- Be aware of hidden complaints that may bring an adolescent in for a "routine physical exam."
- Adolescents tend to respond well to risk behavior questions when asked permission: "As a doctor, I need to ask you some very private and personal questions, is that okay with you?"
- The highest yield from the annual physical exam will be obtained from the medical history.
- Routine laboratory tests for adolescents assist in identifying serious preventable problems.
- Early identification of health risks through history, physical and minimal, well defined lab tests can be a considerable benefit for the adolescent, promoting health and preventing illness.

TEST YOUR KNOWLEDGE ANSWERS

1. C. The AAP no longer recommends routine urinalysis to detect asymptomatic bacteriuria, hematuria and/or proteinuria. A Snellen vision screen is recommended once in early, middle, and late adolescence and risk assessments for vision problems are recommended at other preventive visits. In 2006, the CDC recommended that, "in all healthcare settings, screening for HIV infection should be performed routinely for all patients aged 13–64 years." Healthcare providers should initiate screening unless prevalence of undiagnosed HIV infection in their patients has been documented to be <0.1%. Without existing data for HIV prevalence, healthcare providers should initiate voluntary HIV screening until they establish that the diagnostic yield is <1 per 1,000 patients screened, at which point such screening is no longer warranted. Healthcare providers should subsequently test all persons likely to be at high risk for HIV at least annually. The AAP recommends a fasting lipoprotein profile

(total cholesterol, high and low-density lipoprotein [HDL and LDL] and triglyceride) or total and HDL cholesterol once in late adolescence and earlier for patients at high risk for dyslipidemia. The U.S.Preventive Services Task Force (USPSTF) recommends at least annual screening for Chlamydial infection for all sexually active young women <25 years-old.

2. D. Based on a menstrual period of >5 days, an hemoglobin or hematocrit is indicated. Additional assessment for dietary intake of foods rich in iron should be made with appropriate nutritional counseling. This patient does not meet the criteria for lipid screening with a BMI of 76%, normal blood pressure and negative family history for dyslipidemia. Consider total cholesterol testing (research has shown that many patients without the required risk factors still have high cholesterol levels). Other helpful data include a history of smoking and diet high in saturated fats. A fasting lipoprotein profile is recommended at ages 9–11 and 17–21, or for patients at high risk for dyslipidemia. A Papanicolaou smear is not indicated in this patient as she is <21 years, per American College of Obstetricians and Gynecologists guidelines. STI screening should be ordered including chlamydia, gonorrhea, syphilis and HIV testing. The USPTF has recommended yearly screening for Chlamydia infection for all sexually active women <25 years. The CDC has recommended HIV testing as part of routine clinical care in all health settings for adolescents beginning at age 13.

Table 1. HEEADSSS.

HOME	• **Who lives at home with you?** • **How are your relationships with siblings, parents, other relatives?** • Who do you go to for advice? • What are the rules like at home? • Have you ever been homeless or stayed in a shelter? • Have you ever been in foster care or a group home?
EDUCATION/ EMPLOYMENT	• **What is the name of your school and in what grade are you?** • **What kind of student are you? What are your grades/GPA?** • What are your educational, career and life goals? • How many days were missed in the past year? Why?

(*Continued*)

Table 1. (*Continued*)

	• Have you ever had any educational setbacks? Why?
	• Have there been any recent school changes?
	• Do you have any home chores? Do you receive an allowance?
	• **Do you work after school?**
	  • What type of work do you do? How many hours a week?
	  • Do you help to pay for things at home?
	  • What are your future career interests?

EXERCISE/ EATING	• **Do you exercise? How many hours? days?**
	• Ask about body image:
	  • What is your ideal weight?
	  • What do you like about yourself?
	• **Do you think you eat a healthy well balanced diet?**
	• **Is there enough calcium, iron and fiber in your diet?**
	• How many meals do you eat per day? Do you skip any meals?
	• If thin: Over exercise? Ever vomit, use diuretics or laxatives?
	• Do you drink sugary beverages (i.e. soda, juice or sports drinks)?
	• Do you drink skim, 2% or wholemilk?
	• Do you eat fast food or carryout? If so, how often?

ACTIVITIES	• **How do you like to spend your free time? What are your hobbies?** • **Do you play any sports?** • **How much entertainment media (TV/computer/video games) per day?** • **Is there TV or internet access in your bedroom?** • Do you participate in clubs or religious/spiritual activities?

DRUGS	• **Does anyone you hang out with smoke, drink or use drugs? Do you?** If so, how frequently and how much?
	• **Do you smoke or chew tobacco?**
	• **Do you drink alcohol?**
	  • What kind: beer, wine, hard liquor?
	  • Any blackouts? Ever pass out? Vomit?
	• **Do you use illicit drugs (marijuana, inhalants, cocaine, crack, heroin, pills, LSD, ecstasy, crystal meth, other drugs) or medicines not prescribed?**
	• **Have you ever been in a car with someone who was drinking or used drugs?**
	  • Have you ever done anything you have regretted while high?

(*Continued*)

Table 1. (*Continued*)

	• Context of use: social or alone. • What is your attitude towards cutting back and/or quitting? • Have you ever received drug treatment or counseling? • How is your drug use supported? • Have you ever had any arrests?

SUICIDALITY/ DEPRESSION	• **What is your usual mood: happy, sad or both?**
	• How do you cope with, or relieve stress?
	• Have you ever received counseling and/or therapy?
	• Have you ever been in a psychiatric hospital?
	  • What was the reason?
	  • How long did you stay?
	• **Have you ever thought of hurting yourself?**
	• **Have you ever tried to hurt or kill yourself?**
	  • Whom did you tell?
	• Have you ever tried to hurt or kill someone else?

SEXUALITY	• **Do you have crushes on males, females or both?**
	• **What are the rules of dating in your home?**
	• **Are you dating/going out with anyone?**
	• **Have you ever been intimate with someone (i.e. hugging or kissing)?**
	• **Have you ever had any type of sex (oral, anal, and/or vaginal)?**
	  • How old were you when you first had sex? Include anal, oral and vaginal.
	  • What was the date of your last intercourse?
	  • What kind of protection did you use at last sex?
	  • Condoms? Hormonal contraception?
	• Do you have a current partner?
	  • How long have you been with your partner?
	• How many sexual partners have you had?
	  • Are your partners male, female, or both?
	  • How many sexual partners have you had in the past 3 months?
	• Have you ever had any STIs?
	  • Do you know what the symptoms of STIs are? Tell me.
	  • Have you ever been tested for an STI?
	• Have you ever been pregnant or gotten anyone pregnant? What was the outcome?
	  • Do you have any concerns about fertility?
	  • When (if ever) would you like to have children?

(*Continued*)

Table 1. (*Continued*)

SAFETY	• **Do you wear a seatbelt?**
	• **Is there a working smoke detector and fire extinguisher in your home?**
	• **Do you feel safe at home, school and in your neighborhood?**
	• **Have you ever been in a fight?**
	• **Are there guns at home or do you know someone who has a gun?**
	• Have you ever been locked up/in trouble with the law?
	• **Has anyone ever hurt you on a repeated basis? At home, in school, or in your neighborhood?**
	• **Have you ever been forced to have sex or been touched against your will?**
	  • By whom and is this still going on?
	  • Who did you tell?
	  • How does it affect your day-to-day life?
	  • In what ways does that experience affect your sexual relationships now?

SPIRITUALITY (Optional)	• What do you consider to be your religion? • How often do you participate in religious activities? • How important are your spiritual beliefs in your day-to-day life? • How do your beliefs influence your health and attitudes about sex and contraception?

*Bolded questions should be asked of *all* adolescents. Other questions can be asked when appropriate.

Table 2. Sexual Maturity Rating (SMR).

Females

Developmental Stage	SMR	Pubic Hair	Breasts
Early adolescence	1	Preadolescent	Preadolescent
(10–13 years)	2	Sparse and straight	Small mound
Middle adolescence	3	Dark and curly	Bigger with no contour separation
(12–14 years)	4	Coarse, curly and abundant	Secondary mound of areola
Late adolescence (14–17 years)	5	Triangle pattern that extends to the medial thigh	Nipple projects and areolar complex conforms to breast

Males

Developmental Stage	SMR	Pubic Hair	Penis	Testes
Early adolescence	1	None	Preadolescent	Preadolescent
(10.5–14 years)	2	Scanty	Slight increase	Larger
Middle adolescence	3	Darker and curly	Longer	Larger
(12.5–15 years)	4	Adult, coarse and curly	Larger	Scrotum dark
Late adolescence	5	Extends to thighs	Adult	Adult
(14–16 years)				

Table 3. Recommended Adolescent Medical Screening Tests.

Screening	AAP/Bright Futures	USPTF*	Other Professional Organizations	Recommended Test
Anemia	Risk assessment: • Diets deficient in iron rich foods (i.e. meat, eggs, iron fortified cereals or beans). • Prior diagnosis of iron deficiency anemia. • History of excessive menstrual bleeding or other blood loss. • Periods lasting more than 5 days.	B: Pregnant; adolescents not mentioned.	N/A	Hemoglobin or Hematocrit
Cervical Cancer	Within 3 years of sexual activity.	A: All who have ever been sexually active with a cervix (as of 2003 currently being updated).	*American Congress of Obstetricians & Gynecologists* (Aug 2010): • 21 years for most ♀ & then annually. • Sexual debut for immunocompromised & newly diagnosed HIV. Screen every 6 months for 1st year & then annually.	Papanicolaou test (slide or liquid based)

(Continued)

Table 3. (*Continued*)

Screening	AAP/Bright Futures	USPTF*	Other Professional Organizations	Recommended Test
Diabetes	Not mentioned.	Not mentioned for children.	*American Diabetes Association*: • Start at 10 years or puberty onset. • Frequency: every 3 yrs. • >85%ile BMI + 2 risk factors (family history, race or signs of insulin resistance). • HAIC • Hemoglobin A1C	Fasting plasma glucose every 2 years
Dyslipidemia	Universal screening 9–11 yrs & 17–21 yrs. Screen at other ages if high risk: • Family history of cardiovascular disease or dyslipidemia. • Patient has diabetes, BMI >85%ile, smokes, or has other chronic conditions that can cause 2° dyslipidemia.	I: Children & adolescents.	N/A	Fasting lipoprotein profile OR Non-fasting total cholesterol & high-density lipoprotein (HDL) if unable to fast

(*Continued*)

Table 3. *(Continued)*

Screening	AAP/Bright Futures	USPTF*	Other Professional Organizations	Recommended Test
Gonorrhea (GC) & Chlamydia (CT)	All sexually active.	A: Sexually active ♀ <25 yrs. B: GC for all sexually active ♀ if at risk. I: GC/CT for asymptomatic ♂.	*CDC*: Consider screening sexually active adolescent ♂ in clinical settings associated with high prevalence of Chlamydia (e.g., adolescent clinics, correctional facilities, and STI clinics).	Urine, vaginal, and/or rectal nucleic acid amplification tests
Hearing	Risk assessment: • Trouble hearing on phone, during conversations, in noisy environments. • Ask people to repeat themselves.	Not mentioned.	N/A	Audiometry
HIV	*Bright Futures*: High risk. *AAP*: Universal by 16–18 yrs if prevalence is >0.1% (published Oct 2011).	A: High risk C: Universal screening.	*CDC*: Opt out universal screening; 13–64 yrs should have at least 1 test unless in low prevalence area (<0.1%). At least annual screening for high risk.	HIV antibody test

(Continued)

Table 3. (*Continued*)

Screening	AAP/Bright Futures	USPTF*	Other Professional Organizations	Recommended Test
Pregnancy	Sexually active without contraception, late menses, or amenorrhea.	Not mentioned.	N/A	Urine human chorionic gonadotropin
Syphilis	High risk settings: • STI or Tuberculosis clinics, homeless shelters & correctional facilities. • Clinics serving ♂ who have sex with ♂. • Adolescent health clinics with a high prevalence of STIs.	A: Pregnant or high risk.	N/A	Rapid plasma reagin (RPR)
Tuberculosis	Annual skin test for incarcerated & HIV positive. Screen TB contacts, patients born in or traveled to high risk country. Annual assessment for all others.	Defers to CDC guidelines.	*CDC*: High risk.	Tuberculin skin test

(*Continued*)

Table 3. *(Continued)*

Screening	AAP/Bright Futures	USPTF*	Other Professional Organizations	Recommended Test
Urinalysis	Not mentioned.	*D*: Asymptomatic bacteruria in ♂ & non pregnant ♀. A: Asymptomatic bacteruria in pregnant ♀ at 12–16 weeks gestation or 1st prenatal visit.	N/A	N/A
Vision	Universal: once in early, middle, & late adolescence. Risk assessment if: • Trouble seeing. • Trouble reading. • Squinting. • Failed school vision screen.	Adolescents & young adults not mentioned.	N/A	Snellen test

*USPTF (U.S. Preventive Services Task Force) Recommendations Guide. Evidence-based graded recommendations.

A: Strong recommendation. Good evidence. Benefits > harms.

B: Recommendation. Fair evidence. Benefits > harms.

C: No recommendation for or against. Fair evidence of health improvement. Benefits: harms balance to close to justify general recommendation.

D: Recommends against routine use in asymptomatic patients. Fair evidence of ineffectiveness or harms > benefits.

I: Insufficient evidence to recommend for or against service.

Table 4. Recommended Adolescent Psychosocial Screening Tests.

Screening	AAP/Bright Futures	USPTF*	Other Professional Organizations	Recommended Test
Alcohol/ Drug Use	Universal screening	I: Children & adolescents	N/A	Administer validated alcohol and drug screening tools (i.e. CRAFFT screening).
Depression	Universal screening	B: 12–21 years	N/A	Administer validated screening test for primary care (Patient Health Questionnaire for Adolescents or the Beck Depression Inventory-Primary Care)
Tobacco Use	Universal screening	I: Children & adolescents A: Pregnant and/or adults	N/A	N/A

*USPTF (U.S. Preventive Services Task Force) Recommendations Guide. Evidence-based graded recommendations.
A: Strong recommendation. Good evidence. Benefits > harms.
B: Recommendation. Fair evidence. Benefits > harms.
C: No recommendation for or against. Fair evidence of health improvement. Benefits: harms balance to close to justify general recommendation > benefits.
D: Recommends against routine use in asymptomatic patients. Fair evidence of ineffectiveness or harms > benefits.
I: Insufficient evidence to recommend for or against service.

WEB REFERENCES

- The Affordable Care Act:
  - The Affordable Care Act (2009): www.healthcare.gov: http://www.healthcare.gov/law/full/patient-protection.pdf

- American Academy of Pediatrics Publications (www.aappublications.org):
  - Committee on Adolescence, 'Achieving Quality Health Services for Adolescents', *Pediatrics*, June 2008; 121(6); 1263–1270: http://pediatrics.aappublications.org/content 121/6/1263.full.pdf+html.
  - Committee on Pediatric AIDS, 'Adolescents and HIV Infection: The Pediatrician's Role in Promoting Routing Testing', *Pediatrics*, November 2011; 128(5); 1023–1029: http://pediatrics.aappublications.org/content/128/5/1023.full.pdf+html.
  - Irwin, CE, *et al.*, 'Preventive Care for Adolescents: Few Get Visits and Fewer Get Services', *Pediatrics*, April 2009; 123(4); e565–e572: http://pediatrics.aappublications.org/cgi/reprint/123/4/e565
  - Kavey, RW, *et al.*, 'Expert Panel on Integrated Guidelines for Cardiovascular Health and Risk Reduction in Children and Adolescents: Summary Report', *Pediatrics*, December 2011;128; Supplement 5: http://pediatrics.aappublications.org/site/misc/2009-2107.pdf
- American College of Obstetricians & Gynecologists (http://www.acog.org/):
  - Committee on Adolescent Health Care, 'Cervical Cancer In Adolescents: Screening, Evaluation and Management', Committee Opinion, August 2010;463: http://www.acog.org/~/media/Committee%20Opinions / Committee % 20on % 20Adolescent % 20Health % 20Care /co463.pdf?dmc=l&ts=20130313T1052275427.
- American Medical Association, Guidelines for Adolescent Preventive Services (GAPS), Recommendations Monograph. 1997: http://www.ama-assn.org/resources/doc/ad-hlth/gapsmono.pdf

Additional Clinician and Patient Resources:

- American Diabetes Association: www.diabetes.org
- Bright Futures: www.-brightfutures.-aap.-org
- Centers for Disease Control and Prevention: www.cdc.gov
- Physicians for Reproductive Health and Choice: http://www.prch.org/arshepdownloads
- Teen Screen National Center for Mental Health Checkups at Columbia University:
- www.teenscreen.org
- United States Preventive Services Task Force: http://www.uspreventiveservicestaskforce.org/
  - Child and Adolescent Recommendations-Clinical Categories: http://www.uspreventiveservicestaskforce.org/tfchildcat.htm

2

ADOLESCENT CONSENT AND CONFIDENTIALITY

Kirsten B. Hawkins

TEST YOUR KNOWLEDGE

3. A 15 year old male who attends boarding school in your community comes to your office because of persistent headaches. When alone with the patient, he tells you that he feels depressed and suicidal, and has a plan to kill himself. Of the following, the *BEST* description of your obligation to alert his parents is that:

   A. Parental notification is not required because he is a mature minor.
   B. Parental notification is not required because he is an emancipated minor.
   C. Parental notification is optional.
   D. Parental notification is required due to his serious threats of self-harm.
   E. Parental notification is prohibited by the Health Insurance Portability and Accountability Act.

4. Anna is a 17 year old "A student" who comes in alone for her pre-college physical. Anna and her same age boyfriend are sexually active. She has been taking birth control pills inconsistently and they do not use condoms. She is on her parents' health insurance and does not want her parents to know she is sexually active.

Refer to end of chapter for answers on page 28.

What care can you offer Anna based on her own consent?

A. Screening for sexually transmitted infections (STIs)
B. Human papillomavirus vaccine
C. Pregnancy Test
D. Menactra vaccine
E. A and C
F. All the above

Amy is a 16 year old female who reports being sexually active for the past year with sporadic condom use. She requests a pregnancy test and a refill on her birth control pills that she has used inconsistently in the past but doesn't want her mother to know…

BACKGROUND

- Adolescents can give independent consent for some health services if their capacities for understanding are sufficiently evolved (Mature Minor Doctrine).
- Many legal systems recognize "mature minors" as enjoying adult rights of medical consent for specific situations. Mature minors enjoy confidentiality and the right to treatment according to their wishes rather than their best interests.
- Examples of conditions for which adolescents are capable of giving consent for treatment include pregnancy, sexually transmitted infections (including HIV infection), mental disorders and substance use.
- Minors incapable of self-determination may grant or deny assent to treatment for which guardians provide consent.
- Emancipated minors' self-determination may be judicially recognized, for instance on marriage or military service.
- Psychological research into adolescent decision-making has found that adolescents at least as young as 14 years are capable of making informed decisions. However, such capacities vary based on the intelligence and social experiences of the individual.
- Sometimes clinicians may not recognize the decision-making capacity of their adolescent patients and may not be familiar with local laws. Therefore, clinicians who work with teens must be familiar with local statutes and customs and advocate for the medical rights of minors.

ASSESSMENT

HISTORY:

Developmental Considerations

- Evaluate the developmental stage of the adolescent (early, middle or late adolescent).
- Assess autonomy: What decisions has the teen been allowed to make in the past?
- Assess likelihood of compliance by history of adherence to commitments.
- Determine the capacity to understand alternatives and make voluntary choices. Assess the teen's:
  - Prior ability to cope with illness.
  - Emotional stability.
  - Previous adherence to medications or treatment recommendations.

DISPOSITION

- Guidelines recommend that healthcare providers maintain confidentiality with teens unless the teen consents to disclose or disclosure is necessary to protect their well being.
- Clinicians must be able to identify when a teen can be deemed a mature minor.
- Emphasis placed on the adolescent's growing need for privacy in preliminary attempts at self-determination should not be seen as an abrogation of the role of parents.
- The health care team providing services to the adolescent needs to achieve balance between supporting this important developmental task and encouraging teens to involve parents, guardians or other trusted adults for the wisdom and experience they could contribute to the teen's decision-making.
  - Explain limits of confidentiality to adolescents and parents at their initial visit.

- Be aware of legal requirements and mandatory reporting laws:
  - Child abuse
  - Harm to self or others
  - Public health reporting when applicable
- Exercise professional judgment regarding assessments for abuse and risk of harm.

What is unique about consent and confidentiality in adolescents?

- Adolescent confidentiality recognizes adolescents' developing capacity for autonomous decision making, protects the health of adolescents, avoids negative health outcomes and enhances public health.
- Many adolescents who seek medical care have privacy concerns. They are specifically concerned about the disclosure of information related to sexual behaviors, substance use and mental health to their parents or legal guardians.
- Privacy concerns influence whether, when and where adolescents seek care and if they can talk openly with physicians.
- Minor consent does not always equal confidentiality. Even when minor consent is allowed, it is not a sufficient guarantee of confidentiality. Involuntary disclosure may occur through billing or insurance records and this should be communicated to the teen at the medical visit.
- Parents of adolescents with intellectual deficiencies or with conditions affecting their cognitive abilities (such as brain wasting in severe anorexia or suicidality in a patient with severe depression) need to be involved in decision making.
- Some states and countries have mandatory notification laws for adolescents in need of protection against neglect or abuse.
- Additional exceptions may arise when there is a serious or imminent threat to the life or health of an individual (e.g. suicide) or another person. It is generally best to first discuss the disclosure with the adolescent.

- Adolescents who fear parental reaction to the decisions they are making about their sexuality may resist parental involvement.
  - Reasons for resistance need to be carefully explored with the adolescent.
  - Adolescents who have been granted the ability to consent may then decide whether their confidences can be shared with others, such as their parents or other individuals.
- Unfortunately, confidentiality may be compromised when adolescents are dependent on their parents or other adults for payment of medical services.
  - Involuntary disclosure can occur through billing or insurance records.
  - Most countries and states do not have safeguards in place for prevention of such disclosure.

TEST YOUR KNOWLEDGE ANSWERS

3. D. Disclosure is required when the minor is dangerous to themself or others. Always explain the limits to confidentiality to adolescents and parents ahead of time either through verbal explanation, written office policy statement, or posted notice so that the minor understands the need to breach confidentiality protections. Always try to engage the minor in this process and involve them in the process of notification.
4. E. Many states allow minors to consent for the diagnosis of pregnancy and the diagnosis and treatment of sexually transmitted infections. Some states allow for minor consent to prevent sexually transmitted infections via immunization against Hepatitis B or Human Papilloma Virus; however, most states do not, as immunizations may require parental consent.

WEB REFERENCES

- Ford C, English A, Signman G (2004), 'Confidential Health Care for Adolescents: Position Paper of the Society for Adolescent Medicine', Journal of Adolescent Health, 2004;35; 160–167, Retrieved from http://www.adolescenthealth.org/AM/Template.cfm?Section=Position_Papers&Template=/CM/ContentDisplay.cfm & ContentID=2597
- Guttmacher Institute (www.guttmacher. org)
  - Boonstra H & Nash E, 'Minors and the Right to Consent to Health Care', The Guttmacher Report on Public Policy, August 2000;3(4);4–8: http://www.guttmacher.org/pubs/tgr/03/4/gr030404.pdf

- Dallard, C, 'New Medical Records Privacy Rule: The Interface with Teen Access to Confidential Care', The Guttmacher Report on Public Policy, March 2003;6(l);6-7: http://www, guttmacher. org/pubs/tgr/06/1/gr060106 .html
- Dallard, C & Richardson, CT, 'Teenagers' Access to Confidential Reproductive Health Services', The Guttmacher Report on Public Policy, November 2005;8(4);6–l 1: http://www.guttmacher.org/pubs/tgr/08/4/gr080406.pdf
- English, A& Ford CA, 'The HIPAA Privacy Rule and Adolescents: Legal Questions and Clinical Challenges', Perspectives on Sexual and Reproductive Health, March/April 2004;36(2);80–86: http://www.guttmacher.org/pubs/journals/3608004.pdf
- Guttmacher Institute, 'An Overview of Minors' Consent Laws', State Policies in Brief, as of March 1, 2013: http://www.guttmacher.org/statecenter/spibs/spib_OMCL.pdf

- Center for Adolescent Health and Law (www.cahl.org):
- Morreale, MC, et al. Policy Compendium on Confidential Health Services for Adolescents, Second Edition, 2005: http://www.cahl.org/policy-compendium-2005/

Additional Clinician Resources:

- National Center for Youth Law: http://www.youthlaw.org/
- Society for Adolescent Health and Medicine: Clinical Care Resources on Confidentiality http://www.adolescenthealth.org/Clinical Care Resources.htm#Confidentiality

3

NORMAL NUTRITION THROUGH ADOLESCENCE

Erin Wolf-Barnett

TEST YOUR KNOWLEDGE

5. All the following statements are true *EXCEPT*:

   A. Vegetarians exclude meat, seafood and poultry from their diets.

   B. Lacto-vegetarians exclude meat, seafood, poultry and eggs from their diets.

   C. Vegans exclude meat, seafood, poultry, eggs and dairy products from their diets.

   D. Teens with eating disorders may initially present masked as new vegetarians.

   E. Vegetarian diets are not appropriate for teens because they induce nutritional deficiencies.

Refer to end of chapter for answer on page 37.

"My daughter has decided to become vegan. Is that normal? Won't she miss out on important nutrients?"

BACKGROUND

- Nutrition decisions through adolescence are multifaceted. Adolescents are influenced by peers, family, media and other factors that may affect their nutritional status.
- During the adolescent growth spurt, there is increased appetite and food intake, more prominent in males.
- Common characteristics of adolescent eating behaviors include: snacking more, skipping meals, focusing on body image and dieting.
- To accurately assess estimated nutrition needs, it is important to address a teen's eating behaviors and level of physical activity.

ASSESSMENT

HISTORY

- The nutritional history should include quantity, quality and frequency of food intake.
- Ask about: duration of meals; food allergies and intolerances; stooling patterns; social, economic and environmental circumstances; physical activity; history of vomiting/diarrhea; and dieting or body image concerns.

PHYSICAL

Vital Signs

- Malnutrition may be associated with temperature instability, bradycardia and orthostatic hypotension.
- High salt diets and obesity predispose to hypertension.

Anthropometric Measurements

- The Centers of Disease Control and Prevention (CDC) developed growth charts to plot individual anthropometric data including weight, height and BMI for age.

- These growth charts were designed using a cross-sectional sample of healthy American children with racial and ethnic distribution. Internet access to these charts are listed under Web Resources at the end of the chapter.
- Weight for Age
  - Ensure accuracy of scales and weigh with minimal clothing and no shoes.
  - If possible, use the same scale at each visit for consistent measurement.
  - Weight loss or excessive weight gain should be explored.
- Height for Age
  - Height, or stature, is affected slowly and therefore provides a better representation of long-term nutritional status. Malnutrition may cause poor linear growth and children who grow less than 4.5 cm per year should be evaluated.
  - Female growth spurts begin before the onset of breast development with mean age of 10 years (approximately 8.5–9 cm per year).
  - Male growth spurts begin approximately 2 years after start of testicular development with mean age at 10.5–11 years (9.5–10.5 cm per year).
  - Calculate alternative height measurements for adolescents unable to stand.
    - Arm Span Measurement (approximates vertical length): With back against the wall, have the teen stretch both arms laterally. Measure from the tip of the middle finger on one hand to the tip of the middle finger on the other and repeat the measurement two times for accuracy.
- Body Mass Index (BMI) for Age
  - BMI = Weight (kg)/Height (m)^2 OR BMI = Weight (lbs)/Height (in)^2 × 703.
  - This is a gender and age-specific effective screening tool used to determine underweight or overweight status.
  - BMI calculations do not consider muscle mass and can be misleading in particularly muscular teens.
  - Adolescents who meet criteria for underweight or overweight status should undergo further evaluation.

General

- Assess general appearance looking for signs of muscle wasting or excess fat stores.

HEENT

- Look for signs of dental caries that can occur with high sugar diets or enamel breakdown.

Skin

- Assess skin and nail color.
- Striae can appear with weight gain or loss and can commonly be found on the abdomen, back and upper thighs.
- Lanugo, or thin fine hair growth, can occur with severe malnutrition.

STUDIES

Accurate assessment of dietary intake is facilitated by use of food diaries.

Dietary Intake Assessments Tools

- 24 Hour Food Recall: Adolescents or caregivers provide food intake over the past 24 hours.
- 3–7 Day Food Record: Adolescents or caregivers document 72 hours or more of food intake, typically 1 weekend day and 2 weekdays for more accurate assessment.
- Food Frequency Questionnaire: Adolescents or caregivers complete a questionnaire designed to gather data on the frequency, portion and types of food eaten over the past week, month or year and is typically used in research settings.

Laboratory data may be indicated when screening for malnutrition, nutritional rehabilitation or insufficient nutrient intake.

CBC and Iron

- To evaluate for **iron-deficiency anemia**.

Calcium and Vitamin D Levels

- Teens often have inadequate intake of calcium rich foods.

Total Cholesterol, LDL, HDL, Triglycerides, ALT, and HgA1c, and Fasting or Random Glucose

- These labs should be considered in the overweight or obese adolescent, or in cases where history or physical warrant concern.

DEXA Scan

- To evaluate bone mineralization in patients with acute or chronic weight loss, malnutrition and/or loss of menses for more than 6 months.

Celiac Screening

- Serological testing: transglutaminase antibodies (tTGA) and anti-endomysium antibodies (EMA) are used to establish a diagnosis.
- Intestinal biopsy is the "gold standard" and is usually performed after a positive blood test.

Calprotectin and Occult Blood in Stools

- Consider if screening for granulomatous colitis.

DIETARY TREATMENT CONSIDERATIONS

- Teens engaged in special diets may benefit from consultation with a Registered Dietitian (RD).
- An RD can help determine nutrient needs based on Dietary Reference Intakes (DRIs), the daily nutrient requirements for an individual.
- There is a quick interactive online tool that provides the most up to date calculations for all nutrient reference values requested for an individual patient.
    - To make the calculations, health care providers will need to enter: age, sex, height, weight and activity level: http://fnic.nal.usda.gov/interactiveDRI/.

Vegetarian/Vegan

- There is considerable variability in dietary practices among vegetarians. Adolescents can maintain adequate nutritional status on these diets with education and good planning.

- Terminology:
  - **Pescatarians** exclude meat and poultry.
  - **Vegetarians** exclude meat, seafood and poultry.
  - **Lacto-vegetarians** exclude meat, seafood, poultry and eggs.
  - **Vegans** exclude meat, seafood, poultry, eggs and dairy products.
- Menu Planning Approach:
  - Choose a variety of foods, including whole grains, vegetables, fruits, legumes, nuts, seeds and if desired, dairy products and eggs.
  - Minimize foods high in sweeteners, sodium and fat, especially saturated and trans fat.
  - Consume adequate amounts of vitamin B12. Sources of B12 include: eggs, milk products, fortified cereals, soy based drinks, veggie burgers and nutritional yeast.
  - If sunlight exposure is limited, a source of vitamin D should be considered.
  - Vegetarians and vegans may be low in vitamin B12, C, calcium and zinc and may require regular supplementation.
  - Vegetarians who consume large amounts of carrots and squash tend to have a yellow- orange skin color because of elevated levels of carotenoids. This should not be confused with jaundice.

Lactose Intolerance

- Lactose is a natural sugar found in dairy products. Most people with lactose intolerance do not require a lactose-free diet.
- Patients with problems digesting lactose can usually eat or drink: 1 cup of milk with a meal, yogurt or cheese and/or milk with hot or cold cereal.
- Non-dairy calcium rich food alternatives include:
  - Calcium-fortified soy or rice drinks, juices, cereals or breads.
  - Canned fish (i.e. sardines, salmon with bones).
  - Soybeans, black-eyed peas (cow peas), white beans, and soy products.
  - Some leafy greens (i.e. collard and turnip greens, kale, and bok choy).

Celiac Disease

- Gluten is found in a number of food and non-food products and it is important to get detailed food and nutrient intake (e.g., diet history, diet

experience and macronutrient or micronutrient intake, specifically calcium, iron, vitamin B complex and vitamin D) as well as use of medications and herbal supplements.
- Determine a teen's readiness to change nutrition-related behaviors and assess their knowledge about celiac disease.
- The success of dietary changes is related to social and familial supports.
- Ascertain a teen's access to food. While gluten-free diets are becoming more main stream, they are still not as readily available across all socioeconomic demographics. Limited access can be a barrier to dietary success.

DISPOSITION

Make recommendations based on current dietary guidelines (Table 1).

What is unique when considering nutrition in adolescents?

- Adolescence is a period of remarkable growth and development and teens must match metabolic needs with balanced diet and exercise.
- It is normal for an adolescent to experiment with diet as long as their nutritional needs are met. It is important to reassure parents and closely monitor patients for significant weight changes or nutritional deficiencies.
- Many adolescents do not have well balanced, nutritionally optimized diets. Poor fiber and fluid intake often result in constipation.
- Overweight, obesity and eating disorders may arise or worsen after puberty.

TEST YOUR KNOWLEDGE ANSWER

5. E. Vegetarian diets can be safely embraced by teens who decide to pursue them for philosphical reasons as long as they choose from a variety of foods including whole grains, vegetables, fruits, legumes, nuts, seeds and if desired, dairy products and eggs. It is important to ensure a source of vitamins B12 and D as these can be lower in vegetarian diets.

Table 1. Nutrition Guidelines for Adolescents*.

Food Group	9–13 Years Servings/Day	14–18 Years Servings/Day	Serving Size Examples
Milk and Milk Products	3 cups	3 cups	1 cup = 8 oz $1\frac{1}{2}$ oz cheese 6–8 oz yogurt
Meat and Plant Proteins	5 oz or 34 grams	5–6 oz or 46–52 grams	1 oz meat $\frac{1}{4}$ cup beans 1 egg 1 tablespoon peanut butter
Breads, Cereals and other Starches	6 oz Note: 3 oz should be whole grains	6–7 oz Note: 3 oz should be whole grains	1 slice of bread $\frac{1}{2}$ cup cooked rice or pasta 1 cup dry cereal
Fruits	$1\frac{1}{2}$ cups	$1\frac{1}{2}$–2 cups	1 cup fruit $\frac{1}{2}$ cup dried fruit
Vegetables	2–$2\frac{1}{2}$ cups	$2\frac{1}{2}$–3 cups	1 cup raw or cooked
Fats and Oils	5–6 servings (1 serving = 1 teaspoon)	6–7 servings	1 teaspoon (tsp) oil or butter 1 tsp salad dressing 1 tsp mayo
Discretionary Calories	Use sparingly	Use sparingly	Candy, jams, chips, etc.

*Based on 2010 Dietary Guidelines: www.choosemyplate.gov

WEB REFERENCES

- U.S. Department of Agriculture
  - U.S. Department of Agriculture and U.S. Department of Health and Human Services. Dietary Guidelines for Americans, 2010. 7th Edition, Washington D.C.: U.S. Government Printing Office, December 2010: http://www.health.gov/dietaryguidelines/dga2010/DietaryGuidelines2010.pdf
  - A Brief History of USDAFood Guides (June 2011), http://www.choosemyplate.gov/food-groups/downloads/MyPlate/ABriefHistoryOfUSDAFoodGuides.pdf

- U.S. Department of Health & Human Services, National Institutes of Health:
    - NIH Consensus Development Conference on Celiac Disease (June 2004), http://consensus.nih.gov/2004/2004CeliacDiseasell8html.htm

General Nutrition Resources:

- Centers for Disease Control and Prevention. 2000 CDC Growth Charts: United States: http://www.cdc.gov/growthcharts/cdc_charts.htm
- Maternal and Child Health Bureau. Accurately Weighing and Measuring Infants, Children and Adolescents: http://depts.Washington.edu/growth
- U.S. Department of Agriculture Dietary Guidelines: www.choosemyplate.gov
- U.S. Department of Health and Human Services: www.health.gov

Celiac Resources:

- The National Foundation of Celiac Awareness: www.celiaccentral.org
- Celiac Disease Center at Columbia University: www.celiacdiseasecenter. columbia.edu
- Celiac Disease Foundation: www.celiac.org
- Celiac Sprue Association: www.csaceliacs.org
- Gluten Intolerance Group of North America: www.gluten.net

Diabetes Resources:

- American Diabetes Association: www.diabetes.org
- Juvenile Diabetes Research Foundation International: http://www.jdrf.org/

Food Allergy Resources:

- The Food Allergy and Anaphylaxis Network: www.foodallergy.org
- Kids with Food Allergies: http://www.kidswithfoodallergies.org

Vegetarian Resources:

- Vegetarian Nutrition Dietetic Practice Group: www.vegetariannutrition.net
- The Vegan Society: www.vegansociety.com/food/nutrition/bl2
- The Vegetarian Resource Group: www.vrg.org

Nutrition Resources for Teens

- Dietary Guidelines 2010: www.choosemyplate.gov
- Office on Women's Health: www.girlshealth.gov
- Nemours Center for Children's Health Media: http://kidshealth.org/
- LoveMyBody Non-Profit Organization: www. 1 ovemyb ody. org

4

IMMUNIZATIONS IN ADOLESCENTS

Lawrence J. D'Angelo

TEST YOUR KNOWLEDGE

6. Which adolescent is a candidate for the influenza vaccine?
   A. A 14 year old with cerebral palsy.
   B. A 16 year old with behaviorally acquired HIV infection and a CD4 count of 668 cells/mm^3.
   C. An 18 year old with no significant past medical history presenting for a sports physical exam.
   D. A 13 year old with multiple sclerosis.
   E. All the above.

Refer to end of chapter for answer on page 51.

An 18 year old male presents for his pre-college physical exam. His parents divorced when he was 12 years old and he subsequently moved with his mother to a remote community where his medical care was provided for by a naturopathic physician who did not believe in vaccinations. There are no health records available for the past 6 years. Which vaccines is he likely to need at this time?

BACKGROUND

- The availability of new vaccines and changes in the frequency and scheduling of existing vaccines has made comprehensive adolescent immunization a rapidly evolving part of both clinical and public health practice.
- The focus of this emerging health priority is to:
  - Protect adolescents against infectious diseases that can have lifelong, and even life-threatening complications;
  - Reduce transmission of disease from adolescents to others who are at high risk for infection, from the very young (including infants) to the very old;
  - Provide clinicians an opportunity to promote regularly scheduled healthcare visits to adolescents who have traditionally been among the least frequent consumers of preventive health care.
- For years, adolescents have not figured in the public health agenda for improving immunization rates, as few available vaccines were routinely administered during this age period; this is now changing.

THE NEW GENERATION OF "ADOLESCENT" VACCINES

- In the past ten years, new vaccine products have emerged, targeted towards preadolescents, adolescents, and/or young adults, or have been reformulated to allow use in these age groups (Table 1).
- This has resulted in rethinking about how and when to administer these vaccines and how to overcome barriers clinicians face appropriately vaccinating this age group.
- Below is a description of each vaccine preventable illness and vaccine characteristics.

Meningococcal Disease

- Meningitis is caused by the gram negative diplococcal organism, *Neiserria meningitides*, and this illness is often difficult to diagnose in its early manifestations.
- It may manifest itself as overwhelming sepsis (meningococcemia) or as meningitis.
- From the time of first symptoms, which are often indistinguishable from any other minor infectious prodrome, it can progress to a life-threatening illness within less than 24 hours.
- Of the 1000–2000 cases of invasive meningococcal disease that occur in the United States every year, 10%–14% are fatal.
- Meningococcemia carries a case-fatality rate as high as 40%.
- Adolescents and young adults are at particularly high risk of dying from meningococcal disease. In the U.S., more deaths occur among 15–24 year olds than in any other age group, accounting for 1 in 5 fatalities from meningococcal disease.
- For those who survive, long-term effects may be severe: 11–19% of survivors across all age groups experience sequelae such as hearing loss, neurologic defects or limb amputation.
- Adolescents who survive may experience a disturbing series of deficits, including poorer physical health, mental health, quality of life and academic achievement.

Meningococcal Vaccine

- Currently 3 different meningococcal vaccines are available, but only the two most recent forms of the vaccine (quadrivalent conjugated) are recommended for routine use.
- The vaccines are licensed by the FDA for use in persons aged 11–55 years.
- The Advisory Committee on Immunization Practices (ACIP) recommends the vaccine for all persons aged 11–18 years and for persons aged 2–55 years who are at risk of meningitis.
- Persons at continuing or increased risk of meningococcal disease include:
    - College freshmen living in dormitories

  - Microbiologists who are routinely exposed to isolates of Neiserria meningitides
  - Military recruits
  - Persons who live in or travel to countries where meningococcal disease is hyperendemic or epidemic
  - Persons who have persistent complement deficiencies
  - Persons with anatomic or functional asplenia.
- Both vaccines are available in a 0.5 ml dose meant for intramuscular injecting, preferably into the deltoid.
- Both vaccines are capable of stimulating appropriate immune responses.
- The ACIP recommended age for administration of the initial dose of meningococcal vaccine is 11 to 12 years.
  - A recent recommendation states that all individuals who received an initial vaccine at that age should receive a booster dose at age 16.
  - At the time of this publication, an alternative approach of delaying the first dose until age 14 or 15 is in discussion.

Pertussis

- Persons aged 10–19 years accounted for 25–39% of all cases of pertussis diagnosed in the U.S. between 2003 and 2007.
- Similarly, from 2001 to 2003, more cases of pertussis were reported among 10-19 year olds than in any other age group, totaling one-third of nearly 29,000 cases.
- Pertussis is typically milder in adolescents than in younger children, but morbidity is significant.
  - In one study, nearly half (47%) of adolescents had a cough for more than 9 weeks; paroxysmal cough was present for 3 or more weeks in 73%; 67% had the characteristic whoop; and 71% experienced post-tussive emesis.
  - Adolescents with pertussis miss an average of 5 days of school.
  - Adolescents also represent a source of potential transmission of pertussis to others; in a CDC study, 10-19 year olds accounted for 20% of infant pertussis cases where a source could be identified and for whom the age of the source was known.
  - Infants too young to have been fully immunized are at greatest risk for pertussis-related complications, hospitalizations and death.

Pertussis Vaccine

- Two vaccine products are currently available with slightly different antigenic properties but otherwise appear to be clinically equivalent.
- TDaP, or Tetanus, diphtheria, and acellular pertussis, contains antigens from pertussis ("acellular pertussis" component), tetanus and diphtheria bacteria, mirroring the vaccines administered to infants and children.
- Both vaccines are meant to be used as booster doses in adolescents and young adults who have ideally received an appropriate primary immunization series with one of the pediatric formulations of the vaccine.
- The dose of either product is 0.5 ml administered intramuscularly, preferably into the deltoid muscles.
- In adolescents and young adults, the main adverse side effect is pain at the injection site, although approximately 20–25% of patients will experience redness and/or swelling. Some incidents of headache, fatigue, and gastrointestinal complaints have also been reported.
- The preferred interval between the last tetanus/diphtheria product and a TDaP vaccination is 5 years; however, in outbreak situations, TDaP can be administered two years after the last dose of a tetanus/diphtheria vaccine.

Human Papillomavirus (HPV)

- Genital HPV infection is the most common sexually transmitted infection (STI) in the U.S. and may be the leading STI worldwide.
- While most disease is asymptomatic and self-limited, persistent HPV infection with high risk types of virus is responsible for virtually all cases of cervical cancer and other anogenital cancers as well.
- According to the CDC, each year 6.2 million new HPV infections are diagnosed among males and females 14–44 years of age; 74% of those infections occur in those 15–24 years.
- The prevalence of HPV infection among U.S. females 14–19 years of age is 25%, close to the national average of 27% for all women 14–59 years of age.
- Approximately 40–50% of sexually active females will be HPV-positive within 2–3 years of sexual debut.

HPV Vaccine

- Two vaccines are available for preventing HPV infection.

- Each is composed of "virus like particles" (VLPs) that are made up of the main capsid protein of HPV, L1.
- HPV4, licensed as a quadravalent vaccine, is effective in preventing HPV types 16 and 18 (responsible for 70% of all cases of cervical cancer) as well as types 6 and 11 (responsible for the overwhelming number of cases of genital warts).
- HPV2, which only prevents types 16 and 18, has recently been approved.
- Both vaccines appear to be excellent in preventing type-specific infection with efficacy rates of 86–100% depending on HPV subtype and type of cancerous, precancerous or wart lesions being prevented.
- The ACIP recommends the vaccine be administered to females aged 11–26 years who have not been previously vaccinated. It is preferred that the vaccine be administered to women before potential exposure to HPV through sexual contact.
- The ACIP also recommended vaccination to males aged 11–21 who have not previously been vaccinated or who have not completed the 3 dose series, and males 22–26 years may also receive the vaccine.
- The 3 shot administration schedule is the same for both vaccines (0, 1–2, and 6 months) as is the dose (0.5 mL intramuscularly, preferably in the deltoid).
- The minimum interval is one month between the first and second dose, and four months between the second and third dose.
- It is not necessary to restart the series if the schedule is interrupted.
- These vaccines are classified as inactivated, so either can be administered with other inactivated or live vaccines.
- While it can be administered to lactating women, it is not recommended during pregnancy (although if this happens inadvertently, nothing need be done other than to defer the rest of the series until the completion of the pregnancy).
- When first introduced, there were concerns about potential side effects and safety profile.

    - As of May 31, 2010, over 30 million doses of one or the other of the available vaccines have been administered.
    - While over 16,000 adverse events have been reported, the overwhelming majority have been classified as mild to moderate.
    - The three reported deaths associated with vaccine administration have all had alternative explanations.

- Fainting after vaccine administration has resulted in falls and related injuries; hence, it is recommended that patients be briefly monitored before leaving the clinic.

VACCINES OF ADOLESCENCE

Influenza

- Individuals with chronic health conditions have always been at risk of life-threatening complications secondary to influenza infections. Adolescents contribute to the annual spread of influenza and teens are ideal candidates for annual vaccination.
- In July 2010, ACIP recommended annual influenza vaccination for everyone $\geq$6 months of age.

Influenza Vaccine

- Two vaccine products are available for use in adolescents: Trivalent Inactivated Vaccine (TIV) and Live Attenuated Influenza Vaccine (LAIV).
- The former is administered intramuscularly and the later is delivered by a nasal spray.
- Both have been shown to provide excellent immunity during a particular influenza season but because of the propensity for the flu virus to mutate each year, they must be administered annually with the vaccine specifically manufactured for that year.
- The vaccine should be administered before the expected appearance of influenza in the community (fall in the northern hemisphere and spring in the southern hemisphere).

Varicella

- Adolescents remain susceptible to chickenpox if exposed to the virus. Their course of illness tends to be more severe than that in younger children.
- It is currently recommended that children and adolescents receive two doses of the vaccine.

Varicella Vaccine

- The two shot single-antigen (as compared to the multiantigen vaccine used in children) vaccine series is administered as a dose of 0.5 ml injected subcutaneously.
- Susceptible adolescents can also receive varicella vaccine within 5 days of exposure to an individual with overt disease.
- This is a live attenuated vaccine and should not be administered to immunosuppressed individuals.

Hepatitis Vaccines

- Many adolescents have been vaccinated against both hepatitis A and B; those not previously vaccinated or those who have not received the complete series should be vaccinated.
- Hepatitis B is delivered in a 3 shot series (at 0, 1 and 6 months) and Hepatitis A in a 2 shot series (at 0 and 6 months).
- Both vaccines are available in two slightly different formulations from different manufacturers. A combined form of the vaccines is available for adolescents over 18 years of age.

ASSESSMENT

- Many adolescents have not received appropriate vaccines during childhood or latency age, or may have inadequate documentation of shots received.
- Consider the absence of documentation to be synonymous with a lack of appropriate immunization. Reasonable efforts can and should be made to identify this documentation, but if unable to do so, initiate appropriate immunization protocol.
- If there is a hiatus between vaccine receipt longer than that recommended series schedule, do not restart: merely resume the schedule where it was left off. Luckily, most adolescents will respond well to immunizing antigens even if "off schedule" and additional shots are unnecessary (Table 2).

DISPOSITION

- Unimmunized or underimmunized adolescents should receive vaccines according to the ACIP recommended schedule (Figure 1).

- Provider and system-based innovations can improve immunization rates in teens (Table 3).

Provider Innovations

Providers can take steps to improve coverage rates for vaccines in adolescents.

- Clinicians should screen an adolescent's immunization status and vaccination needs at every clinic visit.
- "Standing orders," may allow different staff members to initiate vaccination reviews and vaccination updates.
- When linked to a systematic recall and reminder system, this can take the onus off the provider to remember to check for vaccinations that are necessary or desirable.
- Immunization systems can be even more effective if augmented by a government run registry. While all states are mandated to have such registries, their accuracy and accessibility vary state to state.
- Personal and patient education about adolescent appropriate vaccines should be a priority for all clinicians.

System-Based Innovations

- Get states to expand the mandates for adolescents entering junior high school or high school. Only slightly more than half the states have such mandates in place, and some of these states exclude "adolescent vaccines" discussed earlier.
- The system should allow for immunization tracking; as an example, centralized registries have been found to work best and improve vaccination rates.
- Improved insurance coverage and overall expansion in funding would assure that vaccines are available through the Vaccines for Children (VFC) program which supports the provision of recommended vaccines to adolescents who have no insurance, or state and/or federal support for their care.
- Expansion in coverage and payment must adequately support the costs that providers assume in storing and administering vaccines.
- Preventive health care for adolescents and young adults must be promoted as the desirable norm for all health care settings.

- Settings other than primary care offices should be considered appropriate venues for administering vaccines such as schools, family planning clinics, emergency departments and pharmacies.
- This could be facilitated by revisiting "consent" and "confidentiality" issues which might otherwise impede utilizing alternative sites for immunization activities.

What is unique about immunizations in adolescents?

- Adolescents face unique barriers to successful immunization.
- Adolescents are the least likely age group to seek or receive health care.
    - If not receiving care, they will likely not have regular review and updates to their vaccination history.
    - Insurance plays a role in this access to care issue. Despite aggressive attempts to get all adolescents some form of health care, many still do not have appropriate health coverage and do not receive the services they need.
- When adolescents do get care, they often do not get a level of care likely to result in appropriate review and administration of vaccines.
    - Vaccines are routinely checked and administered during preventive health visits; however, teens are far less likely to receive appropriate preventive health care than younger children.
    - When medical visits occur, patient and provider are often overwhelmed by the myriad of topics that need to be covered including educational issues, exercise, activities, diet and eating patterns, driving and auto safety, alcohol and drug use, sexuality and reproductive health, mental health and general safety issues.
    - In this litany, vaccines often get pushed down the list of topics that need to be addressed.
- The rapid expansion of available and appropriate vaccines may not be as well appreciated by some providers and patients.

- Additionally, school attendance policies are not often updated to keep pace with new guidelines issued by the ACIP.
- Finally, as adolescents move through the health care system, immunization records may not make the transition with them. Only some states have well functioning centralized immunization registries.

TEST YOUR KNOWLEDGE ANSWER

6. E. In 2010, the ACIP recommended annual influenza vaccines for all persons older than 6 months of age. Adolescents constitute significantly to the unusual spread of influenza and those with chronic health conditions are at risk of life threatening complications secondary to influenza infections. Teens are ideal candidates for annual vaccinations.

Table 1. Newly Released Vaccines Targeted to Protect Adolescents and Young Adults.

Vaccine	Basics
Tetanus, Diphtheria, and Acellular Pertussis (TDaP)	• Two different vaccines available for adolescents: BOOSTRIX and ADACEL • Target age: 11–12 years (range, 11–55) • Interval between last TD and reimmunization with TDaP: 5 years (less for high risk or epidemic situations) • Side effects: Primarily local • Dosage and administration: 0.5 mL, intramuscular
Meningococcal Conjugate	• Two different vaccines available for adolescents: MENACTRA and MENVEO • Target age: 11–12 years (range, 11–55) • Need for previous or booster immunization: None • Side effects: Primarily local. Cases of Guillain-Barre Syndrome have been reported. • Dosage and administration: 0.5 mL, intramuscular
Human Papillomavirus	• Two different vaccines available for adolescents: GARDASIL (quadrivalent) and CERVARIX (bivalent) • Target age: 11–12 years (range, 9–26) • Side effects: Primarily local. Syncope has been reported. • Dosage and administration: 0.5 mL, intramuscular
Pneumococcal conjugate vaccine (PCV13)	• Conjugate vaccine for prevention of invasive pneumococcal disease • Target age: 19 and above with immunocompromising conditions • Side effects: Primarily local • If they have received PPSV23, PCV13 should be given 1 year after

Table 2. Catch-Up Immunization Schedule for Persons Ages 7–18 Years.

Vaccine	Minimum Age for Dose 1	Minimum Interval Between Doses: Dose 1 to Dose 2	Dose 2 to Dose 3	Dose 3 to Dose 4
Tetanus, Diphtheria/ Tetanus, Diphtheria, Pertussis	7 years	4 weeks	4 weeks if first dose administered at younger than age 12 months 6 months if first dose administered at 12 months or older	6 months if first dose administered at younger than 12 months
Human Papillomavirus	9 years	Routine intervals are recommended		
Hepatitis A	12 months	6 months if first dose administered at younger than 12 months		
Hepatitis B	Birth	4 weeks	8 weeks (and at least 6 weeks after 1 dose)	
Inactivated Poliovirus	6 weeks	4 weeks		
Meningococcal	9 months	8 weeks		
Measles, Mumps, Rubella	12 months	4 weeks		
Varicella	12 months	3 months if person is younger than age 13 years 4 weeks if person is aged 13 years or older		

http://www.cdc.gov/vaccines/recs/schedules/downloads/child/catchup-schedule-pr.pdf for more detail.

Figure 1. Recommended immunization schedule for persons aged 0 through 18 years – 2013.
(FOR THOSE WHO FALL BEHIND OR START LATE, SEE THE CATCH-UP SCHEDULE [FIGURE 2]).

These recommendations must be read with the footnotes that follow. For those who fall behind or start late, provide catch-up vaccination at the earliest opportunity as indicated by the green bars in Figure 1. To determine minimum intervals between doses, see the catch-up schedule (Figure 2). School entry and adolescent vaccine age groups are in bold.

Vaccines	Birth	1 mo	2 mos	4 mos	6 mos	9 mos	12 mos	15 mos	18 mos	19–23 mos	2-3 yrs	**4-6 yrs**	7-10 yrs	**11-12 yrs**	13–15 yrs	16–18 yrs
Hepatitis B[1] (HepB)	←1st dose→	←2nd dose→			←3rd dose→											
Rotavirus[2] (RV) RV-1 (2-dose series); RV-5 (3-dose series)			←1st dose→	←2nd dose→	See footnote 2											
Diphtheria, tetanus, & acellular pertussis[3] (DTaP: <7 yrs)			←1st dose→	←2nd dose→	←3rd dose→			←4th dose→				←5th dose→				
Tetanus, diphtheria, & acellular pertussis[4] (Tdap: ≥7 yrs)														(Tdap)		
Haemophilus influenzae type b[5] (Hib)			←1st dose→	←2nd dose→	See footnote 5		←3rd or 4th dose, see footnote 5→									
Pneumococcal conjugate[6a,c] (PCV13)			←1st dose→	←2nd dose→	←3rd dose→		←4th dose→									
Pneumococcal polysaccharide[6b,c] (PPSV23)																
Inactivated Poliovirus[7] (IPV) (<18years)			←1st dose→	←2nd dose→	←3rd dose→							←4th dose→				
Influenza[8] (IIV; LAIV) 2 doses for some : see footnote 8					Annual vaccination (IIV only)						Annual vaccination (IIV or LAIV)					
Measles, mumps, rubella[9] (MMR)							←1st dose→					←2nd dose→				
Varicella[10] (VAR)							←1st dose→					←2nd dose→				
Hepatitis A[11] (HepA)							←2 dose series, see footnote 11→									
Human papillomavirus[12] (HPV2: females only; HPV4: males and females)														(3-dose series)		
Meningococcal[13] (Hib-MenCY ≥ 6 weeks; MCV4-D≥9 mos; MCV4-CRM ≥ 2 yrs.)			see footnote 13											←1st dose→		booster

Range of recommended ages for all children | Range of recommended ages for catch-up immunization | Range of recommended ages for certain high-risk groups | Range of recommended ages during which catch-up is encouraged and for certain high-risk groups | Not routinely recommended

This schedule includes recommendations in effect as of January 1, 2013. Any dose not administered at the recommended age should be administered at a subsequent visit, when indicated and feasible. The use of a combination vaccine generally is preferred over separate injections of its equivalent component vaccines. Vaccination providers should consult the relevant Advisory Committee on Immunization Practices (ACIP) statement for detailed recommendations, available online at http://www.cdc.gov/vaccines/pubs/acip-list.htm. Clinically significant adverse events that follow vaccination should be reported to the Vaccine Adverse Event Reporting System (VAERS) online (http://www.vaers.hhs.gov) or by telephone (800-822-7967).Suspected cases of vaccine-preventable diseases should be reported to the state or local health department. Additional information, including precautions and contraindications for vaccination, is available from CDC online (http://www.cdc.gov/vaccines) or by telephone (800-CDC-INFO [800-232-4636]).

This schedule is approved by the Advisory Committee on Immunization Practices (http://www.cdc.gov/vaccines/acip/index.html), the American Academy of Pediatrics (http://www.aap.org), the American Academy of Family Physicians (http://www.aafp.org), and the American College of Obstetricians and Gynecologists (http://www.acog.org).

NOTE: The above recommendations must be read along with the footnotes of this schedule.

Footnotes — Recommended immunization schedule for persons aged 0 through 18 years—United States, 2013

For further guidance on the use of the vaccines mentioned below, see: http://www.cdc.gov/vaccines/pubs/acip-list.htm.

1. **Hepatitis B (HepB) vaccine. (Minimum age: birth)**
   Routine vaccination:
   At birth
   - Administer monovalent HepB vaccine to all newborns before hospital discharge.
   - For infants born to hepatitis B surface antigen (HBsAg)–positive mothers, administer HepB vaccine and 0.5 mL of hepatitis B immune globulin (HBIG) within 12 hours of birth. These infants should be tested for HBsAg and antibody to HBsAg (anti-HBs) 1 to 2 months after completion of the HepB series, at age 9 through 18 months (preferably at the next well-child visit).
   - If mother's HBsAg status is unknown, within 12 hours of birth administer HepB vaccine to all infants regardless of birth weight. For infants weighing <2,000 grams, administer HBIG in addition to HepB within 12 hours of birth. Determine mother's HBsAg status as soon as possible and, if she is HBsAg-positive, also administer HBIG for infants weighing ≥2,000 grams (no later than age 1 week).

   Doses following the birth dose
   - The second dose should be administered at age 1 or 2 months. Monovalent HepB vaccine should be used for doses administered before age 6 weeks.
   - Infants who did not receive a birth dose should receive 3 doses of a HepB-containing vaccine on a schedule of 0, 1 to 2 months, and 6 months starting as soon as feasible. See Figure 2.
   - The minimum interval between dose 1 and dose 2 is 4 weeks and between dose 2 and 3 is 8 weeks. The final (third or fourth) dose in the HepB vaccine series should be administered no earlier than age 24 weeks, and at least 16 weeks after the first dose.
   - Administration of a total of 4 doses of HepB vaccine is recommended when a combination vaccine containing HepB is administered after the birth dose.

   Catch-up vaccination:
   - Unvaccinated persons should complete a 3-dose series.
   - A 2-dose series (doses separated by at least 4 months) of adult formulation Recombivax HB is licensed for use in children aged 11 through 15 years.
   - For other catch-up issues, see Figure 2.
2. **Rotavirus (RV) vaccines. (Minimum age: 6 weeks for both RV-1 [Rotarix] and RV-5 [RotaTeq]).**
   Routine vaccination:
   - Administer a series of RV vaccine to all infants as follows:
     1. If RV-1 is used, administer a 2-dose series at 2 and 4 months of age.
     2. If RV-5 is used, administer a 3-dose series at ages 2, 4, and 6 months.
     3. If any dose in series was RV-5 or vaccine product is unknown for any dose in the series, a total of 3 doses of RV vaccine should be administered.

   Catch-up vaccination:
   - The maximum age for the first dose in the series is 14 weeks, 6 days.
   - Vaccination should not be initiated for infants aged 15 weeks 0 days or older.
   - The maximum age for the final dose in the series is 8 months, 0 days.
   - If RV-1(Rotarix) is administered for the first and second doses, a third dose is not indicated.
   - For other catch-up issues, see Figure 2.
3. **Diphtheria and tetanus toxoids and acellular pertussis (DTaP) vaccine. (Minimum age: 6 weeks)**
   Routine vaccination:
   - Administer a 5-dose series of DTaP vaccine at ages 2, 4, 6, 15–18 months, and 4 through 6 years. The fourth dose may be administered as early as age 12 months, provided at least 6 months have elapsed since the third dose.

   Catch-up vaccination:
   - The fifth (booster) dose of DTaP vaccine is not necessary if the fourth dose was administered at age 4 years or older.
   - For other catch-up issues, see Figure 2.
4. **Tetanus and diphtheria toxoids and acellular pertussis (Tdap) vaccine. (Minimum age: 10 years for Boostrix, 11 years for Adacel).**
   Routine vaccination:
   - Administer 1 dose of Tdap vaccine to all adolescents aged 11 through 12 years.
   - Tdap can be administered regardless of the interval since the last tetanus and diphtheria toxoid-containing vaccine.
   - Administer one dose of Tdap vaccine to pregnant adolescents during each pregnancy (preferred during 27 through 36 weeks gestation) regardless of number of years from prior Td or Tdap vaccination.

   Catch-up vaccination:
   - Persons aged 7 through 10 years who are not fully immunized with the childhood DTaP vaccine series should receive Tdap vaccine as the first dose in the catch-up series; if additional doses are needed, use Td vaccine. For these children, an adolescent Tdap vaccine should not be given.
   - Persons aged 11 through 18 years who have not received Tdap vaccine should receive a dose followed by tetanus and diphtheria toxoids (Td) booster doses every 10 years thereafter.
   - An inadvertent dose of DTaP vaccine administered to children aged 7 through 10 years can count as part of the catch-up series. This dose can count as the adolescent Tdap dose, or the child can later receive a Tdap booster dose at age 11–12 years.
   - For other catch-up issues, see Figure 2.
5. ***Haemophilus influenzae* type b (Hib) conjugate vaccine. (Minimum age: 6 weeks)**
   Routine vaccination:
   - Administer a Hib vaccine primary series and a booster dose to all infants. The primary series doses should be administered at 2, 4, and 6 months of age; however, if PRP-OMP (PedvaxHib or Comvax) is administered at 2 and 4 months of age, a dose at age 6 months is not indicated. One booster dose should be administered at age 12 through15 months.
   - Hiberix (PRP-T) should only be used for the booster (final) dose in children aged 12 months through 4 years, who have received at least 1 dose of Hib.

   Catch-up vaccination:
   - If dose 1 was administered at ages 12-14 months, administer booster (as final dose) at least 8 weeks after dose 1.
   - If the first 2 doses were PRP-OMP (PedvaxHIB or Comvax), and were administered at age 11 months or younger, the third (and final) dose should be administered at age 12 through 15 months and at least 8 weeks after the second dose.
   - If the first dose was administered at age 7 through 11 months, administer the second dose at least 4 weeks later and a final dose at age 12 through 15 months, regardless of Hib vaccine (PRP-T or PRP-OMP) used for first dose.
   - For unvaccinated children aged 15 months or older, administer only 1 dose.

For further guidance on the use of the vaccines mentioned below, see: http://www.cdc.gov/vaccines/pubs/acip-list.htm.

- For other catch-up issues, see Figure 2.

Vaccination of persons with high-risk conditions:

- Hib vaccine is not routinely recommended for patients older than 5 years of age. However one dose of Hib vaccine should be administered to unvaccinated or partially vaccinated persons aged 5 years or older who have leukemia, malignant neoplasms, anatomic or functional asplenia (including sickle cell disease), human immunodeficiency virus (HIV) infection, or other immunocompromising conditions.

6a. Pneumococcal conjugate vaccine (PCV). (Minimum age: 6 weeks)

Routine vaccination:

- Administer a series of PCV13 vaccine at ages 2, 4, 6 months with a booster at age 12 through 15 months.
- For children aged 14 through 59 months who have received an age-appropriate series of 7-valent PCV (PCV7), administer a single supplemental dose of 13-valent PCV (PCV13).

Catch-up vaccination:

- Administer 1 dose of PCV13 to all healthy children aged 24 through 59 months who are not completely vaccinated for their age.
- For other catch-up issues, see Figure 2.

Vaccination of persons with high-risk conditions:

- For children aged 24 through 71 months with certain underlying medical conditions (see footnote 6c), administer 1 dose of PCV13 if 3 doses of PCV were received previously, or administer 2 doses of PCV13 at least 8 weeks apart if fewer than 3 doses of PCV were received previously.
- A single dose of PCV13 may be administered to previously unvaccinated children aged 6 through 18 years who have anatomic or functional asplenia (including sickle cell disease), HIV infection or an immunocompromising condition, cochlear implant or cerebrospinal fluid leak. See MMWR 2010;59 (No. RR-11), available at http://www.cdc.gov/mmwr/pdf/rr/rr5911.pdf.
- Administer PPSV23 at least 8 weeks after the last dose of PCV to children aged 2 years or older with certain underlying medical conditions (see footnotes 6b and 6c).

6b. Pneumococcal polysaccharide vaccine (PPSV23). (Minimum age: 2 years)

Vaccination of persons with high-risk conditions:

- Administer PPSV23 at least 8 weeks after the last dose of PCV to children aged 2 years or older with certain underlying medical conditions (see footnote 6c). A single revaccination with PPSV should be administered after 5 years to children with anatomic or functional asplenia (including sickle cell disease) or an immunocompromising condition.

6c. Medical conditions for which PPSV23 is indicated in children aged 2 years and older and for which use of PCV13 is indicated in children aged 24 through 71 months:

- Immunocompetent children with chronic heart disease (particularly cyanotic congenital heart disease and cardiac failure); chronic lung disease (including asthma if treated with high-dose oral corticosteroid therapy), diabetes mellitus; cerebrospinal fluid leaks; or cochlear implant.
- Children with anatomic or functional asplenia (including sickle cell disease and other hemoglobinopathies, congenital or acquired asplenia, or splenic dysfunction);
- Children with immunocompromising conditions: HIV infection, chronic renal failure and nephrotic syndrome, diseases associated with treatment with immunosuppressive drugs or radiation therapy, including malignant neoplasms, leukemias, lymphomas and Hodgkin disease; or solid organ transplantation, congenital immunodeficiency.

7. Inactivated poliovirus vaccine (IPV). (Minimum age: 6 weeks)

Routine vaccination:

- Administer a series of IPV at ages 2, 4, 6–18 months, with a booster at age 4–6 years. The final dose in the series should be administered on or after the fourth birthday and at least 6 months after the previous dose.

Catch-up vaccination:

- In the first 6 months of life, minimum age and minimum intervals are only recommended if the person is at risk for imminent exposure to circulating poliovirus (i.e., travel to a polio-endemic region or during an outbreak).
- If 4 or more doses are administered before age 4 years, an additional dose should be administered at age 4 through 6 years.
- A fourth dose is not necessary if the third dose was administered at age 4 years or older and at least 6 months after the previous dose.
- If both OPV and IPV were administered as part of a series, a total of 4 doses should be administered, regardless of the child's current age.
- IPV is not routinely recommended for U.S. residents aged 18 years or older.
- For other catch-up issues, see Figure 2.

8. Influenza vaccines. (Minimum age: 6 months for inactivated influenza vaccine [IIV]; 2 years for live, attenuated influenza vaccine [LAIV])

Routine vaccination:

- Administer influenza vaccine annually to all children beginning at age 6 months. For most healthy, nonpregnant persons aged 2 through 49 years, either LAIV or IIV may be used. However, LAIV should NOT be administered to some persons, including 1) those with asthma, 2) children 2 through 4 years who had wheezing in the past 12 months, or 3) those who have any other underlying medical conditions that predispose them to influenza complications. For all other contraindications to use of LAIV see MMWR 2010; 59 (No. RR-8), available at http://www.cdc.gov/mmwr/pdf/rr/rr5908.pdf.
- Administer 1 dose to persons aged 9 years and older.

For children aged 6 months through 8 years:

- For the 2012–13 season, administer 2 doses (separated by at least 4 weeks) to children who are receiving influenza vaccine for the first time. For additional guidance, follow dosing guidelines in the 2012 ACIP influenza vaccine recommendations, MMWR 2012; 61:613–618, available at http://www.cdc.gov/mmwr/pdf/wk/mm6132.pdf.
- For the 2013–14 season, follow dosing guidelines in the 2013 ACIP influenza vaccine recommendations.

9. Measles, mumps, and rubella (MMR) vaccine. (Minimum age: 12 months for routine vaccination)

Routine vaccination:

- Administer the first dose of MMR vaccine at age 12 through 15 months, and the second dose at age 4 through 6 years. The second dose may be administered before age 4 years, provided at least 4 weeks have elapsed since the first dose.
- Administer 1 dose of MMR vaccine to infants aged 6 through 11 months before departure from the United States for international travel. These children should be revaccinated with 2 doses of MMR vaccine, the first at age 12 through 15 months (12 months if the child remains in an area where disease risk is high), and the second dose at least 4 weeks later.
- Administer 2 doses of MMR vaccine to children aged 12 months and older, before departure from the United States for international travel. The first dose should be administered on or after age 12 months and the second dose at least 4 weeks later.

Catch-up vaccination:

- Ensure that all school-aged children and adolescents have had 2 doses of MMR vaccine; the minimum interval between the 2 doses is 4 weeks.

10. Varicella (VAR) vaccine. (Minimum age: 12 months)

Routine vaccination:

- Administer the first dose of VAR vaccine at age 12 through 15 months, and the second dose at age 4 through 6 years. The second dose may be administered before age 4 years, provided at least 3 months have elapsed since the first dose. If the second dose was administered at least 4 weeks after the first dose, it can be accepted as valid.

Catch-up vaccination:

- Ensure that all persons aged 7 through 18 years without evidence of immunity (see MMWR 2007;56 [No. RR-4], available at http://www.cdc.gov/mmwr/pdf/rr/rr5604.pdf) have 2 doses of varicella vaccine. For children aged 7 through 12 years the recommended minimum interval between doses is 3 months (if the second dose was administered at least 4 weeks after the first dose, it can be accepted as valid); for persons aged 13 years and older, the minimum interval between doses is 4 weeks.

11. Hepatitis A vaccine (HepA). (Minimum age: 12 months)

Routine vaccination:

- Initiate the 2-dose HepA vaccine series for children aged 12 through 23 months; separate the 2 doses by 6 to 18 months.
- Children who have received 1 dose of HepA vaccine before age 24 months, should receive a second dose 6 to 18 months after the first dose.
- For any person aged 2 years and older who has not already received the HepA vaccine series, 2 doses of HepA vaccine separated by 6 to 18 months may be administered if immunity against hepatitis A virus infection is desired.

Catch-up vaccination:

- The minimum interval between the two doses is 6 months.

Special populations:

- Administer 2 doses of Hep A vaccine at least 6 months apart to previously unvaccinated persons who live in areas where vaccination programs target older children, or who are at increased risk for infection.

12. Human papillomavirus (HPV) vaccines. (HPV4 [Gardasil] and HPV2 [Cervarix]). (Minimum age: 9 years)

Routine vaccination:

- Administer a 3-dose series of HPV vaccine on a schedule of 0, 1-2, and 6 months to all adolescents aged 11-12 years. Either HPV4 or HPV2 may be used for females, and only HPV4 may be used for males.
- The vaccine series can be started beginning at age 9 years.
- Administer the second dose 1 to 2 months after the <u>first</u> dose and the third dose 6 months after the <u>first</u> dose (at least 24 weeks after the first dose).

Catch-up vaccination:

- Administer the vaccine series to females (either HPV2 or HPV4) and males (HPV4) at age 13 through 18 years if not previously vaccinated.
- Use recommended routine dosing intervals (see above) for vaccine series catch-up.

13. Meningococcal conjugate vaccines (MCV). (Minimum age: 6 weeks for Hib-MenCY, 9 months for Menactra [MCV4-D], 2 years for Menveo [MCV4-CRM]).

Routine vaccination:

- Administer MCV4 vaccine at age 11–12 years, with a booster dose at age 16 years.
- Adolescents aged 11 through 18 years with human immunodeficiency virus (HIV) infection should receive a 2-dose primary series of MCV4, with at least 8 weeks between doses. See MMWR 2011; 60:1018–1019 available at: http://www.cdc.gov/mmwr/pdf/wk/mm6030.pdf.
- For children aged 2 months through 10 years with high-risk conditions, see below.

Catch-up vaccination:

- Administer MCV4 vaccine at age 13 through 18 years if not previously vaccinated.
- If the first dose is administered at age 13 through 15 years, a booster dose should be administered at age 16 through 18 years with a minimum interval of at least 8 weeks between doses.
- If the first dose is administered at age 16 years or older, a booster dose is not needed.
- For other catch-up issues, see Figure 2.

Vaccination of persons with high-risk conditions:

- For children younger than 19 months of age with anatomic or functional asplenia (including sickle cell disease), administer an infant series of Hib-MenCY at 2, 4, 6, and 12-15 months.
- For children aged 2 through 18 months with persistent complement component deficiency, administer either an infant series of Hib-MenCY at 2, 4, 6, and 12 through 15 months or a 2-dose primary series of MCV4-D starting at 9 months, with at least 8 weeks between doses. For children aged 19 through 23 months with persistent complement component deficiency who have not received a complete series of Hib-MenCY or MCV4-D, administer 2 primary doses of MCV4-D at least 8 weeks apart.
- For children aged 24 months and older with persistent complement component deficiency or anatomic or functional asplenia (including sickle cell disease), who have not received a complete series of Hib-MenCY or MCV4-D, administer 2 primary doses of either MCV4-D or MCV4-CRM. If MCV4-D (Menactra) is administered to a child with asplenia (including sickle cell disease), do not administer MCV4-D until 2 years of age and at least 4 weeks after the completion of all PCV13 doses. See MMWR 2011;60:1391–2, available at http://www.cdc.gov/mmwr/pdf/wk/mm6040.pdf.
- For children aged 9 months and older who are residents of or travelers to countries in the African meningitis belt or to the Hajj, administer an age appropriate formulation and series of MCV4 for protection against serogroups A and W-135. Prior receipt of Hib-MenCY is not sufficient for children traveling to the meningitis belt or the Hajj. See MMWR 2011;60:1391–2, available at http://www.cdc.gov/mmwr/pdf/wk/mm6040.pdf.
- For children who are present during outbreaks caused by a vaccine serogroup, administer or complete an age and formulation-appropriate series of Hib-MenCY or MCV4.
- For booster doses among persons with high-risk conditions refer to http://www.cdc.gov/vaccines/pubs/acip-list.htm#mening.

Additional information

- For contraindications and precautions to use of a vaccine and for additional information regarding that vaccine, vaccination providers should consult the relevant ACIP statement available online at http://www.cdc.gov/vaccines/pubs/acip-list.htm.
- For the purposes of calculating intervals between doses, 4 weeks = 28 days. Intervals of 4 months or greater are determined by calendar months.
- Information on travel vaccine requirements and recommendations is available at http://wwwnc.cdc.gov/travel/page/vaccinations.htm.
- For vaccination of persons with primary and secondary immunodeficiencies, see Table 13, "Vaccination of persons with primary and secondary immunodeficiencies," in General Recommendations on Immunization (ACIP), available at http://www.cdc.gov/mmwr/preview/mmwrhtml/rr6002a1.htm; and American Academy of Pediatrics. Immunization in Special Clinical Circumstances. In: Pickering LK, Baker CJ, Kimberlin DW, Long SS eds. Red book: 2012 report of the Committee on Infectious Diseases. 29th ed. Elk Grove Village, IL: American Academy of Pediatrics.

U.S. Department of Health and Human Services
Centers for Disease Control and Prevention

Table 3. Provider and Community Actions to Promote Adolescent Immunization.

Provider Actions	• Use all patient interactions to screen for immunization status. • Use "standing orders" to review status and initiate immunization of adolescents who need them. • Initiate a recall system to assure that adolescents return when they are supposed to for appropriate immunizations. • Require and use up to date centralized registries. • Prioritize personal, staff, and patient education concerning proper immunizations.
System-Based (Community/ Government) Actions	• Mandate appropriate proof of vaccination for junior and senior high school students. • Assure that a functioning and available central vaccine registry is in place and mandate its use by providers. • Mandate private and public insurance coverage for all ACIP approved and recommended vaccines for adolescents and preadolescents. • Promote preventive health care for adolescents. • Allow alternative sites for immunizing adolescents such as schools, family planning clinics, emergency departments, pharmacies, etc.

WEB REFERENCES

- American Academy of Pediatrics (http://www.aap.org/healthtopics/immunizations.cfm)
  - Recommended Immunization Schedules (Last Updated 2/28/2013), http://www.healthychildren.org/English/safety-prevention/immunizations/pages/Recommended-Immunization-Schedules.aspx

- Centers for Disease Control and Prevention (http://www.cdc.gov/vaccines/)
  - CDC. Advisory Committee on Immunization Practices (ACIP) 'Recommended Immunization Schedules for Persons Aged 0 Through 18 years and Adults Aged 19 Years and Older-United States,'2013. MMWR2013;62(Suppl 1):1–19: http://www.cdc.gov/mmwr/pdf/wk/mm62eO128.pdf
  - CDC. 'Prevention of Pneumococcal Disease Among Infants and Children-Use of 13-Valent Pneumococcal Conjugate Vaccine and 23-Valent Pneumococcal Polysaccharide Vaccine.' MMWR2010;59(RRll);l-18: http://www.cdc.gov/mmwr/preview/mmwrhtml/rr5911al.htm
  - CDC. 'Recommendations on the Use of Quadrivalent Human Papillomavirus Vaccine in Males — Advisory Committee on Immunization Practices (ACIP).' MMWR 2011;60(50); 1705–1708: www.cdc.gov/mmwr/preview/mmwrhtml/mm6050a3.htm

- Ipp LS, Breuner CC, Middleman AB (2012) 'Meningococcal Vaccine: A Position Statement of the Society for Adolescent Health and Medicine', Journal of Adolescent Health 2012;50;211-212, Retrieved from http://www.adolescenthealth.org/AM/Template.cfm?Section=Position_Papers&Template=/CM/ContentDisplay.cfm&ContentID=3569
- Middleman AB, et al. (2006) 'Adolescent Immunizations: A position paper of the Society for Adolescent Medicine', Journal of Adolescent Health 2006;38;321-327, Retrieved from http://www.adolescenthealth.org/AM/Template. cfm?Section=Position_Papers&Template=/CM/ContentDisplay.cfm&ContentID=1479

Additional Clinician Resources:

- Centers for Disease Control and Prevention, Vaccine Schedules: http://www.cdc.gov/vaccines/schedules/index.html
- Immunization Action Coalition: http://www.immunize.org/
- Medline Plus: http://www.nlm.nih.gov/medlineplus/immunization.html
- Quackwatch: http://www.quackwatch.org/03HealthPromotion/immu/immu00.html

5

TAKING CARE OF ADOLESCENT MALES

Daniel E. Korin

TEST YOUR KNOWLEDGE

7. The *MOST* important purpose of the annual physical exam in adolescent males is to:

   A. Identify high blood pressure.
   B. Auscultate heart for murmurs.
   C. Complete a genital exam for testicular masses.
   D. Clear athletes to play sports.
   E. Ascertain and intervene for risky behaviors.

Refer to end of chapter for answer on page 62.

Joel is a 14 year old male in your office for routine PE. He has noticed that all his friends are growing taller while he is not. At the end of the visit, he asks "How tall am I going to be?"

BACKGROUND

- Most adolescent males are in good health and rarely seek medical attention unless it is mandatory (i.e. athlete physical) or there is an acute problem (i.e. fracture).
- Nevertheless, there are important considerations to make when evaluating an adolescent male.

ASSESSMENT

HISTORY

- Males tend to be more reluctant to seek medical advice and reticent during medical visits; nevertheless, a good psychosocial history can identify problem areas.

PHYSICAL

Pubertal Development (Table 1)

- Sexual maturity rating (SMR), or Tanner staging, correlates highly with physical maturity by bone age.
- SMR for the male is based on changes in pubic hair, testes and penis. SMR for pubic hair and penis are closely correlated.
- The changes of puberty follow a predictable sequence although the timing is highly variable and differs by racial and ethnic groups.
- Puberty sequence begins with gonadarche (enlargement of the testes) at age 11 to 12 (SMR 2). Pubic hair starts about six months later, followed by enlargement of the penis (hallmark of SMR 3). Presence of sperm in the ejaculate (spermarche) begins 12 to 18 months after testicular enlargement during SMR 3, when nocturnal emissions ("wet dreams") are also expected. Growth spurt takes place about 2 to 2.5 years after gonadarche. The whole pubertal sequence lasts about three to four years.

Other changes:

- Voice changes and growth of facial as well as body hair occur during SMR 4.
- Changes to physical appearance start with the hands, feet and extremities, and then the trunk.
- Males grow an a average of 28 cm (11 inches) during puberty.
- They have two more years to grow at a prepubertal rate than do girls, and gain 3 cm more than girls during the growth spurt.
- Papules on the border of the penile glans are also normal and are referred to as **pink pearly papules.**

Stature

- Concern about stature is often a presenting complaint of adolescent males.
- It is important to remind patients that their estimated adult height is based on parental heights (Figure 1).
- Normal growth variants
  - **Constitutional delay of growth and adolescence** (CDGA): "Late bloomer"
    - These teens tend to reach their pubertal stages later than most.
    - They typically reach target height later.
    - Confirm diagnosis by assessing bone age. Films show a delay in bone development compared to chronologic age.
  - **Familial short stature**
    - There is a family history of short stature.
    - Bone age is consistent with chronologic age.

Gynecomastia

- An increase in the glandular and stromal tissue of the male breast is a normal variant of puberty known as **gynecomastia** (see Chapter 21).
  - Unilateral or bilateral gynecomastia is common in middle adolescence.
  - It affects up to 20% of adolescent males and is usually mild, less than 3–4 cm in size.

- It can be worse in obese males because of **pseudogynecomastia,** or accumulation of fatty tissue that may not resolve with weight loss. Surgical correction after weight loss may be indicated but should be done after puberty.
- Reassure! Many of your patient's peers have the same condition, and it will resolve in one or two years without any treatment.
- Rarely related to testicular tumors, Klinefelter's Syndrome, psychotropics, H2 blockers, drug use (i.e. anabolic steroids, heroin or heavy marijuana use) or scrotal pathology.

What is unique about caring for adolescent males?

- Create a safe space for adolescent males to open up while respecting their need for privacy.
- Recognize normal male pubertal development, such as gynecomastia and penile pink pearly papules as well as abnormal physical findings. Bodily concerns ("Am I normal?") are frequently addressed during routine visits.
- Know that morbidity and mortality are closely related to life style, compounded by the fact that role models of masculinity can lead young men to risk-taking behaviors.
- Understand the socio-cultural and economic context in which males construct their masculinity, and recognize the diversity among adolescent males (rural vs. urban, sexual orientation, socioeconomic class, race and ethnicity, indigenous youth, incarcerated youth, adolescent fathers, adolescents in foster care, etc.).

TEST YOUR KNOWLEDGE ANSWER

7. E. While it is important to identify high blood pressure, auscultate the heart for murmurs, clear adolescents to play sports and examine the testicles at the time of the annual physical exam, the most important part of the visit is to take a developmentally appropriate psychosocial history to identify risky health behaviors. The major causes of morbidity and mortality in the adolescent population are unintentional injuries, many of which are related to alcohol and drug use. Lifelong health habits are formed during this time,

creating a unique window for healthcare providers and health educators. During routine healthcare visits, providers have an opportunity to screen for risk and provide health education.

$$\text{Final Adult Height} = \frac{[\text{Mother's height (inches)} + 5 \text{ inches}] + [\text{Father's height (inches)}]}{2}$$

Add 13 to mother's height if heights are provided in centimeters

Figure 1 Estimated Adult Height.

Table 1. Normal Male Puberty and Development.

Pubic Hair	SMR1	No hair or presence of fine hair (represents adrenarche, not pubarche).
	SMR2	Hair is sparse, long, straight, slightly pigmented and downy at the base of penis.
	SMR3	Hair is darker, coarser, curled and spread over the pubic synphisis.
	SMR4	Hair completely fills the pubic triangle.
	SMR5	Adult pattern, with hair extending to inner thighs and the navel.
Testes/Penis	SMR1	Pre-pubertal.
	SMR2	Testes enlargement marks first sign of puberty (gonadarche).
	SMR3	Lengthening of penis, and continued growth of testicles. Scrotal skin starts to wrinkle and becomes thinner in appearance and darker in pigmentation.
	SMR4	Testes continue to grow to a volume of 10 to 15 ml, and penis lengthens to 11 to 17 cm when flaccid.
	SMR5	Adult genital size and shape with testes volume of about 20–25 ml. Left testis usually hangs lower than right.

WEB REFERENCES

- American Medical Association, Guidelines for Adolescent Preventive Services (GAPS), Recommendations Monograph. 1997: http://www.ama-assn.org/resources/doc/ad-hlth/gaps mono.pdf
- Marcell AV, Bell DL, Joffe A (2011) 'The Male Genital Examination: A Position Paper of the Society for Adolescent Health and Medicine, Retrieved from http://www.adolescenthealth.org/AM/Template.cfm?Section=Position_Papers&Template=/CM/ContentDisplay.cfm&ContentID=3566
- Marcell AV, Wibbelsman C, Seigel WM (2011), 'Male Adolescent Sexual and Reproductive Health Care', Pediatrics, 128(6);el658–el676, Retrieved from http://pediatrics.aappublications.org/content/128/6/el658.full
- The National Campaign to Prevent Teen Pregnancy (www.thenationalcampaign.org):
  - Suellentrop, K. 'Adolescent Boys' Use of Health Services.' Science Says. 2006;26;l–5: http://www.thenationalcampaign.org/resources/pdf/SS/SS26_BoysHealthSvcs.pdf
- Westwood M, Pinzon, J. 'Adolescent Male Health.' Paediatrics & Child Health. 2008;13(l): 31–36: http://www.ncbi.nlm.nih.gov/pmc/articles/PMC2528816/

Additional Clinician and Patient Resources:

- Healthy Teen Network, Making a Difference in the lives of Teens and Young Families. Young Men: http://www.healthyteennetwork.org/index.asp?Type=B_BASIC&SEC=%7B7D35294E-AE5A-441A-BE60-75FDA3D9F5D8%7D&DE=%7B51D108FD-53FD-47A2-B232-782817FE01BF%7D
- New York: Presbyterian: Puberty, Adolescent Male: NYP.ORG/health/puberty-adolescent-male.html
- Teens Health from Nemours: http://www.kidshealth.org/teen/question/just_guys/boy brst.html
- Young Men's Health: Health Information for young men around the world, Children's Hospital Boston: www.voungmenshealthsite.org

6

TAKING CARE OF LESBIAN, GAY, BISEXUAL, TRANSGENDER AND QUESTIONING (LGBTQ) TEENS

William M. Barnes and
David S. Reitman

TEST YOUR KNOWLEDGE

8. Michael, a 17 year old patient in your practice comes in for his annual physical examination. While taking a sexual history, he reveals that he is gay and that he has had two boyfriends over the past year. He has been "sexually active" with both of them. After counseling him on safer sex practices, which of the following screening tests would you *NOT* recommend?
   A. Gonorrhea culture of the pharynx and rectum
   B. HIV ELISA test
   C. Herpes culture of the rectum
   D. Rapid Plasma Reagent test
   E. Urine screen for chlamydia and gonorrhea

Refer to end of chapter for answer on page 74.

John is a 16 year old male patient who recently returned home after running away. His parents bring him to clinic for a "check up" and reveal that he might have "caught HIV."

BACKGROUND

- Lesbian, gay, bisexual, transgender and questioning (LGBTQ) adolescents face many of the same somatic health concerns as their non-LGBTQ contemporaries; nevertheless, LGBTQ-specific sexual health issues should be addressed as part of preventive care for these teens.
- Many adolescents may be burdened by not being able to be themselves and often struggle with acknowledging their sexual identities.
- This can lead to withdrawal, conflict and estrangements with family and friends.

RISK FACTORS

- LGBTQ teens in supportive environments have risks similar to their non-LGBTQ counterparts.
- The risk considerations listed below are often the result of societal perceptions and discrimination against LGBTQ teens.
  - **Violence:** LGBTQ youth are often the victims of bullying or are threatened with violence because of their sexual orientation. LGBTQ victimization has been associated with truancy, depression, anxiety and substance abuse.
  - **Mental health issues:** Increased risk of depression and suicidality exist when an individual's sexual orientation is rejected by friends, family or community institutions.
  - **Drug use:** LGBTQ youth are at increased risk of experimentation with drug and alcohol use. In particular, providers should inquire about "club drugs" such as MDMA, Ketamine and Methamphetamine.
  - **Disordered eating and body image:** Eating disorders are seen more frequently in gay male adolescents than in straight male adolescents.
  - **HIV/AIDS:** Providers must inquire and counsel regarding condom use, especially for receptive anal sex.

ASSESSMENT

HISTORY

- Establish where the adolescent falls in their cognitive development. This will determine how much you can expect them to comprehend and what level of language to use.
- Teens may be chronologically young but more developed in experience and exposure.
- History taking need not be lengthy but it should be rich with content. A relaxed, open-minded clinician will create an environment for open and honest dialogue.
- Clinicians need to become comfortable talking about sensitive issues and should not pass judgement on a teen's lifestyle choices or values as this may limit the discussion.
- Components of a HEEADSSS exam provide general information about teens, their strengths and support systems. It can also highlight "red flags" that may arise during the discussion.
- Health issues specific to transgendered teens should also be considered (Table 1).

Home Situation

- Discuss current living arrangements. Do not assume that the teen is living with family. Ascertain how long a teen has lived and anticipate living at their current "home."
- Who are the members of the teen's support network and to what extent are they involved in the teen's life?
- Can the teen identify a person with whom they can discuss personal health issues including their sexual orientation or gender identity? If possible, obtain consent to communicate with this person, who may be a liaison to the patient in the future.
- Are members of the teen's support network aware of his or her current living situation? Is the teen uncomfortable with anyone knowing his or her living situation, including family members?

- How involved are members of the teen's biological family in his or her life? Are they aware of the teen's sexual orientation? Are there any family members with whom teen feels comfortable or safe.
- Explore safe addresses and phone numbers for communicating with patients in the future. Identify where they prefer mail to be sent and primary as well as back up phone numbers for contact. Inquire whether messages can be left at a given phone number.

Education

- Is the teen currently enrolled in school? Do they identify educational strengths and future academic or career plans.
- Explore peer dynamics at school and/or in the community. To what degree is the teen integrated versus marginalized from their peer set, and does this affect daily functioning?
- This information may be a marker for mental health problems such as depression, a diagnosis which can significantly impact a teen's ability to participate in their health care.
- Distress in this population is extremely important to ascertain as they are vulnerable to many negative consequences: bullying and teasing from peers, adverse reactions from family members, rejection and isolation, threats and possible physical assault.
- When warranted, it is important to offer mental health services that are tailored and sensitive to this population.

Employment/Financial Support

- Is the teen currently employed? Does the teen have financial support? Establish whether payment for health services is a barrier to care or medications.
  - For example, many teens avoid engaging the healthcare system for fear that a bill for services will be sent home, raising questions from parents or other family members.
  - This may limit the amount of information teens disclose to clinicians, to retain secrecy of their sexual orientation.

Sexual History

- A detailed sexual history can help assess potential health risks for teens. Some tips for taking an appropriate sexual history follow.
- When appropriate, identify current relationship status. How stable has the relationship been and how satisfied is the patient in the relationship?
- Clinicians should inquire about sexual activity or sexual attractions in an open and nonjudgmental manner rather than using labels such as "gay" or "lesbian."
- Many LGBTQ teens are unsure of their identity and may be developmentally unready to be labeled. Avoid labels such as "gay," "bisexual," or "homosexual." Instead, phrases like "a guy who has sex with guys" can be used.
- Be comfortable talking about issues such as oral-genital, anal-genital, oral-anal sex, bisexuality and transgender health concerns.
- Avoid making assumptions about current or future sexual activity based on past-reported activities. A female with a boyfriend may also have sex with females.
- When discussing oral and anal sex, inquire whether the patient is the "inserter" and/or the "receiver." For men who have sex with men (MSM), the slang for the insertive anal sex partner is "top" while the receptive partner is "bottom."
- With transgendered youth, avoid making assumptions whether the patient is sexually active with either or both genders: ask the patient.

PHYSICAL

HEENT

- Individuals engaging in insertive oral sex are at risk for **oropharyngeal gonorrhea (GC)**, **herpes simplex** and **human papillomavirus** infections of the mouth and throat.
- Consider a sexually transmitted infection (STI) work up in patients with pharyngitis, concerning clinical history and/or negative strep test results.

Abdomen

- As many women who have sex with women (WSW) have had a male sexual partner in the past, they generally share the same STI risk as their heterosexual counterparts.
- Assess for tenderness, especially in lower quadrants, as this may indicate more serious infection such as **pelvic inflammatory disease (PID).**

Genital

- Females: Assess for inguinal adenopathy, signs of abnormal vaginal discharge or evidence of STIs. WSW have increased rates of **bacterial vaginosis (BV).**
- Males: Assess for inguinal adenopathy. Observe for any penile or testicular lesions or penile discharge that could indicate an underlying STI.

Pelvic

- A pelvic exam including bimanual evaluation may be warranted in suspected cases of **PID.**

Anal

- Males or females who engage in unprotected receptive anal sex may be at risk for anorectal tears or localized trauma to the anus.
- They are also at risk for **anorectal GC, chlamydia, herpes** and **anal warts.**
- Proctitis with lymphadenopathy might indicate **lymphogranuloma venereum.**

STUDIES

<u>WSW</u>

Wet Prep

- Consider collecting a vaginal swab for microscopic evaluation in cases of suspected BV.

HIV and STI Screening

- Follow current STI screening practices as recommended by the CDC.
- Consider screening for chlamydia, gonorrhea, HIV, and syphilis.
- If symptomatic, consider testing for herpes simplex virus.

PAP Smears

- Guidelines established by the American College of Obstetrics and Gynecology (ACOG) assert that women have annual routine PAP smear evaluations starting at age 21 regardless of age of sexual debut; however, if the patient has HIV or is immunocompromised, routine testing is still recommended annually starting at 3 years post sexual debut.

MSM

STI Screening

- MSM should be tested at least annually for the following (those with multiple partners may require more frequent testing, every 3–6 months):
  - Oral GC, urethral GC and chlamydia, and rectal GC and chlamydia
  - Syphilis

HIV Testing

- Rates of HIV transmission are especially high in patients who engage in unprotected, receptive anal sex; however, oral and insertive anal sex without condom use also place individuals at increased risk for HIV transmission.
- MSM should be tested for HIV at least annually.

Hepatitis B

- Transmitted through semen, tends to be of higher risk in MSM.
- All patients should be immunized against the Hepatitis B virus. Testing should be considered in unimmunized symptomatic patients.

Hepatitis A

- Heptatis A can be transmitted via oral-anal contact, and all patients should be immunized against this infection.
- Consider testing in unimmunized, symptomatic patients.

What is unique about LGBTQ adolescents?

- LGBTQ teens may hide their sexual orientation or gender identity from clinicians for fear of being judged or treated differently. This often results in unmet health needs as this population is at higher risk of not accessing medical care as needed. It is especially important that clinicians provide a safe, open-minded and nonjudgmental environment for teens.
- LGBTQ adolescents experience the same stages of development as other adolescents.
- Behaviors such as defiance of authority figures and resistance to direct communication are likely typical adolescent behaviors and should not be construed as the result of the teen's sexual orientation or gender identity.
- Recognize developmental stages along a continuum of establishing a sexual identity for all teens, but particularly for this population, as stereotypes and discrimination may negatively affect this process.
- Issues faced by LGBQT youth may affect their willingness to engage in health care, treatment and/or follow through on health care recommendations.
- For teens, issues that affect daily life or function may take precedence over health concerns.
- An adolescent living in circumstances where disclosing health status (i.e. on anti-retrovirals for the treatment of HIV) could have adverse implications (i.e. loss of housing), may refrain from bringing medications home, thereby becoming non-adherent with the prescribed medication regimen.

TEST YOUR KNOWLEDGE
ANSWER

8. C. A random herpes culture of the rectum is not indicated in a patient who is asymptomatic and has never had a prior outbreak; however, if the patient complained of rectal pain or if lesions were noted on external rectal exam,

then a herpes culture would be appropriate. As pharyngeal gonorrhea (GC) can be asymptomatic, a screening culture should be offered. Similarly, GC and chlamydia cultures of the rectum should be obtained in patients who have receptive anal sex. Urinary GC and chlamydia, HIV and RPR screens are indicated as part of health maintenance.

Table 1. Health Issues Specific to Transgendered Individuals.

Transgendered teens...	• feel that their internal sense of gender is incompatible with their biologically assigned physical gender. • may experience significant distress about their body's wrong gender as they develop secondary sex characteristics during puberty. In many cases, this may lead to depression, anxiety and oppositional-defiant behavior.

- While some transgendered youth are content wearing clothing of the opposite gender, others may desire hormonal or surgical therapy for phenotypic gender change.
- The World Professional Organization for Transgender Health (WPATH) standards of care states that transgendered teens may undergo hormonal therapies at age 16 and may be eligible for surgical treatments after age 18.
- The standards suggest that therapies begin once the individual and his or her family have worked in consultation with a mental health professional for at least 6 months.

Treatments to correct phenotypic gender may include:

- Fully reversible therapies, such as LHRH agonists to prevent further development of secondary sex characteristics.
- Partially reversible hormonal therapies:
  - For male to female conversions, estrogen causes breast development, female body fat distribution and decreased muscle mass.
  - For female to male conversions, testosterone facilitates muscle mass growth, vocal deepening, facial and chest hair growth and male fat distribution.
- Irreversible therapy typically involves surgical procedures such as mastectomy, orchiectomy and genital reconstruction to create an artificial penis or vagina.

Clinicians working with adolescents should be familiar with a mental health provider who has expertise working with gender-variant youth.

WEB REFERENCES

- Institute of Medicine (www.iom.edu/lgbthealth)
  - IOM. 'The Health of Lesbian, Gay, Bisexual, and Transgender People: Building a Foundation for Better Understanding.' March 2011, Retreived from http://www.iom.edu/~/media/Files/Report%20Files/2011/The-Health-of-Lesbian-Gay-Bisexual-and-Transgender-People/LGBT%20Health%202011 %20Report%20Brief.pdf
- Just the Facts Coalition. (2008). Just the Facts about Sexual Orientation and Youth: A Primer for Principals, Educators and School Personnel. Washington, DC: American Psychological Association. Retrieved from http://www.apa.org/pi/lgbt/resources/just-the-facts.pdf
- Mayer, KH *et al.* 'Sexual and Gender Minority Health: What We Know and What Needs to Be Done.' American Journal of Public Health. 2008;98(6);989-995: http://www.lmunet. edu/dcom/hec/PDFs/Sexual%20and%20Gender%20Minority%20Health.pdf
- 'Practice Parameter on Gay, Lesbian, or Bisexual Sexual Orientation, Gender Nonconformity, and Gender Discordance in Children and Adolescents', Journal American Academy of Child Adolescent Psychiatry. 2012;51(9):957-974, retrieved from http://download.journals.elsevierhealth.com/pdfs/journals/0890-8567/PIIS089085671200500X.pdf

Additional Clinician and Patient Resources:

- Advocates for Youth (2008), www.advocatesforyouth.org/glbtq.htm
- American Psychological Association:
  - www.apa.org/topics/orientation.html
  - www.apa.org/pi/lgbc/publications/justthefacts.html
- Child Welfare League of America: www, cwla. org/programs/culture/glbtq.htm
- Family Equality Council (2013), www.familyequality.org/index.html
- Gay and Lesbian Alliance Against Defamation: www.glaad.org
- Gay, Lesbian and Straight Education Network: www.glsen.org/cgi-bin/iowa/all/home/index.html
- GLBT National Help Center, National Youth Talkline: www.glnh.org/talkline/index.html
- The National Coalition for LGBT Health: www.lgbthealth.net
- National Youth Advocacy Coalition: www.nyacyouth.org/nyac/resources.html
- Parents, Families and Friends of Lesbians & Gays: www.pflag.org
- Safe Schools Coalition: www.safeschoolscoalition.org/safe.html
- Youth and AIDS Projects: www.yapmn.com/index.php
- Youth Resource: www.youthresource.com

Transgender and Intersex Focus

- American Psychological Association: www.apa.org/topics/intersx.html
- American Psychological Association: www.apa.org/topics/transgender.html

- CDC Lesbian, Gay and Transgender Health: http://www.cdc.gov/lgbthealth/youth.htm
- Gay and Lesbian Medical Association: www.glma.org
- WPATH: World Professional Organization for Transgender Health: www.wpath.org

Two-Spirit Focus

- NorthEast Two-Spirit Society: www.ne2ss.org\
- The Red Circle Project: wwwapla.org/native_american/RCP

Spanish Language

- Ambientejoven: www.ambientej oven.org
- American Psychological Association: www.apa.org/topics/orientacion.html
- Gay & Lesbian Alliance Against Defamation: www.glaad.org/espanol/bienvenido.php

7

THE PRE-PARTICIPATION SPORTS PHYSICAL

Nailah Coleman

TEST YOUR KNOWLEDGE

9. Which of the following clearance determinations would you use for an athlete with exercise-associated syncope, murmur that increases with Valsalva and otherwise normal exam?
   A. This is a variant seen in elite athletes. Clear without restrictions for any sport.
   B. This may be associated with a mild to moderate valvular dysfunction. Clear with recommendations and/or limitations.
   C. Clearance deferred pending cardiology consult.
   D. Order an exercise stress test.
   E. Disqualify from all sports.

Refer to end of chapter for answer on page 89.

Jane, a 16 year old competitive cross country runner, presents for a pre-participation evaluation before joining the varsity team. She has a cold.

BACKGROUND

- The purpose of the pre-participation physical evaluation (PPE) is to promote the health and safety of physically active teens.
- The primary purpose is to reveal risk factors for life-threatening and/or disabling conditions that may preclude sports participation.
- Ideally, the PPE should be performed 6 weeks before the start of sports season, allowing for necessary follow-up visits and/or rehabilitation, if required.
- States and schools vary widely in the frequency, content, allowed providers and required documentation for the PPE.

ASSESSMENT

HISTORY

- A complete history can identify 65–77% of problems affecting athletes.

History of Present Illness

- Does the teen report any pain related to a recent injury?
- Has the athlete had rehabilitation or treatment for any sports or non-sports related injuries?
- Does the teen report any viral illness or other communicable diseases?

Past Medical History

- Does the teen have any medical condition that could impair or limit physical activity such as:
  - Exercise-related chest pain, dyspnea, palpitations or syncopal episodes that suggest underlying **cardiomyopathy** or **arrhythmia**? Has the teen had an abnormal EKG?
  - Allergies, urticaria or anaphylaxis?
  - **Asthma**, breathing problems or shortness of breath with exercise?
  - Heat-related illness (cramps or feeling ill with exercise in the heat)?

  - Sickle cell trait or disease? Exertional sickling can lead to **rhabdomyolysis, acidosis, acute renal failure, multi-system organ failure** and **death**.
  - **Neurologic injury or disorder,** such as a head injury, concussion, seizures or headaches with exercise?
- Has the teen had a history of **musculoskeletal injury**? If so, what was the nature of that injury (e.g. stress fracture, dislocation, sprain or strain)?
- Has the teen had prior studies for musculoskeletal injury, such as an x-ray, CT or MRI?
- Has the athlete missed practices or games and why?
- Has the teen had prior sports restrictions and why?
- Does the teen have any unpaired organs (i.e. only one kidney)?

Family History

- Is there a family history of heart disease or sudden death under the age of 40, or other condition of concern?

Dietary History

- Is the teen taking any dietary supplements?
- Determine if the athlete is loading or restricting calories to meet a specific goal weight. Some sports (i.e. wrestling or boxing) have weight divisions that athletes strive to reach through less than healthy methods.
- Female athletes with a severely restricted diet (e.g. not enough calories to support level of activity), menstrual dysfunction and low bone mineral density should raise concern for **female athlete triad.**

Medications

- Has the teen ever been prescribed an inhaler for asthma treatment?
- Determine if the teen is taking any medications, supplements, herbs or minerals.
- Clinicians should routinely ask about all herbal or supplemental substances that the athlete may be taking to enhance skill and stamina. Many athletes may be unaware that the substance they are taking is banned and could impact their sports participation, as well as future scholarship potential.

Social History

- Is the teen taking any banned substances or substances of abuse?

Review of Systems

- Any recent or current fever that suggests an underlying infection?
- Chest pain or palpitations that suggest cardiopathy?
- Shortness of breath or difficulty breathing suggesting asthma or other respiratory condition?
- Headache, numbness, tingling or weakness suggesting concussion?

PHYSICAL

Vital Signs

- Heart rate and sitting brachial blood pressure should be documented.
  - Bradycardia can be seen in competitive athletes but may warrant further evaluation.
  - Athletes with pre-hypertension should not be restricted from competitive athletics.
  - Teens with **stage 1 hypertension** warrant frequent follow up, but should not be limited from sports participation.
  - Those diagnosed with **stage 2 hypertension** should be restricted from high static sports until their blood pressure normalizes.

Anthropometric Measurements

- Height, weight and body mass index should be measured and documented.

HEENT

- Assess for visual acuity (no correction needed for better than 20/40 in both eyes), pupil symmetry and response.
- Noting *unequal pupils at baseline* is important, should the pupil exam become necessary after a **head injury**.

Cardiac

- Assess rate and rhythm, note any murmurs (and response to provocation) and check femoral pulses.

- Squat-to-stand and valsalva maneuvers: murmur increases in cases of **hypertrophic cardiomyopathy** and decreases with **aortic stenosis** and **mitral regurgitation.**

Chest

- Observe for chest symmetry, pectus excavatum/carinatum and chest expansion.
- Auscultate for clear breath sounds and good air entry.

Abdomen

- Is there any tenderness, evidence of mass or signs of organomegaly?
- Is there an enlarged spleen? A recent sore throat or viral illness should raise concern for **mononucleosis**, which would limit contact sports participation while symptomatic.

Genital

- A testicular exam will reveal presence of a **single, undescended testis** or any evidence of **mass.** Check for **inguinal hernias.**

Skin

- Observe for presence of rashes or concerning lesions (i.e. herpes).

Musculoskeletal

- Assessment should be brief, unless there is a specific joint concern.
- Assess contour, symmetry, range of motion, stability and strength of joints.

STUDIES

Diagnostic testing may be necessary based on history and physical exam findings.

X-ray

- Warranted in cases of musculoskeletal injury when anomalies or fractures are suspected.

- For example, consider an x-ray of the c-spine/atlanto-occipital area in Special Olympics sports participants with Down Syndrome or an x-ray of the spine in cases of suspected **spondilolysis** or **spondilolysthesis.**

Electrocardiogram (EKG)

- Is not a universal recommendation.
- Indicated in a teen with a history of chest pain, exertional syncope, palpitations, a new onset heart murmur or suspected dysrrhythmia.

Urine or Serum Drug Test

- May be required in some competitive sports and/or college level athletics.

DISPOSITION

Clearance determination will depend upon the history, exam, study results, the static and dynamic demands of the sport, and the level of contact of the sport (Table 1).

CLEARANCE CONSIDERATIONS

Acute Febrile Illness

- Athletes with acute febrile illnesses risk worsening their condition during play, dehydration (due to ongoing fluid losses), thermoregulatory problems and spreading their illness to other players.
- Although rare, the possibility of a **viral myocarditis** is always a concern: athletes with any viral illness should be restricted from play.

Ophthalmologic Conditions

- Restricting conditions include: **one functional eye**, a detached retina, prior eye surgery or a serious eye injury.
- Visual acuity disturbance is one of the most common abnormalities on the PPE. Evaluation is recommended in cases of visual acuity worse than 20/40, eye injury or prior eye surgery.
- Eye guards are available for protection in most sports.

Cardiovascular Conditions

- **Structural heart disease** or symptomatic cardiac conditions require cardiology referral and evaluation before clearance can be determined.
- **Hypertension** is one of the most common abnormalities on the PPE. Athletes should be restricted from participation if they have stage 2 hypertension (greater than 99th percentile) or evidence of end-organ damage.
- Asymptomatic teens with benign **functional murmurs** are allowed full participation.
- Asymptomatic teens with **dysrrhythmias** are allowed full participation.
- **Hypertrophic cardiomyopathy**, the most common cause of sudden death in U.S. athletes, requires restriction from all but low-intensity sports.

Respiratory Conditions

- Patients with upper respiratory infections require assessment to determine clearance.
- **Asthmatics** are allowed full sports participation with proper education and medication unless their disease is severe.
- Teens with **environmental allergies** have an increased risk of exercise-induced bronchospasm.
- Beware that beta-agonists are on the banned substances list unless true exercise-induced bronchospasm can be documented with formal testing (i.e. a treadmill test, a methacholine challenge or similar study).
- Teens with cystic fibrosis are permitted full sports participation, provided their oxygenation remains adequate after a graded exercise stress test.
- Acclimatization and adequate hydration are required to prevent heat illness.

Abdominal Organomegaly

- Participation should be avoided in those with **acute organomegaly** due to the increased risk of organ rupture.
- Athletes with **chronic organomegaly** require further evaluation before clearance to participate in collision, contact or limited-contact sports.
- Splenomegaly is present in all teens with **mononucleosis**. Spleen guards are recommended. The risk of rupture is rare after 28 days of illness. If the date of disease onset is unknown, use the date of diagnosis. According to current

recommendations, if an athlete has no symptoms at 21 days past the start of infection or the date of diagnosis, they can begin light activity and resume full activity at 28 days.

Genitourinary Conditions

- Teens with asymptomatic **inguinal hernias** may participate fully. In symptomatic athletes, pain may limit participation and must be assessed.
- Teens with a **solitary kidney**, planning to participate in contact, collision, and limited-contact sports should be evaluated by nephrology or urology; the decision to participate must be made on an individual basis.
- Female athletes with a **single ovary** are permitted full participation.
- Male athletes with a **single testis** are permitted full participation with use of a protective cup for certain sports. Those with an undescended testis require referral to surgery as they are at increased risk of cancer of the testicle.

Metabolic and Hematologic Conditions

- **Obesity** presents a concern for heat illness. Counsel on appropriate acclimatization when the teen is participating in an unfamiliar environment.
- Teens diagnosed with **diabetes mellitus** may fully participate when their disease is well-controlled. The level of participation may vary depending on the presence or absence of diabetic complications (i.e. neuropathy).
- Teens with **sickle cell disease** may participate in all but high-intensity, exertion, collision and contact sports, so long as their illness status permits participation.

Dermatologic Conditions

- If contagious (e.g. uncontrolled infection or unable to be covered adequately), participation is not permitted in mat-based sports, collision, contact or limited-contact sports.
- Examples of concerning conditions include herpes simplex, community-acquired methacillin-resistant *Staphylococcus aureus* (CA-MRSA), scabies, lice infestation, molluscum contagiosum, tinea corporis, impetigo, furuncles, and carbuncles.
- Teens with recurrent herpes should consider maintenance medication (i.e. acyclovir) to prevent recurrence.

Bloodborne Pathogens

- Pathogens of concern include HIV, hepatitis B, and hepatitis C:
    - The risk of transmission of **HIV** is rare (less than 1/85 million games) and is associated with blood contact.
    - Although **Hepatitis B** is more contagious, widespread immunization prevents spread.
    - The risk of **Hepatitis C** transmission has not been documented in sports participation.
    - Asymptomatic individuals with bloodborne pathogens may participate, as long as consideration is given to the type of activity, the risk of transmission to others and the teen's current health status.
    - Some sports have mandatory testing requirements (e.g. boxing).

Neurologic Conditions

- Burners and stingers are a **transient neuropraxia** affecting the upper extremity after an injury (e.g. after a tackle in football), either due to traction (more common in high school) or compression (with degenerative disk disease; more common in college). Multiple repeated episodes could signal an anatomic concern (i.e. cervical spinal stenosis, degenerative disk disease or osteophytes) and warrant further investigation, such as an electromyelogram.
- Asymptomatic athletes with a history of burners or stingers are allowed full participation once full strength and normal sensation are restored.
- **Cervical spinal cord neuropraxia**, also known as transient quadriplegia, has been associated with **cervical spinal stenosis**. Return to play should not occur in the presence of ligamentous instability, cord injury, cord edema or prolonged symptoms. Permanent sports restriction may need to be considered.
- Teens with **well-controlled seizures** can participate fully in most sports; however, their participation should be limited (i.e. no contact-collision, limited-contact, hazardous non-contact) if seizures are not well-controlled. High-risk sports (i.e. high diving, gymnastics) should be avoided.

- Teens with **migraine headaches** can participate fully when well. There are two categories of exercise-associated headaches:
  - **Benign exertional headaches** (i.e. cough headaches) are associated with increased intracranial pressure; be sure to rule out an **aneurysm** or **Arnold-Chiari malformation** before allowing participation.
  - **Primary exertional headaches** (i.e. effort headaches) are associated with aerobic exercise and result in a pounding pain; be sure to rule out **subarachnoid hemorrhage, arterial dissection, concussion** or **post-concussion syndrome.**
- For concussion and mild traumatic brain injury, refer to chapter 52 on Concussion and Post-Concussion Syndrome.

Teens with Special Needs

- Receive similar benefits from physical activity as able-bodied or mentally competent teens.
- As physical and mental disability can be related to more global issues, these athletes should be evaluated for seizures, hearing or vision loss, cardiorespiratory disease, renal disease and atlanto-axial instability.
- Determine if the special needs athlete is at increased risk of injury. Ask about a history of heat related illness, fractures or dislocations, use of prostheses or special equipment, use of an indwelling catheter and pressure sores.
- The exam of the athlete with special needs is similar to that of an able-bodied or mentally competent athlete, with the addition of a functional assessment to determine that the teen is able to compete safely.

What is unique about the PPE in adolescents?

- Adolescents underutilize health care and for many teens, the PPE may be the entry point into medical care: it may be the only opportunity for clinicians to ask HEEADSSS screening questions and provide anticipatory guidance and preventive counseling.
- Sports are an essential part of many adolescents' lives and restrictions may be devastating.
- Not "making the team" is a significant stressor and to many teens, emotionally equivalent to failing a grade or experiencing parental divorce.

- Be prepared to provide emotional support and watch for **depressive symptoms** or non-adherence to restrictions.
- Athletes who choose not to adhere to sports restrictions should be counseled on the potentially damaging results of playing when not fully recovered or cleared to participate. Relatively minor injuries that would otherwise heal with time may worsen, or there may be further injury.
- When determining an athlete's ability to participate safely in a physical activity, consider the type of activity to be played (contact or collision, limited contact, non-contact), the demands the activity may place on the body (static versus dynamic) and the athlete's skill and competition level.
- If the athlete cannot participate fully and when the situation allows, consider clearing him/her for limited participation.
- Clinicians should routinely ask about all herbal or supplemental substances that a teen may take to enhance skill and stamina (see Chapter 8 on sports supplements). Many athletes may be unaware that the substance they are taking is banned and could impact their sports participation as well as future scholarship potential.

TEST YOUR KNOWLEDGE ANSWER

9. C. Adolescents with exercise-associated syncope should be suspected of having a serious cardiac condition such as an anomalous coronary artery, aortic stenosis, arrhythmias or hypertrophic cardiomyopathy. Adolescents with a heart murmur that increases with valsalva may indeed have hypertrophic cardiomyopathy. All patients with exercise-associated syncope need to have their clearance deferred, pending a cardiology consultation.

Table 1. Clearance Classifications.*

Clear without restriction for any sport.
Clear with recommendations or limitations.
Clearance deferred pending consult, further evaluation, treatment or rehabilitation.
• Female athletes with a concern for female athlete triad may require multidisciplinary care.
• Pregnancy clearance should be determined by the physician providing prenatal care.
Restricted from certain or all sports.
• Athletes disqualified may need follow-up to ascertain the effect of restriction on their psyche: young athletes who do not "make the team" may experience significant stress.

*Reprinted and modified from Mitchell JH, Haskell W, Snell P and Van Camp SP, Task Force 8: classification of sports, *J. Am. Coll.* 45(8): 1364–1367 (2005), with permission from Elsevier.

WEB REFERENCES

- American Academy of Family Physicians (www.aafp.org):
  - Kurowski, K. and Chandran, S. The Preparticipation Athletic Evaluation. American Family Physician. 2000; 61(9):2683–2690: http://www.aafp.org/afp/2000/0501/p2683.html
- American Academy of Pediatrics (AAP) (pediatrics.aappublications.org)
  - Demorest, RA, Washington RL and Councel on Sports Medicine and Fitness. 'Athletic Participation by Children and Adolescents Who Have Systemic Hypertension.' Pediatrics 2010;125;1287, http://pediatrics.aappublications.Org/content/125/6/1287.full.html
  - Rice, SG and the Council on Sports Medicine and Fitness. 'Medical Conditions Affecting Sports Participation'. Pediatrics 2008; 121(4);841-848: http://pediatrics.aappublications.org/content/121/4/841.full.pdf+html\
- American Orthopedic Society for Sports Medicine (www.sportsmed.org)
  - Consensus Statement: Psychological Issues Related to Injury in Athletes and the Team Physician. 2008, Retrieved from http://stopsportsinjuries.reingoldweb.com/files/pdf/Psychological-Issues.pdf
  - Consensus Statement: Selected Issues for the Adolescent Athlete and the Team Physician. 2009, Retreived from http://stopsportsinjuries.reingoldweb.com/files/pdf/Adolescent-Athlete.pdf

Additional Clinician and Patient Resources:

- American College of Sports Medicine: www.acsm.org
    - Patient Information on Pre-Participation Physical Examinations: http://www.acsm.org/docs/ brochures/pre-participation-physical-examinations.pdf
- American Medical Society of Sports Medicine: www.amssm.org
- Stop Sports Injuries: http://www.stopsportsinjuries.org/
- Wheeless' Orthopaedics Online Textbook: http://www.wheelessonline.com/

8

SPORTS SUPPLEMENTS

Gregg Joseph Montalto

TEST YOUR KNOWLEDGE

10. Which one of the following statements is true?
    A. Dietary sports supplements never improve performance in the teen athlete.
    B. Creatine has a long track record of safety and efficacy for improving burst strength in adults; therefore, it is safe for adolescent use.
    C. There is evidence that a combination of ephedrine and caffeine may lead to weight loss.
    D. All the above.
    E. None of the above.

11. An 18 year old high school football player has a history of premature ventricular contractions that has been successfully treated with a beta blocker medication. Which of the following sports supplements should he *absolutely* avoid?
    A. Creatine (only) products.
    B. Synephrine-containing weight-loss products.
    C. Multiple-ingredient sports supplements.
    D. B & C.
    E. All the above.

Refer to end of chapter for answers on page 101.

"Hey doc, a friend of mine takes protein and creatine, and says it helped him become a better football player. What do you think?"

BACKGROUND

- Many adolescents (athletes and non-athletes), look for ways to improve their appearance, enhance performance, gain strength, lose weight or sharpen their mental focus.
- Modern adolescence is highly competitive both on and off the field of play.
- The use of dietary sports supplements is common in teens trying to gain the competitive edge.
- The dietary and sports supplement industry is an evolving, multi-billion-dollar industry that often caters to an adolescents' desire to improve.
- Product sales are boosted by eye-catching marketing campaigns, often touting putative benefits based on little scientific data.
- Scientific uncertainty and shifting market forces leave many medical professionals unable to adequately answer questions about dietary supplements posed by their patients.

ASSESSMENT

HISTORY

Ask Questions About Current Use:

- What is hoped to be gained by using the product? (e.g. to become stronger or faster, lose or gain weight, gain focus, and/or improve energy)?
- How will these goals be achieved?
- Determine if the teen has already tried the supplement or any other supplements.
- If yes, what were the results?
- If using a supplement, does the teen feel that it is working for him or her?

- How did the teen first learn of the supplement (e.g. gym, infomercial, or a website)?
- Where was the supplement bought (e.g. supermarket or supplement store, at the gym, from a friend or on the internet)?
- Using a "food first" methodology, obtain a dietary history to determine areas for improvement, if supplementation is necessary or if its use may be harmful.
- Has the teen experienced any side effects from supplements?
- Is the teen subject to drug testing for his or her sport?

Past Medical History

- Does the teen have a medical condition such as renal disease, hypertension, headaches, asthma, arrhythmia or other heart disease, liver disease or obesity?
- Is there a history of exertional heat injury (i.e. heat exhaustion, heat stroke), chest pain or syncope?

Family History

- Is there a family history of sudden cardiac death or premature cardiac disease?

Medications

- Does the teen take any over-the-counter or prescription medications, herbs or other dietary supplements?

Social History

- Has the teen tried any **illegal supplements or substances?**
- Does the teen use **nicotine products** (e.g. "dip" is commonly used by adolescent athletes for an energy "buzz") or drink alcoholic products?

Review of Systems

- Has the teen gained or lost a significant amount of weight or are there red flags for an **eating disorder** (ED)?
- If a teen taking supplements presents with nausea, vomiting, dizziness, or mental status changes consider **exertional heat injury** (EHI).

PHYSICAL

Anthropometric Measurements

- Assess height and weight and calculate BMI.
- Plot trends over time on a growth curve with the aid of old records.

Vital Signs

- Tachycardia or arrhythmia raise concerns for use of **sympathomimetic supplements.**
- Hypertension can occur with **renal disease.**
- A rectal (core) temperature reading will be necessary if a patient taking supplements presents with signs of **EHI.**

HEENT

- Observe for mydriasis (as occurs with **sympathomimetic supplements**) and evaluate dentition and oral mucosa for signs of **tobacco use** or **ED** (i.e. enamel erosion).

Abdomen

- Evaluate liver for tenderness or hepatomegaly.

Genital

- Low testicular volume occurs with use of **anabolic compounds.**
- Females may have clitoromegaly with use of **anablolic** or **androgenic compounds.**

Skin

- Teens using **anabolic** or **androgenic compounds** may have acne or worsening acne.
- Assess skin for jaundice.

Neurologic Exam

- Assess for tremor as can occur with **sympathomimetic and other supplements.**

- Patients presenting with headaches, changes in mental status, or weakness warrant full neurological examination as these symptoms may be related to **supplement use or abuse**, or a sports related injury such as **concussion** or EHI.

STUDIES

Complete Blood Count

- Elevated hemoglobin and hematocrit can indicate hemoconcentration due to significant **dehydration** or **anabolic compound use.**

Comprehensive Metabolic Panel

- Changes in *electrolytes* can occur in those patients who are **dehydrated** or those with **EHI.**
- *BUN* may be high due to **dehydration** or **large dietary protein intake.**
- *Creatinine* can be mildly elevated in patients taking **creatine**. It can be pathologically elevated in patients with **EHI, rhabdomyolysis** or underlying **renal disease** (a contraindication to supplemental creatine use).
- *Liver enzymes* may be abnormal due to **anabolic compound use.**
- Many other sports supplements can cause similar stress on the liver.
- It is well-known that many sports supplements are contaminated with substances not listed on the label, many of which can be associated with a **chemical hepatitis.**
- Liver-associated enzymes are frequently elevated in cases of **EHI.**
- *Creatine kinase (CK)* may be massively elevated in a patient with **rhabdomyolysis.**
- *Cholesterol* can be elevated in those taking **anabolic compounds.**
- LDL can be elevated, while HDL is decreased.
- *Prealbumin*, with a much shorter half life than albumin, is a good marker for very recent fasting or dieting, a concern in those patients on **weight-loss ("fat burner") supplements.**

Urinalysis

- Patients with **EHI** often develop **rhabdomyolysis**, and will have a false positive chemical assay (dipstick) for blood.

- A positive urine dip for blood with a negative microscopy for RBCs is suspicious for **myoglobinuria.**
- *Ketonuria* may follow the use of **weight loss supplements.**

Coagulation Studies

- Coagulation studies are a test of liver synthetic function.
- Numerous supplements and contaminants have been associated with elevations in liver-associated enzymes.
- Severe **EHI** can lead to multi-organ failure.

Electrocardiogram (EKG)

- Rule out arrhythmias and measure QT interval (particularly important for patients taking **weight loss, energy** or **"fat burner" supplements).**

SPECIAL TESTS

Testosterone Glucuronide to Epitestosterone Glucuronide Ratio (T/E Ratio)

- Typically elevated in patients taken exogenous steroids.

Urine Testosterone to Luteinizing Hormone Ratio

- Elevated in patients taking exogenous steroids due to a negative feedback loop generated by high circulating testosterone levels.

DISPOSITION

Support the adolescent's reasonable athletic goals.

- Educate patients, parents, trainers and coaches about healthy diet and exercise for athletes.
- Incorporate a nutritionist when available, and use a "food first" approach.
- Instead of discounting supplement use, work with patients to positively effect outcomes.

Strongly recommend against the use of weight loss or "fat burner" supplements.

- They have not been shown to be effective in well-designed studies.

- They can lead to **arrhythmias**, especially in patients who have a predisposition for arrhythmias or in patients who are on sympathomimetic medications such as albuterol.
- Note: **Ephedrine**, in combination with caffeine, has been shown to lead to weight loss. Ephedrine was pulled from the U.S. market in 2004 after it was linked to multiple deaths.

Multiple-ingredient supplement products should generally be avoided.

- The sports supplement industry is extremely competitive, and producers often market products with "proprietary blends" that have not been tested for safety or efficacy.
- **"Nitric oxide" creatine products** have been linked to multiple adverse events, and have not been shown to be more effective than creatine alone.

Mega-dose vitamins should also be avoided.

- Doses higher than U.S. RDA have no ergogenic potential, and can potentially be harmful, particularly fat-soluble vitamins in large doses.

Anabolic steroids should always be avoided.

- Patients who are found to be using anabolic steroids should be referred for drug counseling (dependence has been reported).
- Consideration should be given to screening for other drug use including tobacco, alcohol or illicit substances and referrals to substance use counseling made as needed.

Recommend limited daily protein intake.

- A growing adolescent athlete can utilize up to 2.2 grams/kg/day of dietary protein (equates to 1 gram/pound/day).
- Any more will not be utilized by the body and in theory, can have negative effects on the kidney, and may lead to gastrointestinal distress.

Monitor supplement use closely.

- Creatine has been found to be safe in adults at recommended doses (typically 5 grams/day), and is efficacious if the goal is to *sprint faster* or to *improve short-burst strength* (no more than 20–30 seconds).

- It should not be used by anyone who has or is at risk for renal insufficiency.
- Safety in *older* adolescents is extrapolated from adult data and it would be prudent to recommend against its use in younger adolescents.

What is unique about sports supplement use in adolescents?

Adolescents are influenced by the role models around them as they work toward self-actualization.

- They may turn to parents, coaches and teammates, some of whom may have taken supplements themselves.
- Many adolescents will try supplements that others are using in the gym.

Adolescents who play sports that monitor weight may be at increased risk for use and abuse of "fat burners" in combination with a restrictive diet.

- These teens are at risk for arrhythmias or EHI from the sympathomimetic supplement ingredients (e.g. ephedrine, synephrine).
- They also need to be monitored for the development of eating disorders.

Adolescents are generally very web-savvy.

  - Internet sales of sports supplements is immense.
  - Website chat rooms discuss the putative benefits of sports supplements in a misleading fashion, discussing "scientific evidence" when none is truly available.
- Many competitive athletes are offered college scholarships for their sport and may not be aware that many supplements consist of products that if picked up on spot drug testing, could compromise their future academic and athletic success (i.e. anabolic steroids).
- Since most adolescents are not asking their medical providers or a nutritionist about supplement use, it is important for the clinician to become familiar with common sports supplements and develop safe plans for their teen patients.

TEST YOUR KNOWLEDGE ANSWERS

10. C. There is reasonable evidence that some dietary supplements can lead to improved athletic performance (ergogenic potential). Of those that have the most evidence, creatine is one of the most tested. It does have a long track record of safety and efficacy in otherwise healthy adult patients, but there is little data on adolescent patients. It should be used with caution in adolescents, particularly younger adolescents. Ephedrine with caffeine did lead to weight loss in studies; however, it also was associated with numerous adverse events, including death. It was officially banned by the FDA in 2004.
11. D. Synephrine, a sympathomimetic naturally-occurring chemical, has arrhythmogenic potential, and should be strictly avoided in patients who may be prone to arrhythmias. These products should be strictly avoided by patients who are on sympathomimetic medications such as albuterol. In fact, "fat burner" products that contain synephrine have little evidence to back efficacy, and although there are fewer adverse event reports when compared to ephedrine, there are many anecdotal reports of ischemic events. Multiple-ingredient products should be avoided by all patients. As a rule, these products have many untested ingredients and combinations of ingredients. For patients such as this 18 year old who want to safely use creatine, it is best to use a creatine-only supplement.

WEB REFERENCES

- Australian Institute of Sport: Supplements (2012), Retrieved from http://www.ausport.gov.a/aisnutritionsupplements
- Food and Drug Administration: Dietary Supplements (2013), Retrieved from http://www.fda.gov/Food/DietarySupplements/default.htm
- Shekelle P, Morton SC, Maglione M, et al. 'Ephedra and Ephedrine for Weight Loss and Athletic Performance Enhancement: Clinical Efficacy and Side Effects.' Rockville (MD): Agency for Healthcare Research and Quality (US); 2003 Mar. (Evidence Reports/Technology Assessments, No. 76) Available from: http://www.ncbi.nlm.nih.gov/books/NBK36915?

Additional Clinician and Patient Resources:

- Human Performance Resource Center: http://humanperformanceresourcecenter.org/dietary-supplements

- National Center for Complementary and Alternative Medicine (NCCAM), Using Dietary Supplements Wisely (March 2010), Retrieved from http://nccam.nih.gov/health supplementswiseuse.htm#safety
- National Institutes of Health Office of Dietary Supplements: http://ods.od.nih.gov/
- National Library of Medicine: http://dietarysupplements.nlm.nih.gov/dietary/
- Natural Medicines Comprehensive Database: https://www.naturaldatabase.com

  - Setting family restrictions and punishments for violations.
  - Influencing vehicle selection.
  - Instructing and supervising driving.
  - Being a role model for safe driving.
- Parents tend to place more restrictions on details of the trip (i.e. permission, destination and time home) than on dangerous driving conditions (i.e. night driving with teen passengers).
- Graduated Driver Licensing (GDL) systems may help parents better enforce driving rules.
- Parent-teen driving contracts, which clearly delineate rules and consequences may result in better communication, more restrictions and safer parent and teen attitudes (Figure 1).

Legal Interventions

Graduated Driver Licensing Systems (GDLs)

- Delays full licensure allowing new drivers to gain experience under lower risk conditions.
- Consists of 3 stages:
  - Learner's Permit: Optimal minimum age is 16 and this stage lasts at least 6 months, during which parents must certify at least 30–50 hours of supervised driving.
  - Intermediate License (provisional or junior license): Optimally lasts until 18 years and includes both a night driving restriction starting at 9 or 10 p.m. and a strict teen passenger restriction allowing no more than one teen passenger.
  - Full License: Unrestricted license.
- 49 states and the District of Columbia (DC) have now adopted a 3-level GDL system for new drivers. North Dakota is the only state without an intermediate stage.
- Progression through the stages is based on time and achievement as opposed to age.
- Studies have found crash reductions of 10–30% in U.S. states that have adopted elements of graduated licensing.

Nighttime and Passenger Restrictions

- Associated with crash reductions of 40–60% during restricted hours.
- 48 states and DC have nighttime driving restrictions for teens.
- Many states exempt school, work and religious activities from nighttime driving restrictions.
- 42 states and DC have restrictions on the number of passengers for a driver with an intermediate license.
- Family members are usually exempt from the restrictions on passengers.
- Unfortunately, many teens do not comply with passenger restriction, many parents do not support it and police frequently don't enforce it.

Alcohol-Related Measures

- Two existing alcohol-related regulations are: minimum drinking-age laws and drunk-driving laws. The drunk-driving laws include "zero-tolerance" policies and regulations for licensure suspension or revocation.
- By 1998, all states had passed zero-tolerance laws for drinking and driving.
- These laws deter youth through fear of losing their driver's license if they drink and drive and by reinforcing community disapproval of drinking and driving.
- However, there is also evidence that drunk driving is influenced more by friends' approval or disapproval than by fear of arrest or loss of license.

Improved Safety Belt Laws

- Primary laws: Allow an officer to issue a citation when an unbelted occupant is observed.
- Secondary laws: Allow an officer to issue a safety belt citation only after the car has been stopped for another infraction.
- 32 states and DC have primary seat belt laws and only one state (New Hampshire) has no seat belt law at the time of publication.

<u>Ineffective Intervention</u>

Driver Education

- Traditional programs involve 30 hours of classroom and 6 hours of on-road instruction.

  - These programs are *not* effective in creating safe drivers or decreasing crash risk.
  - High school driver education programs may encourage early licensure of the youngest, most dangerous drivers, resulting in more crashes, injuries and deaths.

DISPOSITION

- Know the state laws regarding teen drivers and the driver-licensing process.
- Distribute educational materials about local GDL programs and driver safety to adolescent patients (Table 1).
- Encourage safety belt use.
- Discourage distractions when driving (i.e. eating, drinking, music, texting and cell phone use).
- Encourage teen-parent written contracts that place restrictions on the teen driver (Figure 1).
  - At a minimum, parents should be encouraged to place restrictions on night time driving and the number of adolescent passengers in the car.
  - The rules should start out strict and can become relaxed as the teen grows older and gains more experience.
- Encourage parents to require that the vehicle driven by the teen is safe and in good condition.
- Advise parents that in many states, they have the authority to request that the driver's license of their minor child be revoked.
- Encourage parents to be positive driving role models.
- Counsel adolescents about the dangers of driving while impaired (e.g. under the influence of alcohol, drugs, or medications or feeling ill, tired, depressed or angry).
- Encourage a "safe-ride" agreement in which the teen agrees to call the parent instead of driving impaired. Parents should promise to arrange the ride home in a nonjudgmental manner.

What is unique about adolescents and driving?

- *Inexperience*: Adolescents are less skilled in detecting and responding to hazards, controlling automobiles, integrating speed and performing many of the complex tasks of driving.

- *Propensity to Take Risks:*
  - Teen drivers are more likely to be influenced by peer group pressures, emotional lability and other stresses.
  - Males are especially at high risk, possibly secondary to media images and social norms that equate driving fast and performing difficult driving maneuvers as masculine.
  - Teen immaturity manifests in risky driving practices such as running red lights, making illegal turns, tailgating and speeding.
  - MRI research has shown evidence that the prefrontal cortex (area of the brain responsible for executive functions, judgments and values, ability to set long-term goals and weigh risks versus consequences) does not fully mature until the early to mid-20s.
- *Distractions*: Cellular phone use including text messaging is estimated to increase crash rates fourfold; hands free models are not significantly lowering the risk. Eating, drinking, and adjusting radio or climate controls cause more crashes than cellular phone use.
- *Teen Passengers*: can distract a new driver and/or lead to greater risk-taking behaviors.
  - Distractions such as laughter, music and food increase with the number of passengers in the automobile and can interrupt a driver's concentration.
  - 16 to 17 year olds have a 40% increased risk of crashing when they have 1 friend in the car, double the risk with 2 passengers, and almost 4 times the risk with 3 or more teen passengers.
- *Nighttime Driving*: is difficult for drivers of all ages. Fatigue and lack of practice may play a greater role for teens.
  - The majority of fatal crashes for teens occur between 9 p.m. and 6 a.m.
  - Late night teen outings tend to be recreational. Under these circumstances, adolescents are more likely to become easily distracted, which is associated with multiple teenage passengers, speeding and alcohol use.
- *Alcohol, Drugs, and Medications:*
  - Adolescents' driving abilities are more impaired by small amounts of alcohol than are those of older drivers.

  - Drugs other than alcohol are involved in 10–15% of teen motor vehicle fatalities.
  - A single 50 mg dose of diphenhydramine (Benadryl) has been shown to have a greater affect on driving performance than a blood alcohol content (BAC) of 0.10%. It is important to warn patients about the effects of medications on driving.

- *Low Safety Belt Use Rate*
  - Teens aged 10–20 years use safety belts only about 35% of the time.
  - The risk of injury to teen occupants in a severe crash more than triples if restraints are not used.
  - Safety belt use is lower in high-risk situations (i.e. alcohol use, multiple teen passengers, nighttime driving, older car, male driver, or suspended or no license).

- *Type of Vehicle Driven*
  - Teens are more likely to drive smaller, older-model cars, especially if they are the owner of the vehicle.
  - Smaller cars provide less crash protection than larger vehicles, and older-model cars often have fewer safety features.
  - When adolescents drive sports utility vehicles, they are more likely to have a rollover than drivers older than 24 years.

- *Attention-Deficit/Hyperactivity Disorder (ADHD)*
  - Adolescent drivers with ADHD are 2–4 times more likely to be injured in MVA's than their peers without ADHD.
  - They are also more likely to have repeat traffic citations and to have their licenses suspended or revoked.
  - Psychostimulants improve the driving performance of teens with ADHD.
  - Adolescents with ADHD should remember/be reminded to take their medications when driving, including weekends.

- *Seizure Disorder*: can limit driving for teens who are not well controlled with medications.
  - If well-controlled, states have different laws regarding the length of the seizure free period before a teen is allowed to drive.

TEST YOUR KNOWLEDGE ANSWERS

12. D. Teens tend to have a low rate of safety belt use, which triples the adolescent's risk of injury in a severe crash. Safety belt use also tends to be lower in higher risk conditions such as driving at night, carrying teenage passengers and driving under the influence of alcohol.
13. B. In an optimal GDL, progression through the stages is based on time and achievement as opposed to age. Studies have found that the prefrontal cortex (area of the brain responsible for weighing risks and consequences) does not fully mature until the early to mid-20s. The longer a teen takes to progress through the stages, the more likely he/she will be mentally ready to handle challenging driving conditions.

Table 1. Essential Features That Should Be Mandated in GDL Systems.

- A learner-permit that starts no earlier than 16 years and lasts at least 6 months.
- A minimum of 30 hours (preferably 50 hours) of adult-supervised, on-road driving during the permit stage (at least 5–10 of these supervised practice hours should be at night).
- A provisional (intermediate) stage, with restrictions, that lasts until 18 years.
- A nighttime driving restriction (9:00 PM to 5:00 AM until driving with provisional license for 6 months, followed by a midnight to 5:00 AM restriction until 18 years).
- Passenger limits (unless supervised by an adult)
  - No teen passengers during the first 6 months on a provisional license.
  - No more than 1 teen passenger until driver has reached 18 years.
- Prompt imposition of fines, remedial driver's classes, or license suspension for violation of passenger or curfew restrictions.
- Use of safety belts and appropriate child restraints by all occupants.
- No cellular phone use while in the provisional stage.
- Zero tolerance for alcohol and provisions for administrative license revocation for drunk driving, excessive speeding or reckless driving.
- Documented safe driving record before full licensure is granted.

It is suggested that states also consider a requirement for additional supervised driver experience or education (focused on hazard recognition and risk avoidance) during the provisional stage and a requirement for an additional on-road test to graduate from provisional to full licensure.

It is understood that having a driver's license and driving a motor vehicle are privileges. This privilege has to be earned, and it must be earned on a continuing basis. Driving privileges will be revoked if the following rules are not complied:

I will only use the car with permission. Permission will be granted in most cases unless mom/dad need the car.

I will obey all traffic laws and rules, including speed limits.

I will not carry any passengers younger than 18 in my car (family members excluded).

I, and all my passengers, will always wear seatbelts.

I will not drive unsupervised between 9 pm and 5 am until age 18.

I will participate in a minimum of 50 hours of supervised driving while in the learner stage of the graduated licensing system.

I will not allow others to drive the car. I will not drive someone else's car without my parent's knowledge and permission.

I will never leave the car without gas in it. I will always lock the car when I leave it.

I will not play the radio or CD player so loudly that it interferes with my concentration and ability to drive. I will use common sense concerning this at all times.

I will not talk or text on a cellular phone at any time while driving the car.

I will pay for any parking or other traffic tickets I may incur.

I will take the car to be inspected each year before the date required.

Anytime I take the car I will tell at least one of my parents what time I will be home, and will be on time so they do not worry. If I find I am going to be late, I will call and let them know.

I will not drink or use other illegal substances, since by law I am not allowed to do so. If, on some occasion my better judgment and common sense leave me and I have been drinking, I will not drive the car. I will call my parents and one of them will come and get me, no questions asked.

I will remember at all times that the car is a lethal weapon, both to myself and to others. I will accept the responsibility for driving carefully and safely.

Signature of Teen Driver	*Signature of Parent(s)/Guardian(s)*
Date	Date

Figure 1 Sample Teen Driving Contract.

WEB REFERENCES

- Allstate Foundation Teen Safe Driving Program (www.allstate.com/foundation/teen-safe-driving.aspx)
  - Teen Driving Facts Sheet (2012), Retrieved from http://www.allstatefoundation.org/sites/default/files/Teen_Driving_Facts.pdf
- American Academy of Pediatrics
  - Committee on Injury, Violence, and Poison Prevention, Committee on Adolescence. 'The Teen Driver', Pediatrics. December 2006; 118(6); 2570–2581, Retrieved from http://pediatrics.aappublications.org/content/ll8/6/2570.full
- D'Angelo L, Halpem-Felsher BL, Abraham A (2010), 'Position Paper: Adolescents and Driving: A Position Paper of the Society for Adolescent Health and Medicine', Journal of Adolescent Health, 2010;47(2);212-214, Retrieved from http://www.adolescenthealth.org/AM/Template.cfm?Section=Position_Papers&Template=/CM/ContentDisplay.cfm&ContentID=3223
- Insurance Institute for Highway Safety (www.iihs.org)
  - McCartt AT, Teoh ER, Fields M, Braitman KA, and Hellinga LA. 'Graduated Licensing Laws and Fatal Crashes of Teenage Drivers: A National Study', Traffic Injury Prevention, June 2010, 11(3); 240–248, Retrieved from http://www.iihs.org/research/topics/pdf/rll22.pdf
  - Summary table: young driver licensing systems in the U.S. (February 2013), Retrieved from http://www.iihs.org/laws/GraduatedLicenseCompare.aspx

Additional Clinician and Patient Resources:

- Insurance Institute for Highway Safety (2013): www.iihs.org/research/topics/teenagers.html
- National Highway Traffic Safety Administration: www.nhtsa.gov/Teen-Drivers
- Triple AAA Foundation for Traffic Safety: www.aaafoundation.org

10

THE TRANSITION TO COLLEGE

Isabel Goldenberg and
Harshita J. Saxena

TEST YOUR KNOWLEDGE

14. The following vaccines are all advisable for college students *EXCEPT*:

    A. Tetatus, diptheria and acellular pertussis booster.
    B. Meningococcal vaccine if the first dose was given 5 years ago.
    C. Human papillomavirus vaccine for males and unvaccinated females.
    D. For any vaccine series that has not been completed, the series should be started anew.
    E. Yearly influenza vaccine.

Refer to end of chapter for answer on page 119.

Jack just graduated from high school and plans to go to college in August. He comes over the summer for a physical and to have health forms completed for school.

BACKGROUND

- The prematriculation health care visit is a good opportunity to address many issues.
- Absent chronic health conditions, the physical exam is often the only time a student is seen in a physician's office, so it is an ideal time to engage in a dialogue that addresses the full range of physical and emotional concerns specific to this life change.
- Physician-patient confidentiality is an important part of this process so that young adults feel protected and safe discussing personal matters with a trusted professional.
- Many practical issues need to be addressed during the pre-college health visit including the completion of mandatory school forms, verifying and updating vaccination status, documentation of health insurance and transitioning health care with recommendations specific to the teen's medical concerns and needs.

ASSESSMENT

HISTORY

- Complete a thorough history including HEEADSSS risk assessment.
- This assessment should also include a complete review of immunization status. Recommended institutional immunizations include:
  - Tetanus-Diphtheria-Pertussis vaccine.
  - Quadrivalent Meningococcal conjugate vaccine (Menactra or Menveo) or a booster if the last dose was five years ago or more; some schools allow this vaccine to be waived even though the American College Health Association (ACHA) highly recommends it for students living in dormitory populations).
  - HPV vaccine series (for men and women, three doses at 0, 1–2, and 6 months).

- Hepatitis B vaccine series (three doses at 0, 1, and 6 months at any age or two adult doses at 0 and 4–6 months). Some schools require confirmation of vaccine status through titers.
- Polio vaccine series.
- Measles-Mumps-Rubella (MMR) vaccine series (two doses after the age of 1).
- Varicella vaccine series (two doses or history of disease that may have to be verified by titer status depending on university).
- Annual Influenza vaccine.
- Pneumococcal polysaccharide (PPV) vaccine is recommended for young adults with chronic health conditions and smokers.
- Hepatitis A vaccine series (two doses at 0 and 6 months) is especially recommended for students who will be studying abroad.

- It is necessary to check each school's immunization form to comply with their immunization policy and to sign all completed forms.
  - If additional vaccine doses are needed, inform students of the schedule to follow.
  - Students can often have their vaccines updated at their college's student health center.

PHYSICAL

- A complete physical exam should be performed including vital signs, anthropometric measurements and Tanner staging.

STUDIES

History and physical exam findings should guide laboratory screening tests ordered. Laboratory tests ordered may include:

- Annual gonorrhea and chlamydia testing.
- HIV testing.
- Tuberculosis testing for at-risk groups.
- Anemia screening for females or vegetarians/vegans.
- Lipid screening.
- Vaccine titer status may be required for Hepatitis B and/or Varicella.
- Pap smears are not recommended for most adolescents until age 21 unless they have a weakened immune system (i.e. HIV).

DISPOSITION

Entry Requirements

- Many colleges and universities have student health centers, and health related entrance requirements vary school to school.
- Documents to be completed may include a health inventory and physical exam form, an immunization record and/or an athletic department sports related health inventory and physical exam.

Health Insurance

- Determine the patient's insurance status once he or she starts college. Many colleges and universities may offer mandatory or voluntary student health insurance.
  - Mandatory insurance without a waiver:
    - A fee is included in the tuition and the student is unable to opt out of the insurance.
  - Mandatory insurance with a waiver:
    - After submitting proof of their own insurance and if approved by the school, parents can opt out of the school insurance.
  - Voluntary insurance plans:
    - Families should verify that their insurance plan offers coverage in the geographical region where the teen will attend college.
    - The policy chosen should best suit the teen's needs.
    - If the parents' insurance is an HMO, they should check and see if there is reciprocity with another HMO in the area.
- Students should have copies of their insurance cards (both sides).

Transition of Health Care

- Provide medical records or a discharge summary to the teen to ensure continuation of care at the school student health center.
  - This is especially important when the teen has ongoing medical issues or has been diagnosed with a chronic medical condition.

  - In these situations, it may be necessary to communicate with the student health center clinician or to a specialist near the college to ensure continuity of care.
- Provide a 3 month supply of current prescriptions to cover any possible gaps in care.
  - Students receiving allergy desensitization treatments can request the vials and continue their treatment at school. Most student health centers offer this service.
- Schedule follow-up visits for the next time the student will be home on vacation if there are any health issues that need to be monitored.

Issues to Discuss with the Patient

- Students should be advised to become familiar with the student health center on campus as early as orientation week.
  - Specifically, know where this center is located and what services are routinely offered.
  - Students with chronic medical conditions should determine where their medical needs can best be met. For example, will their student health center address issues that arise such as medication refills or will they have to be referred to a specialist.
- If the teen has been diagnosed with a psychiatric disorder for which they are receiving ongoing therapy and/or medications, it would also be imperative for them to find out about counseling services offered at their school. These services are often offered at a reduced rate that is more affordable.
- Students should receive their semi-annual dental check up if due.
  - Suggest ordering extra retainers for students receiving orthodontic treatment.
- Offer suggestions for a first aid kit for the student to have in his or her room.
  - This kit may contain items such as acetaminophen, lozenges, over the counter decongestants, Maalox, a thermometer, bandages and disinfectant.

What is unique about the pre-college visit with adolescents?

- The college-bound teen has likely never lived on his or her own. With this in mind, it is important to provide guidance on issues pertaining to the teen's newfound independence.
- The teen is now responsible for his or her own health care and should schedule appointments and follow ups with clinicians as needed while away from home.
- Teens may be unaccustomed to communal bathroom arrangements in many dormitories. They may be sharing a bathroom with a roommate or roommates and should prepare accordingly.
- Most colleges offer meal plans and dining services. Many college campuses also have gyms and work-out facilities built into tuition costs for students. Teens should be advised to maintain healthy diets and exercise regimens while away at school.
- Student athletes often need to maintain minimum grade point averages to maintain scholarship and/or team status.

    - Advise athletes to consult with clinicians if considering sports supplements (Chapter 8).
    - Products may not be screened by the FDA and may be adulterated and unsafe.
    - Many sports enhancing products are illegal. If used, these could affect the student's scholarship and/or team status. Colleges often perform random drug screening among their student athletes.

- Many teens may experiment with alcohol and drug use, often with easier access when away from parental supervision.

    - Teens should be aware of the dangers of alcohol and drug use, including sharing of stimulant medications, and potential repercussions if caught (legal ramifications and affect on matriculation status).
    - Teens should be prepared with designated drivers in all situations. Consider advising that they carry a small amount of cash if needed for cab fare.

- Teens should drive responsibly, including always wearing a seat belt.

- Encourage good organizational skills. Teens will need to maintain regular class attendance and develop time management skills to ensure college success.
- Teens and parents should be aware of the emotional aspects of leaving home and adjusting to college life as well as knowing how and where to seek help on campus.
- Teens should understand the importance of healthy and safe sexual practices to prevent unintended pregnancies and the transmission of sexually transmitted infections.
- Many teens will be dating or start dating during college. Both males and females should be advised on dating violence and rape prevention.

TEST YOUR KNOWLEDGE ANSWER

14. If a vaccine series is incomplete, it is appropriate to give the missing immunization: it is not necessary to restart the series. Universal HPV is recommended to reduce the burden of illness. Tdap and Meningococcal boosters better protect from diseases that can break out on campus than primary immunization alone. Annual influenza vaccine is recommended.

WEB REFERENCES

- American College Health Association (www.acha.org):
  - ACHA Vaccine Preventable Diseases Committee 2012, 'Recommendations for Institutional Prematriculation Immunizations', Apil 2012, Retrieved from http://www.acha.org/Publications/docs/ACHA_RIPI_Apr2012.pdf
  - ACHA Tuberculosis Guidelines Task Force with revisions by Emerging Public Health Threats and Emergency Response Coalition 2012, 'Tuberculosis Screening and Targeted Testing of College and University Students', April 2012, Retrieved from http://www.acha.org/Publications/docs/ACHA_Tuberculosis_Screening_Apr2012.pdf
- American College of Obstetricians & Gynecologists (http://www.acog.org/):
  - Committee on Adolescent Health Care, 'Cervical Cancer In Adolescents: Screening, Evaluation and Management', Committee Opinion, August 2010;463: http://www.acog.org/~/media/Committee%20Opinions/Committee%20on%20Adolescent%20Health%20Care/co463.pdf?dmc=l&ts=20130313T1052275427

Additional Clinician and Patient Resources:

- Center for Young Women's Health, Boston Children's Hospital, 'College Health', patient handout (last updated 2/1/2013), retrieved from http://www.youngwomenshealth.org/PDFs/Full%20PDF's%20of%20Broken%20Out%20Guides/College%20Health_Full.pdf
- Centers for Disease Control and Prevention, Information on Tuberculosis (2013): www.cdc.gov/tb
- Centers for Disease Control, Preteen and Teen Vaccinations (2012): www.cdc.gov/vaccines/recs/schedules/teen-schedule.htm
- Centers for Disease Control, Vaccine Safety (2011): www.cdc.gov/vaccinesafety/Vaccines/HPV/iama.html

11

THE ADOLESCENT TRAVELER AND IMMIGRANT

Natwarlal Shah

TEST YOUR KNOWLEDGE

15. Which one of the following statements is true? Adolescents who return from a trip abroad or immigrate to the United States should:
    A. Tell their physician of any foreign travel dating back a couple of years whenever they seek medical attention.
    B. End their malaria prophylaxis when they return from their trip abroad to avoid any unnecessary side effects.
    C. Be considered protected against tuberculosis (TB) if they received the BCG vaccine.
    D. All the above.
    E. None of the above.

Refer to end of chapter for answer on page 126.

A 19 year old Afghan student studying in the U.S. presents to his college health center with a three week history of an ulcer on his forearm. He is treated for an insect bite with secondary infection but the ulcer persists. Frustrated, he calls his physician in Afghanistan who recommends testing for Leishmaniasis.

BACKGROUND

- Adolescents frequently travel abroad, often to underdeveloped regions or remote areas of developing countries.
- Clinicians should be prepared to make recommendations to traveling teens to prevent or minimize exposure to potentially life threatening infections and situations.
- It is important to appropriately diagnose and promptly treat sick adolescent globetrotters returning from their trips abroad. They, as well as immigrants to the U.S., may develop infections and ailments unique to the regions of their travels.
- Adolescents may import illnesses or export them, developing symptoms after they arrive at their final destination.

PRE-TRAVEL RECOMMENDATIONS

- Review and update most currently recommended vaccines and prophylactic medications:
  - Advise vaccines based on specific travel destination considering diseases such as yellow fever, typhoid, Japanese encephalitis, etc.
  - Offer malaria prophylaxis if traveling to endemic regions and remind patients to start medications pre-travel depending on regimen chosen.
  - In travel medicine, most of the focus is on imported diseases such as malaria, dengue fever and typhoid, but physicians also need to educate the traveling adolescent what diseases one may be exporting, such as influenza and whooping cough.
- Educate adolescents about appropriate travel precautions as follows:
  - Prepare for the trip by packing a basic first aid kit, disposable gloves, toilet seat covers and general hygiene items such as hand sanitizer.

- Use sunscreens and insect repellents to protect skin and prevent insect spread infections.
- Do *not* drink the tap water in developing countries.
- Use caution when buying bottled water, often filled with tap water by unscrupulous vendors.
    - Drink only certified bottled water from a reliable source.
    - Consider packing chlorine or iodide tablets if certified bottled water is unavailable.
    - Many food products are prepared with tap water and handled by unhygienic utensils. Consider avoiding raw fruits, vegetables and salads to avoid water borne illnesses.
- Stay hydrated and consider packing oral hydrating powder packs.
- Teens with chronic medical conditions need to remember to pack their medications to prevent disease related complications while abroad.
    - Medications should be packed in original pharmacy containers with proper labels.
    - Medications often go by different names in other countries and may not be readily available, or the quality of medication may be substandard or unreliable.
- Avoid use of contact lenses in dusty areas, as there is an increased potential for corneal injury and eye infections. Pack an extra pair of prescription eyeglasses.
- In their excitement, traveling teens on "vacation" mode may forget important safety precautions that they would normally use at home.
    - Do not venture out alone at night.
    - Stay only at reputable hotels or youth hostels.
    - If sexually active, always engage in safe sex practices. Abstain from sex or use condoms to prevent the spread of sexually transmitted infections (STI's).
    - Follow the legal standards of the destination country. Alcohol age limit laws vary from country to country and some countries have strict legal codes and severe punishments for drug possession.
    - Be aware of dress codes and appropriate expressions/displays of emotion in public.

  - While uncommon, rape, kidnapping and even murder can occur. Political enemies and sex traders may target traveling teens-ALWAYS maintain safety precautions.

- Even with the best precautions, illness or injury may occur. Become familiar with local medical clinics and establish a local physician especially during prolonged stays (i.e. semester, internship or exchange programs abroad).
  - Seek medical care promptly when a concern arises.
  - Contact parents back home. Teens may postpone calling parents for fear of causing worry, but parents can assist the teen and the treating physician.
  - Families should consider buying travel medical insurance, including Medical Evacuation, in case of serious illness or injury.
- Traveling teens should always carry some form of identification with them.
  - Identification information should include both local and home base contact information, that could prove useful in cases of vehicle accident, other accidents, serious illness, natural disaster (i.e. earthquake, flood) or terrorism attack.
- Advise the teen to carry the contact information for the U.S. embassy, consulate and state department.
- Before travel, check USA State Department and CDC web sites for travel alerts due to geopolitical turmoil or disease outbreak.
- Do not rely on cell phones, laptops or other devices to carry identification or contact information because these expensive items can be stolen: maintain back up emergency contact information.

POST-TRAVEL RECOMMENDATIONS

- After returning home to the U.S., the teen may need to maintain precaution regimens as follows:
  - Complete malaria prophylaxis if it was prescribed at the pre-travel consult.
  - A teen who returns home sick or becomes ill shortly thereafter, should contact their primary care physician and mention *recent foreign travel history.*

- If the teen seeks urgent medical care at their clinician's office or an Emergency Department, they should mention foreign travel dating back 2 years. Urge patients to proactively tell health care professionals of their travel history.
- Whenever symptoms are confusing, or there is no response to treatment, clinicians should research infectious diseases prevalent in the countries visited by the patient (e.g. malaria, Dengue fever, Chikyngunya and chancroid).
- Ask teens about their sexual activity and screen for STIs, HIV and Hepatitis C when indicated. Consider Hepatitis B if a vaccine record is unavailable or the vaccine series was not received.

THE ADOLESCENT IMMIGRANT

- Immigrant adolescents should have a complete physical examination including HEEADSSS and screening for HIV and other STIs. In doing so, be cognizant of cultural norms and respectful of patient preferences.
- For recent immigrants, review vaccines administered, as many teens may not have received full vaccine schedules and some vaccines may not have been available in their country of origin. These teens will need their vaccines updated.
- Many countries may not have the same at birth screening standards as the U.S. Consider screening for sickle cell disease and G6PD deficiency.
- Those coming from tuberculosis (TB) endemic regions are screened for TB and may require treatment of latent TB infection.

    - BCG, or Bacillus Calmette-Guérin, is a TB vaccine that many foreign born individuals may have received at birth or a later date. It can cause false-positive reactions to TB intradermal skin tests. The size of the reaction does not predict if the BCG vaccine protects against TB.
    - A strongly positive skin test many years after BCG is more likely to be due to tuberculosis than to the vaccine and a chest x-ray is required.
    - Blood test (Quantiferon®) to detect TB is not affected by prior BCG vaccination and will not give false-positive results. Clinicians may want to consider blood testing for TB detection if available to determine prior exposure.

- Malaria can incubate for up to 2 years so it is important to consider the infection in any adolescent arriving from a malaria endemic country.
- If indicated by geographical area, consider stool exam for ova and parasites.
- If indicated, advise on genetically inherited diseases.
- Adolescents that come as refugees or from countries in political turmoil may have been victims of rape or witnessed rape and/or horrific violence. They may suffer from anxiety, depression, PTSD or other mental illness and should be screened.

What is unique about the adolescent traveler?

- Adolescents are curious, adventurous, free-spirited and relatively inexperienced as they embark on travels including study abroad programs, cultural tours, internships and volunteer programs. These endearing characteristics can also place them in dangerous situations.
- As travelers who are used to being protected by their parents, teens are often unprepared for the basic medical precautions of travel and physicians need to educate them about how to travel healthy.
- Many adolescent immigrants arrive in the U.S. every day for study, exchange programs and visits. They can also get sick from illnesses prevalent in their countries of origin of which physicians in the U.S. may not be as familiar. Research about illnesses known to the region then becomes necessary.

TEST YOUR KNOWLEDGE ANSWER

15. A. Malaria prophylaxis needs to continue once patients return from travel abroad to endemic regions for up to 1 to 4 additional weeks depending on the medication. Disease can manifest initial symptoms after the teen returns to the U.S. and in some cases, (i.e. parasites) may be indolent. Adolescents should be advised to let doctors know about foreign travel of the past couple of years. A strongly positive skin test many years after the BCG vaccine has been administered is more likely to be due to TB than due to the vaccine and a chest x-ray will be required to rule out active TB infection.

WEB REFERENCES

- American Academy of Pediatrics Publications (http://pediatrics.aappublications.org):
    - Committee on Community Health Services 2005, 'Providing Care for Immigrant, Homeless, and Migrant Children', Pediatrics, 2005;115;1095-1100, Retrieved from http://pediatrics.aappublications.org/content/ll5/4/1095.full.pdf+html?sid=b98779ab-7ce2-4311-98cc-0048079b61fd
    - Worley CW, Worley KA, Kumar PL 2000, 'Infectious Disease Challenges in Immigrants From Tropical Countries,' Pediatrics, 2000;106;e3, Retrieved from http://pediatrics.aappublications.org / content/ 106/l/e3.full.pdf+html?sid=03bea794-d854-460d-8587-0efcdfl70a7e
- American Academy of Family Physicians (www.aafp.org)
    - Dick, L 1998, "Travel Medicine: Helping Patients Prepare for Trips Abroad', American Family Physician, 1998 Aug l;58(2);383–398, Retrieved from http://www.aafp.org/afp/1998/08017p383.html
- Kozarsky, P. 'CDC Commentary: The Pre-Travel Consultation-What Providers Should Know', Medscape. Jun 07, 2010, Retrieved from http://wwwnc.cdc.gov/travel/page/presentations-health-pros.htm
- Kozarsky, P. 'CDC Commentary: Clues to Diagnosis in the Patient with Posttravel Illness.' Medscape. Jun 21,2010, Retrieved from http://wwwnc.cdc.gov/travel/page/presentations-health-pros.htm

Additional Clinician and Patient Resources:

- Centers for Disease Control (www.cdc.gov)
    - Adventure Travel Campaign: http://m.cdc.gov/en/MobileCampaigns/adventure
    - Immigrant and Refugee Health: http://www.cdc.gov/immigrantrefugeehealth/
    - Travelers' Health information: www.cdc.Gov/travel/.com
    - Your Survival Guide to Safe and Healthy Travel: http://wwwnc.cdc.gov/travel/page/survival-guide.htm
    - Vaccines & Immunization Information: www.cdc.gov/vaccines
- Immunization Action Coalition: www.immunize.org
- Passport Health: www.passporthealthusa.com
- Travel.State.Gov, Current Travel Warnings: www.travel.state.gov/travel
- U.S. Department of State:
    - International Travel: http://travel.state.gov/travel/travel_1744.html
    - Tips for Traveling Abroad: http://travel.state.gov/travel/tips/tips_1232.html

SECTION II

COMMON PROBLEMS

12

SHORT STATURE/DELAYED ONSET OF PUBERTY

Karen Bernstein

TEST YOUR KNOWLEDGE

16. The *BEST* initial step in the assessment of the cause of delayed puberty is to obtain:

    A. Serum gonadotropin measurement
    B. Karyotype
    C. Bone age
    D. Growth curve and assessment of sexual maturity
    E. Thyroid stimulating hormone (TSH) measurement

17. What is the *MOST* likely diagnosis for a 16 year old tall thin male who has small testes and Tanner stage 5 pubic hair?

    A. Kallman syndrome
    B. Hypothyroidism
    C. Kleinfelter's Syndrome
    D. Constitutional Delayed Puberty
    E. Functional Gonadotropin Deficiency

Refer to end of chapter for answers on page 138.

"Joey is the shortest boy in his class. Will he ever grow ? Do you think we should start growth hormone?"

BACKGROUND

- The hypothalamic-pituitary-axis, quiescent from about 6 months of age, resumes activity during puberty prompting increased height velocity, development of secondary sex characteristics, and maturation of the seminiferous tubules and ovarian follicles leading to sperm and oocyte production.
- An increase in hypothalamic gonadotropin-releasing hormone (GnRH) triggers the release of luteinizing hormone (LH) and follicle-stimulating hormone (FSH) from the pituitary. LH and FSH then stimulate gonadal production of sex steroids.
- In females, this usually begins between the ages of 9–12 years, starting with breast enlargement, then pubic hair growth, followed by the "growth spurt" and menarche.
- In males these changes start between 10–13 years, beginning with testicular enlargement, then pubic hair growth, followed by penile enlargement, and peak height velocity growth.
- The majority of adolescents are found to have no pathology causing their growth delay, and when puberty begins, it progresses normally. However, there are many causes of delayed puberty that warrant further investigation (Table 1).

DEFINITIONS

- Delayed puberty is defined as no evidence of breast growth in girls by age 13, and failure of testicular enlargement in boys by age 14.
- In addition, the diagnosis of delayed puberty can be made in girls who have not achieved menarche by age 16, or the absence of menarche within 5 years of pubertal onset.
- Failure at any point along the hypothalamic-pituitary-gonadal axis can lead to delayed puberty.

ASSESSMENT

HISTORY

Neonatal/Past Medical History

- Congenital lymphedema suggests **Turner Syndrome.**
- Consider chronic diseases, previous surgeries, radiation exposure, chemotherapy or congenital anomalies.

Growth History

Pattern of growth and changes in the pattern, plotted appropriately on a growth curve, are key factors in leading to a diagnosis:

- A greater decline in weight than height is usually seen in nutritional deficiencies such as **eating disorders, inflammatory bowel disease (IBD), celiac disease** or other **chronic illnesses.**
- A greater slowing in height than weight is usually associated with an endocrinopathy such as **hypothyroidism** or **gonadal dysgenesis.**
- Teens growing consistently at or just below the third percentile may have **constitutional growth delay.**
- Girls whose growth curve has been below the third percentile may have **Turner's Syndrome** even without usual clinical findings. This is especially so if parents are of normal height.
- Males with small testicles whose growth curves show tall stature and relatively thin body habitus may have **Kleinfelter's Syndrome.**

Family History

- Determine parental and sibling heights, age of puberty onset and age of attained adult height. Adolescents with **constitutional delayed puberty** will often have a family history of "late bloomers."
- Is there a history of medical problems or familial congenital anomalies. Anosmia or growth delay in male relatives on the mother's side of the family suggests **Kallmann syndrome.** Consider **hypothyroidism** with a family history of autoimmune disorders.

Medications

- Methylphenidate or other stimulants may decrease appetite and cause weight loss or failure to grow.
- Psychotropic drugs such as antipsychotics frequently cause **hyperprolactinemia.**

Review of Systems

- A history of constipation or cold intolerance suggests **hypothyroidism.**
- Weight changes or dieting behaviors suggest an **eating disorder.**
- Excessive exercise or environmental stress may contribute to **functional delayed puberty.**
- Headaches or loss of peripheral vision suggest a **pituitary adenoma.**
- Sudden slowing down of growth and headaches can be due to a **craniopharingioma.**
- Anosmia is seen with **Kallmann Syndrome.**

PHYSICAL

Anthropometric Measurements

- Plot height and weight on a patient's growth curve.
- Calculation of target height (Table 2):
- Most teens achieve an adult stature within 10 cm of their target height.
- A teen whose height percentile differs greatly from his/her genetic potential is considered inappropriately short and deserves a thorough evaluation.

General Appearance

- Dysmorhic features should be noted, including abnormal facies, ear placement, webbed neck, cubitus valgus and the size and shape of hands and feet.
- General examination of the heart, lungs, and abdomen should be performed looking for signs of chronic medical conditions.
- Dull dry skin, hair loss, decreased pulse rate, and/or goiter suggest **hypothyroidism.**

Breast

- Breast development should be noted and appropriately staged (Chapter 1, Table 2).

Genital

- Pubertal development is usually described by Tanner stage (Chapter 1, Table 2). The clinician must assess pubic hair, clitoris size, penis length, testicle volume and vaginal appearance (estrogen effect).
- Examination of the external genitalia is essential.
- A pelvic exam is unnecessary in most teens but should be considered for females with normal pubertal development and delayed menarche.

Neurologic Exam

- A neurologic exam should be performed to help rule out intracranial pathology.
- Visual field defects might be seen in a **pituitary adenoma.**

STUDIES

If chronic illness is suspected, consider:

Complete Blood Count

- Anemia may indicate blood loss such as in **IBD.**

Sedimentation rate and C-Reactive Protein

- Useful as a screening test for chronic illness.

Basic Metabolic Panel

- BUN and creatinine may be abnormal in **chronic renal disease.**
- Electrolyte abnormalities such as hypokalemia, hyponatremia, hypochloremia and alkalosis may occur with **eating disorders.**

Albumin, Pre-Albumin

- Useful as a screen for malnutrition caused by diseases such as **IBD.**

Urinalysis

- Hematuria or proteinuria may occur with chronic renal disease.

Anti-tissue Transglutaminase/Celiac Panel

- Send if **celiac disease** is suspected.

Calprotectin

- If granulomatous colitis is suspected.

For an otherwise healthy adolescent, consider:

TSH and Free T4

- Low T4 and an elevated TSH indicate **hypothyroidism.**
- A low T4 and normal TSH may indicate **hypopituitarism** (patients often have severe short stature).
- A low T3 and normal TSH is seen in malnutrition (e.g. anorexia nervosa).

Luteinizing Hormone (LH) and Follicle Stimulating Hormone (FSH)

- By adolescence (10–12 years), individuals with gonadal failure (primary or secondary) will have markedly elevated LH/FSH.
- Low LH/FSH would be consistent with **constitutional delayed puberty** or **functional gonadotropin deficiency.**
- Rarely, low LH/FSH may suggest an isolated gonadotropin deficiency (i.e. **Kallmann syndrome**).

Prolactin

- Elevated prolactin occurs with **pituitary adenomas** or certain medications.

Testosterone

- Expect levels less than 40 ng/dl in males with delayed puberty.
- Patients with **Klinefelter's Syndrome** have normal testosterone levels. Their small testicles are due to a deficit of Sertoli cells.

Estradiol

- Expect low levels in females with delayed puberty and/or primary amenorrhea.

Karyotype

- Send a karyotype to rule out **Turner syndrome** (in females with elevated LH/FSH) or **Klinefelter's Syndrome** (in males with elevated LH/FSH and small testes).

SPECIAL TESTS

Bone Age

- A single radiograph of the left hand and wrist is useful in assessing how much growth potential remains.
- Delayed bone age can be seen in patients with **hypothyroidism, chronic disease** and **constitutional growth delay.**
- Bone age is often normal with **Turner syndrome** and in constitutional small stature.

MRI

- Consider when there is a clinical suspicion of a CNS tumor.

TREATMENT

- Management of pubertal delay should address the underlying cause.
- Constitutional delay of puberty can usually be managed with close monitoring and reassurance.
- If a male adolescent is very distressed, three to four monthly intramuscular injections of testosterone 50 mg may accelerate growth and "jump start" puberty.
- If hypothalamic dysfunction is related to exercise, eating disorders or chronic illness, these underlying issues must be resolved to allow puberty to proceed.
- Patients with primary gonadal failure will require estrogen or testosterone replacement, and should be referred to an endocrinologist.

- Hypothyroidism should be treated with levothyroxine until TSH is in the normal range.
- Estrogen, testosterone and growth hormone may help attain secondary sexual characteristics, and induce a growth spurt. However, there is a concern that such treatments may result in some loss of adult height.

What is unique about treating adolescents with short stature/delayed puberty?

- Special attention should be given to the psychological consequences of delayed puberty.
- Significant delays may lead to poor body image, low self-esteem, teasing, bullying and decline in academic performance.
- Males seem to be affected more adversely than females.
- Occasionally, hormonal therapy (testosterone) is used in cases of constitutional pubertal delay to accelerate puberty when psychosocial distress to the patient is significant.

TEST YOUR KNOWLEDGE ANSWERS

16. D. As with any diagnostic evaluation, the history and physical exam is often the key factor in determining the etiology. Anthropometric measurements and Tanner staging are key to diagnosis. Patients are often unaware that early signs of sexual development are present, and often do not require a costly evaluation. In the case of delayed puberty, laboratory evaluation is guided by the findings on physical exam. All other choices should be considered in SOME patients depending on the findings on physical exam.
17. C. The described patient meets criteria for Kleinfelter's syndrome. Patients with Kallman syndrome also have small testes but are usually not tall, and have associated anosmia. Patients with hypothyroidism, constitutional delayed puberty or functional gonadoptropin deficiency are usually short and those with hypothyroidism usually have normal or slightly increased weight.

Table 1. Causes of Delayed Puberty.

	Acquired	Congenital
Normal or Low Serum Gonadotropins	Constitutional delay of puberty Hypothalamic dysfunction (functional gonadotropin deficiency) Malnutrition Strenuous exercise Chronic illness Eating disorders Central nervous system tumors Hypopituitarism Panhypopituitarism Hypothyroidism Hyperprolactinemia Pituitary adenoma Drug-associated Infiltrative disease Hemochromatosis Granulomatous disease Histiocytosis Head trauma Drugs: Marijuana	Isolated gonadotropin deficiency Kallmann syndrome Idiopathic isolated growth hormone deficiency Lawrence-Moon-Bardet-Biedel syndrome Obesity, polydactaly, retinitis pigmentosa, genital hypoplasia and developmental delay Prader-Willi syndrome Extreme obesity, developmental delay, small hands and feet Chromosome 15 deletion
Increased Serum Gonadotropins	Bilateral gonadal failure Irradiation Cytotoxic therapy Trauma Infections Post cryptorchidism surgery Autoimmune ovarian failure	Turner syndrome (gonadal dysgenisis) Kleinfelter's syndrome Small testes but adequate androgen production Bilateral Gonadal Failure Primary testicular failure Anorchia (vanishing testes syndrome)
Other Conditions	Anatomic abnormalities Mayer-Rokitansky-Kuster-Hauser syndrome: Normal puberty, absent menses Androgen receptor defects Congenital androgen insensitivity 46,XY; phenotypic female No menarche Bloom syndrome Noonan syndrome	

Table 2. Formulas to Calculate Target Height.

Final Male Adult Height	$\frac{[\text{Mother's height (inches)} + 5 \text{ inches}] + [\text{Father's height (inches)}]}{2}$
Final Female Adult Height	$\frac{[\text{Mother's height (inches)}] + [\text{Father's height (inches)} - 5 \text{ inches}]}{2}$

WEB REFERENCES

- American Family Physician
  - Blondell RD, Foster MB, Dave KC (1999), 'Disorders of Puberty', American Family Physician, 60(l);209-218, Retrieved from http://www.aafp.org/afp/1999/0701/p209.html
  - Nwosu BU and Lee MM (2008), 'Evaluation of Short and Tall Stature in Children', American Family Physician, 87(5);597–604, Retrieved from http://www.aafp.org/afp/2008/09017p597.html
- The Pediatric Orthopaedic Society of North America (POSNA), Short Stature, Retrieved from http://www.posna.org/education/StudyGuide/shortStature.asp

Additional Clinician and Patient Resources:

- American Academy of Pediatrics, Healthy Children: www.healthychildren.org
  - Delayed Puberty (updated May 11, 2011), Retrieved from http://www.healthychildren.org/English/ages-stages/gradeschool/puberty/Pages/Delayed-Puberty.aspx
  - When a Child is Unusually Short or Tall (updated November 5, 2012), Retrieved from http://www.healthychildren.org/English/ages-stages/gradeschool/puberty/Pages/When-a-Child-is-Unusually-Short-or-Tall.aspx
- KidsHealth from the experts of Nemours: www.kidshealth.org
  - Delayed Puberty, Retrieved from http://kidshealth.org/teen/sexual_health/changing_body/delayed_puberty.html
  - What is Growth Disorder?, Retrieved from http://kidshealth.org/parent/medical/endocrine/growthdisorder.html
- The Magic Foundation: www.magicfoundation.org
- Medline Plus: Short stature (updated 8/2/2011), Retrieved from http://www.nlm.nih.gov/medlineplus/ency/article/003271.htm
- The Human Growth Foundation: www.hgfound.org

13

TALL STATURE

Karen Bernstein

TEST YOUR KNOWLEDGE

18. Patients with Marfan Syndrome may have each of the following characteristics *EXCEPT*:

    A. Dislocated lens
    B. Height greater than 2.5 standard deviations for age
    C. Arachnodactyly
    D. Mental retardation
    E. Scoliosis

19. Which of the following statements is true?

    A. Patients with tall stature generally need extensive laboratory evaluation.
    B. Patients with constitutional tall stature are likely to have at least one tall parent.
    C. Females with tall stature should be treated with estrogen to promote growth plate closure.
    D. Patients with Sotos syndrome have delayed bone age.
    E. All the above.

Refer to end of chapter for answer on page 146.

Your 14 year old patient has always been above the 97th percentile in height. She asks you, "Doctor, is there anything that can be done to stop me from getting taller? I am worried I will never get asked out on a date!"

BACKGROUND

- The mean adult height of men and women in the United States has increased over past decades.
- An individual is "tall" if he or she is greater than 2.5 standard deviations above the mean for their age and gender. In adults, this is more than 192 cm for males or 179 cm for females.
- The generally accepted heights for treatment of tall stature in females has changed over time ranging from 175 cm in the 1950's to 188 cm in 1999.
- The most common cause of tall stature is genetic (familial or constitutional tall stature).
- Less common causes include: excess growth hormone, anabolic steroid excess, hyperthyroidism, Marfan syndrome, homocystinuria, androgen insensitivity, Klinefelter's syndrome and Sotos syndrome.

ASSESSMENT

HISTORY

Growth History

- Determine patient's age at puberty onset.
- Overall pattern of growth and changes in pattern as plotted appropriately on a growth curve can help lead to a diagnosis.

Family History

- Ascertain age of puberty onset and final adult height of parents and siblings.
- Patients with one tall parent are likely to have **constitutional tall stature.**
- If there are family members with gigantism and macrocephaly, consider **Sotos Syndrome** (autosomal dominant).

- If there are family members with heart murmurs and/or cardiac problems with tall stature, consider **Marfan Syndrome** (autosomal dominant).

Review of Systems

- A history of thromboembolic phenomena suggests **homocystinuria**.
- In patients with tall stature and developmental delay, consider **Klinefelter's Syndrome, 47 XYY, Sotos Syndrome or homocystinuria.**

PHYSICAL

Anthropometric Measurements

- Height measurements plotted on a growth curve are essential.
- Assess genetic potential using a calculation of target height to help differentiate familial from pathologic tall stature (Chapter 12, Table 2).
  - Most children achieve an adult stature within 10 cm of their target height.

General Appearance

- Evaluate body proportions to distinguish **constitutional tall stature** (normal upper to lower body segment ratio and arm span) from syndromes such as **Kleinfelter's Syndrome** or **Marfan Syndrome** (patients might have increased arm span).
- Hypersecretion of growth hormone or "gigantism" is usually associated with a **pituitary adenoma.**
  - These patients have extremely long extremities due to unfused epiphyses.
  - They have acromegaly and continue growing (including hands and feet) into their 4th decade.
- Tall stature, lean body, elongated extremities, arachnodactyly and heart murmur suggests **Marfan Syndrome.**
  - These patients may also have pectus excavatum or pectus carinatum, arm span to height ratio of greater than 1.05 and scoliosis.
- Patients with **homocystinuria** have a similar body habitus to those with Marfan sydrome; in addition, they may have mental retardation and joint contractures.

- Males with eunuchoid proportions, diminished upper-lower segment ratio and low sitting height compared to length may have **sex hormone deficiency or insufficiency.**
- Small testes, gynecomastia and expressive language delays suggests **Kleinfelter's Syndrome.**
- Males with tall stature, delayed motor or language development, acne, large teeth, tremor and incoordination may have 47, **XYY.**
- Consider **Sotos Syndrome** in patients with macrocrania, acromegaly and mental retardation.
- Obese children may be taller than average, possibly due to higher levels of insulin.

STUDIES

- No studies are indicated if there is a family history of tall stature and a normal physical exam.
- If exam findings are abnormal, consider:

TSH and T4

- Assess for **hyperthyroidism.**

Insulin-Like Growth Factor (IGF)-1, IGF Binding Protein-3 and Random Growth Hormone

- Exclude excess growth hormone secretion as a cause.

Urine Homocystine

- Rule out **homocysteinuria.**

FSH and LH

- Elevated if tall stature is eunuchoidal as in the hypogonadic patient with Klinefelter's Syndrome.

Karyotype

- If considering **Kleinfelter Syndrome** or 47, **XYY.**

SPECIAL TESTS

Slit-Lamp Exam

- A slit-lamp exam may be helpful in diagnosing the lens dislocation sometimes seen with **Marfan Syndrome**.

Bone Age

- Can assist in determining growth potential.
- Advanced skeletal maturation occurs with overgrowth syndromes such as **Sotos Syndrome**.

Echocardiogram

- May show mitral valve prolapse, aortic root dilatation or aortic dissection in patients with **Marfan Syndrome**.

MRI

- Should be done in patients with acromegaly/excess growth hormone to rule out pituitary adenoma.

TREATMENT

- In the past, high doses of estrogen were used in females to accelerate epiphysial fusion, and therefore limit growth when the predicted height was above average.
- Currently, estrogen treatment is seldom used due to increased social acceptability of tall stature and unacceptable side effects including nausea, hypertension and blood clots.
- Decisions to intervene with treatment for tall stature should be considered balancing patient's goals and desires with the side effects of treatment (typically hormonal therapy).
- Tall stature in boys due to constitutional tall stature is typically not treated.

What is unique about tall stature and adolescents?

- Although tall stature is as common as short stature, teens are less likely to present with complaints to their physician.

- While adolescent males rarely complain about tall stature, females may occasionally express concern even though tall stature in women has become more accepted over time.
  - Counseling is a more appropriate treatment than high dose estrogen.
- Tall stature may be due to a genetic condition: the physical examination may direct the need for further investigation.

TEST YOUR KNOWLEDGE ANSWERS

18. D. Patients with Marfan syndrome have normal intelligence. On the other hand, patient's with homocystinuria may have a "marfanoid" body habitus and often have some degree of mental retardation. Tall stature, long fingers and ectopic lentis are common findings in Marfan's Syndrome.
19. B. Patients with tall stature are likely to have at least one tall parent. Constitutional or familial tall stature is the most common cause of tall stature and a family history will usually reveal at least one parent who is tall. A positive family history and normal physical exam, makes extensive "lab work-up" unnecessary. The exception would be if the adolescent develops acromegaly. As tall stature has become more accepted in society, it is less likely to be a presenting complaint of patients, and adolescents are less frequently treated with estrogen. Sotos syndrome is an "overgrowth" syndrome and bone age is often advanced.

WEB REFERENCES

- American Family Physician
  - Nwosu BU and Lee MM (2008), 'Evaluation of Short and Tall Stature in Children', American Family Physician, 87(5);597-604, Retrieved from http://www.aafp.org/afp/ 2008/09017p597.html
- Drop SLS, et al. (1998) 'Sex Steroid Treatment of Constitutionally Tall Stature', Endocrine Reviews, 19(5);540–558, Retrieved from http://edrv.endojournals.org/content/19/5/540.full.pdf+html

Additional Clinician and Patient Resources:

- American Academy of Pediatrics, Healthy Children: www.healthychildren.org

- When a Child is Unusually Short or Tall, (updated november 5, 2012), Retrieved from http://www.healthychildren.org/English/ages-stages/gradeschool/puberty/Pages/When-a-Child-is-Unusually-Short-or-Tall.aspx
- KidsHealth from the experts of Nemours: www.kidshealth.org
- The Magic Foundation: www.toosoon.com
- The Human Growth Foundation: www.hgfound.org

14

ABNORMAL WEIGHT GAIN

Harshita J. Saxena

TEST YOUR KNOWLEDGE

20. A 15 year old teen presents to the office for his annual physical exam. His BMI is noted to be above the 99th percentile. He appears severely obese and his skin exam is significant for acanthosis nigricans on the nape of his neck as well as abdominal striae. He is normotensive and his exam is otherwise normal. He has a strong family history of type 2 diabetes mellitus. Of the following studies, which would be *LEAST* helpful:

    A. Lipid Panel
    B. Hemoglobin A1c
    C. Alanine Transaminase (ALT)
    D. 24 hour Urinary Cortisol Levels
    E. All the above should be ordered.

Refer to end of chapter for answer on page 160.

A 16 year old female comes into the office for her annual physical exam. Her BMI is calculated to be at the 94th percentile. On history, you learn that the patient is doing well in school and has a positive peer group. However, she reports eating carry out or fast food several times a week and watching 4–5 hours of television daily.

BACKGROUND

- There are an increasing number of adolescents worldwide who are being diagnosed as overweight or obese and are at risk of medical conditions that were once considered diseases of adulthood such as hypertension and type 2 diabetes mellitus.
- Most cases are due to exogenous obesity but there are a wide variety of causes (Table 1).
- Body Mass Index (BMI), a measure used to define adolescent overweight and obese status, is a reasonable indicator of body fat content, though it does not directly measure body fat.
  - Overweight: BMI at or above the 85th percentile and lower than the 95th percentile for teens of the same age and sex.
  - Obesity: BMI at or above the 95th percentile for teens of the same age and sex.
  - Severe obesity: BMI at or above the 99th percentile for teens of the same age and sex.

ASSESSMENT

HISTORY

History of Present Illness

- Determine how much weight was gained and over what time?
  - A lifelong history of being overweight or obese may indicate **primary obesity** but the possibility of obesity associated with a **genetic disorder** should be considered.

What is the teen's self-assessment?

- Do they believe they have a weight problem?
- How do they feel about their body when they look in the mirror?

Obtain a detailed dietary history. It may be helpful to obtain a 3 day food diary from the patient or at least a 24 hour recall.

- Does the teen frequent fast food restaurants? What types of foods or drinks are ordered? How many times a week does the teen eat fast food or order carry out?
- Is the teen a frequent snacker? What types of foods are chosen for snacks?
- Does the teen eat "junk food" often?
- Does the teen drink non-diet sodas or sugary drinks such as juice or ice teas?
- Is the teen eating 3 meals a day? Does the teen ever skip meals such as breakfast because of morning time constraints, or lunch because they don't like school food?
- Is portion control an issue? Does the teen eat healthy foods but is still gaining weight? Does the teen frequently load the plate up and go back for seconds and/or thirds? Does the teen eat quickly?
- Who makes household grocery purchases or prepares meals for the family?

Does the teen lead an active or sedentary lifestyle?

- Determine if the teen exercises (e.g. no exercise, exercise through gym class, exercise through school sports with daily practice) and what are his or her preferred routines (e.g. weight lifting, sports, running, etc.).
- For how long does the teen exercise and how often?
- How long does the teen engage in physical inactivity including amount of t.v., video games or computer time daily?

Has the teen ever attempted to lose weight in the past?

- How successful were past attempts at weight loss?
- What did the teen do to try to lose weight? Diet? Exercise? Use supplements?

Does the teen think his or her eating habits are healthy or unhealthy?

- **Bulimia Nervosa** is characterized by binge eating episodes followed by purging. These teens can be of normal weight or overweight.
- **Binge Eating Disorder** is distinct in that there is no associated purging behavior.

- **Nocturnal eating** is characterized by prolonged evening eating or waking up during the night to eat large meals.

Past Medical History

- Recent weight gain over short duration may suggest a more serious underlying etiology.
  - Obesity has often been thought to be caused by hypothyroidism but this is not actually the case. **Hypothyroidism** is usually associated with a small amount of weight gain (i.e. 5–10 pounds) due to myxedema.
  - Rapid weight gain of 3–5 pounds over a couple of days associated with other symptoms such as cough or extremity swelling suggests **congestive heart failure**, especially in teens with known chronic medical conditions.
- Does the patient have a history of brain tumor or trauma that could disturb the hypothalamic satiety center?
- Has the patient been diagnosed with a genetic disorder?
  - Obesity since infancy, poor vision (especially at night), polydactyly, hypogonadism, renal problems and/or learning disabilities are characteristic features of **Laurence-Moon-Bardet-Biedl Syndrome.**
  - Long-standing obesity caused by insatiable and uncontrolled appetite, reduced muscle tone, developmental delays and hypogonadism suggest **Prader-Willi Syndrome.**
  - Short stature, rounded face, bone deformities of the hands and feet (shortened 4th metacarpals) and dental hypoplasia associated with obesity suggests **Pseudohypoparathyroidism.**
  - Poor vision or blindness, sensorineural hearing loss, dilated cardiomyopathy, short stature and weight gain suggests **Alstrom Syndrome.**

Family History

- There may be a genetic component to overweight and obesity.
  - Are there family members with weight issues who may be overweight or obese?
  - Has anyone in the family had gastric bypass surgery?
- Is there a family history of inheritable congenital disorders?
- Is there a family history of type 2 diabetes mellitus, hypercholesterolemia or hyperlipidemia, hypertension, heart disease, obstructive sleep apnea, thyroid disease or menstrual disorder?

Medications

- Is the teen taking any medications that could potentially stimulate their appetite?
- There are numerous medications with weight gain as a known side effect.
  - A number of antidepressants have been associated with weight gain including amitriptyline, amoxapine, desipramine, doxepin, imipramine, phenelzine, remeron, tranylcypromine and trazadone.
  - Antipsychotics such as haloperidol are associated with weight gain, as are anticonvulsants such as carbamazepine or valproate.
  - Contraceptives such as depo-provera (medroxyprogesterone) can stimulate appetite.
  - Hormonal therapy containing estrogens (combined oral contraceptives) may cause fluid retention which can be perceived by some teens as causing weight gain.
- Has the teen ever taken weight loss supplements in an attempt to lose weight?
  - Were they successful losing weight on supplements?
  - What happened when they stopped taking the supplements?

Social

- Does the teen report any recent life stressors? Any bullying, teasing or name calling from family members, peers or others?
- In what type of community does the teen live and what are the food resources available? Is there food insecurity?
  - Families with limited resources from underserved communities may not have access to healthier food choices.
  - In these circumstances, fast food may be their most convenient and economic option.
- Has the teen recently quit smoking cigarettes? Nicotine is an appetite suppressant and many individuals experience weight gain when they quit smoking.
- Is there any suspicion that the teen could be using or abusing anabolic steroids which can cause weight gain.

Review of Systems

- Does the teen report irregular or missed periods? Teens who are overweight or obese are at higher risk of developing **polycystic ovarian syndrome (PCOS).**
- Do parents report snoring or mouth breathing at night and does the teen admit to daytime sleepiness, all characteristic of **obstructive sleep apnea (OSA).**
- What is the teen's overall mood? Has the teen ever been diagnosed with and/or treated for depression?
- Teens living with **depression** or experiencing life stressors may gain weight from compensatory self soothing eating behaviors.
- Unexplained weight gain along with poor growth, delayed puberty, fatigue, cold sensitivities, constipation, dry skin and brittle nails or hair suggest **hypothyroidism.**
- Consider **Cushing's Syndrome** in patients who complain of weight gain, facial fullness ("moon facies") and upper back ("buffalo hump"), truncal and/or abdominal obesity while their limbs remain thin. The suspicion is even higher if there is concomitant hypertension and relatively short stature.

PHYSICAL

Vital Signs

- Elevated blood pressure may be found in overweight or obese teens.
- High blood pressure can also be found in patients with **Cushing's Syndrome.**
- "Pseudohypertension" can be seen when a cuff size is too small for an above average arm size.

Anthropometric Measurements

- It is essential to calculate weight and height measurements so that the body mass index (BMI) can be calculated.
  - Teens with a BMI between the 85th and 95th percentiles are considered overweight while those above the 95th percentile are considered obese.
  - Many obese adolescents have an early growth spurt. Whenever short stature is noticed, a secondary cause of weight gain should be suspected.

- Some athletic teens with high BMI's have significant lean muscle mass contributing to their high body weight to height calculations. In these special cases, a high BMI does not indicate obesity.

General Appearance

- Does the teen appear overweight or obese?
- Are there any dysmorphic features that suggest underlying genetic or endocrine disorder? Does the patient have short stature?

HEENT

- Enlarged tonsils and associated snoring can occur with excessive weight and raises concern for **obstructive sleep apnea**.

Neck

- Palpate for enlarged thyroid which can occur in hypothyroidism.

Chest

- **Pseudogynecomastia** is due to increased subcutaneous fatty breast tissue in males.

Abdomen

- Central adiposity is a poor long term prognosticator for overweight and obese teens.
- Assess for any tenderness. Right upper quadrant tenderness may be associated with fatty steatohepatitis or gallbladder pathology (e.g. stones).

Back

- Observe for the characteristic "buffalo hump," or fat pad of the upper back, which is characteristic of Cushing's Syndrome. However, this can also be present in severely obese patients with no underlying endocrine disorder.

Male Genitalia

- True hypogonadism is rare. Pseudohypogonadism can occur in obese males when most of the penile shaft is hidden in subcutaneous suprapubic fat. Testicles are of normal size.

Skin

- Observe for acanthosis nigricans on the nape of neck, axilla or under breasts which is a sign of **insulin resistence**.
- Striae may be observed on the abdomen, back or other areas of the body where weight has recently been gained.
- Thin skin, hair loss, easy bruising and abdominal striae occur with **Cushing's Syndrome**.
- Pale dry skin and brittle nails and hair can be seen with **hypothyroidism**.
- Acne and/or hirsutism may occur with **PCOS**.

STUDIES

Complete Blood Count (CBC)

- Teens may be overweight or obese due to poor dietary habits and iron deficiency anemia is common.

Lipid Panel

- A non-fasting lipid panel will give an accurate assessment of total cholesterol, HDL and LDL levels. Overweight and obese teens are at greater risk of hypercholesterolemia and/or hyperlipidemia.
- Triglyceride levels are affected by fasting status. Elevated levels can lead to pancreatitis and should be treated.

Glucose and Hemoglobin A1c

- Any overweight or obese teen with signs of insulin resistance such as acanthosis nigricans is at greater risk of developing type 2 diabetes mellitus and screening with a fasting blood sugar should be done every two years.

Alanine Transaminase (ALT)

- Consider if there is central adiposity or if obesity presents with right upper quadrant pain.
- This test screens for steatohepatitis. Further work up is warranted if elevated.

Basic Metabolic Panel

- Consider testing in teens that have elevated blood pressure.
- BUN and creatinine are good measures of kidney function and could indicate underlying renal disease.

Thyroid Studies including TSH and Free T4

- Consider only if the patient has other symptoms of hypothyroidism.
- In this situation, T4 levels would be low while TSH is elevated.

Urine Pregnancy Test

- Consider testing in teens who have recently gained weight and admit to being sexually active or who report a missed period. In obese individuals, pregnancy may not "show" for many months.

Urinalysis

- Consider testing in teens who are overweight or obese, especially if they have elevated blood pressure. Proteinuria may indicate underlying renal disease.
- Glucosuria would indicate type 2 diabetes mellitus.

SPECIAL TESTS

Sleep Study

- Test in obese patients who snore, especially if they have daytime somnolence, as they may have obstructive sleep apnea.

Diagnostic Imaging

- Abdominal Ultrasound or CT scan is indicated in patients with right upper quadrant pain to identify cholelithiasis.
- Abdominal Ultrasound is also indicated when there is an elevated ALT, as it may detect steatohepatitis.

Liver Biopsy

- Consider when there is steatohepatitis confirmed by ultrasound.

TREATMENT

- The task of treating overweight and obese teens remains challenging. Ideally, a multidiciplinary team including a clinician, registered dietician and exercise consultant should work closely with a teen and teen's family to help them manage their weight loss goals. The clinician can also:
  - Remaining non-judgemental towards patients and their families and work to promote an office setting that is accommodating to overweight and obese teens.
    - Promote sensitivity training among staff to decrease potential stigma experienced by overweight and obese teens.
    - Provide overweight and obese friendly accommodations including appropriately sized seating, gowns and equipment (e.g. blood pressure cuffs).
  - In cases where patients are receptive to making diet and lifestyle changes, establish simple and achievable goals in manageable increments.
  - Refer severely obese patients that may benefit from bariatric surgery (Table 2).
- Whenever an underlying medical condition is found to be the cause of abnormal weight gain, treatment should be targeted at managing that condition. Consultation with a specialist such as endocrinology or genetics may be warranted.

DISPOSITION

- Teens who are obese or severely obese are at risk of developing medical conditions such as OSA, heart disease, hypertension, type 2 diabetes mellitus, non-alcoholic steatohepatitis (NASH), proteinuria and menstrual disorders. Consultation with sleep medicine, cardiology, endocrinology, gastroenterology and/or nephrology may be warranted to co-manage these co-morbid conditions.
- If the teen is found to have an elevated manual blood pressure measurement with an appropriately sized blood pressure cuff, outpatient follow up will

be needed to establish persistence in blood pressure elevations to make the diagnosis of essential hypertension. Cardiology and/or nephrology consultation may become necessary.

- If the patient has signs of insulin resistance on exam, with elevated blood glucose and hemoglobin A1c, refer to endocrinology for consultation and/or further management.
- Metformin may be initiated and has been shown to promote weight loss in overweight/obese teens who have signs of insulin resistance with or without a diagnosis of type 2 diabetes mellitus.
- Metformin is also known to improve glucose, lipid abnormalities, and hyperandrogenism in obese adolescents with insulin resistance so it may also be of benefit to teens with PCOS.
- Metabolic acidosis is an uncommon but deadly side effect of metformin. It can be triggered by alcohol consumption and teens should be warned.
- Overweight or obese teens who snore, report mouth breathing or daytime sleepiness should be evaluated for obstructive sleep apnea and referred for sleep study.
- If these teens have large tonsils or adenoids, a referral to Otolaryngology is warranted for surgical consideration.
- Teens with signs of PCOS or hyperandrogenism benefit from use of combined hormonal therapy to relieve symptoms and prevent endometrial cancer.

What's unique about abnormal weight gain in adolescents?

- Treating overweight and obese teens is daunting and associated with poor success rates, although family interventions and bariatric surgery seem promising.
- Teasing and bullying can seriously affect self esteem and lead to social withdrawal, isolation, depressed mood and even suicidality.
- Adolescent obesity is often a precursor to adult obesity and may mark the beginning of hypertension, atherosclerosis and type 2 diabetes as well as many other health problems associated with obesity.

TEST YOUR KNOWLEDGE ANSWER

20. D. Of the studies listed, a 24 hour urine cortisol level would be least helpful. Although the patient has abdominal striae, he doesn't have any of the other classic symptoms of Cushing's syndrome. This finding is also commonly seen in exogenous obesity. A lipid panel should be ordered in a severely obese teen who is at higher risk of hyperlipidemia. This patient also has acanthosis nigricans, a sign of insulin resistance, and an elevated hemoglobin A1c can be diagnostic of type 2 diabetes mellitus. ALT should also be ordered in an obese teen to screen for steatohepatitis, or fatty liver.

Table 1. Causes of Abnormal Weight Gain in Adolescents.

Genetic Syndromes	Alström
	Beckwith-Wiedermann
	Borijeson-Forssman-Lehmann
	Cohen
	Familial lipodystrophy
	Laurence-Moon-Bardet-Biedl
	Prader Willi
	Sotos'
	Turner's
Endocrine Disorders	Cushing's syndrome
	Hypothyroidism (myxedema)
	Primary hyperinsulinism
	Pseudohypoparathyroidism
Behavioral or Psychiatric Disorders	Major depression
	Binge eating disorder
	Nocturnal eating disorder
Other Causes	Primary or exogenous obesity
	Hypothalamic tumors
	Congestive heart failure
	Nephrotic syndrome
	Liver/Cirrhosis (ascites)

Table 2. Criteria for Bariatric Surgery.[1,2]

Tanner Staging	Reached physiologic maturity, at least Tanner stage IV or V.
Skeletal Maturity	Reached at least 95% of estimated growth.
Lifestyle	At least 6 months of weight loss attempts that have failed.
BMI	• Severely obese with BMI >40 with associated serious health problems related to obesity. • BMI >50 with less severe health problems related to obesity.
Commitment	• Demonstrates understanding of the commitment to lifestyle changes that will be needed post-operation including diet and exercise. • Commits to comprehensive medical and psychological evaluations pre and post operation. • Agrees to avoid pregnancy for at least one year post operation as rapid weight loss would place a developing fetus at risk. • Adheres to strict nutrition program post-operation. • Has a supportive family. • Demonstrates the ability to make sound decisions.

Contraindications to Bariatric Surgery in Adolescents
The adolescent:

- has a medically correctable cause of obesity.
- has a substance abuse problem in preceding year.
- is unable to understand or unwilling to commit to the surgery as well as pre and post surgical regimen.
- is pregnant, plans to become pregnant soon after surgery, or is lactating following a recent pregnancy.

[1]Inge TH, Krebs KF, Barcia VF *et al.*, Bariatric surgery for severely overweight adolescents: concerns and recommendations, *Pediatrics.* **11**: 217–223 (2004), http://www.pediatricsdigest.mobi/content/114/1/217.full
[2]Mann, Denise. 'Adolescent Obesity and Weight Loss Surgery: Special Report', Consumer Guide to Bariatric Surgery, Retrieved from http ://www.yourbariatricsurgeryguide.com/obesity-teens

WEB REFERENCES

- American Academy of Pediatrics (http://pediatrics.aappublications.org)
  - Barlow, SE and the Expert Committee (2007), 'Expert Committee Recommendations Regarding the Prevention, Asssessment, and Treatment of Child Adolescent Overweight and Obesity: Summary Report', Pediatrics, 2007; 120(Supplement4);sl64-sl92, Retrieved from http://pediatrics.aappublications.org/content/120/Supplement_4/S164.abstract?ijkey=4c8d0ef2f651bb52f2falf6e98dad9635743644d&keytype2=tf_ipsecsha

- Inge TH, Krebs KF, Barcia VF, et al. Bariatric surgery for severely overweight adolescents: concerns and recommendations. Pediatrics. 2004; 11: 217–223: http://www.pediatricsdigest.mobi/content/114/1/217.full
- Krebs, NF, et al. (2007) 'Assessment of Child and Adolescent Overweight and Obesity', Pediatrics. 2007;120(Supplement4);sl93–s228, Retrieved from http://pediatrics.aappublications.org/content/120/Supplement_4/S193.full?sid=2e641523-60fd-4d8b-9fdb-d4dcf56d22fa
- Spear, BA, et al. (2007) 'Recommendations for Treatment of Child and Adolescent Overweight and Obesity', Pediatrics. 2007;120(Supplement 4);s254–s288, Retrieved from http://pediatrics.aappublications.org/content/120/Supplement_4/S254.fullsid=2e641523-60fd-4d8b-9fdb-d4dcf56d22fa
- Story, MT, et al. (2002) 'Management of Child and Adolescent Obesity: Attitudes, Barriers, Skills, and Training Needs Among Health Care Professionals', Pediatrics. 2002;110(Supplementl); 210-214, Retrieved from http://pediatrics.aappublications.org/content/110/Supplement_l/210.full?sid=2e641523-60fd-4d8b-9fdb-d4dcf56d22fa
- Strasburger, VC (2011) 'Policy Statement: Children, Adolescents, Obesity and the Media', Pediatrics 2011;128(l);201–208, Retrieved from http://pediatrics.aappublications.org/content/128/l/201.full.pdf+html?sid=2e641523-60fd-4d8b-9fdb-d4dcf56d22fa
- U.S. Preventive Services Task Force (2010), 'Screening for Obesity in Children and Adolescents: US Preventive Services Task Force Recommendation Statement', Pediatrics, 2010; 125(2); 361–367, Retrieved from http://pediatrics.aappublications.org/content/125/2/361.full?sid=2e641523-60fd-4d8b-9fdb-d4dcf56d22fa

- August GP, et al. (2008) 'Prevention and Treatment of Pediatric Obesity: An Endocrine Society Clinical Practice Guidelines Based on Expert Opinion', Journal of Clinical Endocrinology & Metabolism, December 2008;93(12);4576-4599, Retrieved from http://www.endo-society.org/guidelines/final/upload/FINAL-Standalone-Pediatric-Obesity-Guideline.pdf
- Centers for Disease Control and Prevention (CDC), The National Health and Nutrition Examination Survey (updated February 28, 2013), Retrieved from http://www.cdc.gov/nchs/nhanes.htm
- CDC, Childhood Overweight and Obesity (updated April 27, 2012), Retrieved from http://www.cdc.gov/obesity/childhood/index.html
- Kohn M, et al. (2006) 'Preventing and treating adolescent obesity: A position paper of the Society for Adolescent Medicine', Journal of Adolescent Health June 2006;36(6);784–787, Retrieved from http://www.j ahonline.org/article/Sl 054-139X(06)00079-6/fulltext
- National Institutes of Health, National Heart, Lung, and Blood Institute. 'How are Overweight and Obesity Diagnosed?', Bethesda, MD: National Institutes of Health; 2010, Retrieved from http://www.nhlbi.nih.gov/health/health-topics/topics/obe/diagnosis.html
- Pub Med Health, Prader Willi Syndrome (last reviewed May7, 2012), Retrieved http://www.ncbi.nlm.nih.gov/pubmedhealth/PMH0002572/
- U.S. Department of Health and Human Services. 'The Surgeon General's Vision for a Healthy and Fit Nation', Rockville, MD: U.S. Department of Health and Human

Services, Office of the Surgeon General, January 2010, Retrieved from http://www.surgeongeneral.gov/initiatives/healthy-fit-nation/obesityvision2010.pdf

- Yale Rudd Center for Food Policy and Obesity (2013) Retrieved from http://www.yaleruddcenter.org/

Additional Clinician and Patient Resources

- American Thyroid Association, Thyroid and Weight (2012), Retrieved from http://www.thyroid.org/patients/brochures/Thyroid_and_Weight.pdf
- Mann, Denise. 'Adolescent Obesity and Weight Loss Surgery: Special Report', Consumer Guide to Bariatric Surgery, Retrieved from http ://www.yourbariatricsurgeryguide.com/obesity-teens
- Endocrine Web, Hypothyroidism (updated 10/18/12), Retrieved from http://www.endocrineweb.com/conditions/thyroid/hypothyroidism-too-little-thyroid-hormone
- KidsHealth from the experts of Nemours: www.kidshealth.org
  - Overweight and Obesity, Retrieved from http://kidshealth.org/parent/general/body/overweight_obesity.html and http://kidshealth.org/teen/diseases_conditions/obesity/obesity_overweight.html
- Troubled Teen 101, Teen Obesity Statistics, Retrieved from http://www.troubledteen101.com/articles42.html

15

ABNORMAL WEIGHT LOSS/MALNUTRITION

Tomas J. Silber

TEST YOUR KNOWLEDGE

21. Which one of the following statements is true?

    A. Patients with Anorexia Nervosa (AN) have accelerated gastric emptying.
    B. Superior Mesenteric Artery (SMA) syndrome can mimic AN, purging type.
    C. Hyperphosphatemia is a complication of refeeding that can lead to peripheral edema.
    D. All the above are true.
    E. None of the above is true.

22. Which one of the following statements is true?

    A. Microhematuria and proteinuria in a patient with an eating disorder may suggest abuse of diuretics.
    B. A patient with anorexia nervosa, restrictive type, has mild jaundice with a bilirubin of 2.5 mg%. Her liver enzymes are not elevated. These laboratory results indicate that she has "liver burnout" with rapid onset fatty liver infiltrate placing her at high risk for liver failure.
    C. An adolescent has sustained abnormal weight loss and her laboratory results reveal an elevated cholesterol and a very low T3. This rules out anorexia nervosa and requires an endocrine consult.
    D. All the above are true.
    E. None of the above is true.

Refer to end of chapter for answers on page 175.

"My daughter has lost 15 pounds in the past month. I never see her eating, she is constantly exercising and is complaining about being cold all the time…"

BACKGROUND

- Normally there is rapid weight increase during puberty. Weight loss or the lack of appropriate weight gain should be cause for concern.
- There is a wide range of illnesses that cause weight loss in teens (Table 1) and the most common cause is an eating disorder (Table 2).
- A good way of discerning the cause of weight loss is to determine whether there is a caloric deficit, and if there is, determine if it is due to poor intake, excessive output or both.

ASSESSMENT

HISTORY

History of Present Illness

- Ascertain the degree of malnutrition: over what time has the weight loss occurred and what is the patient's current intake and level of activity?
- Food disappearing at home, frequent bathroom visits post-meals and/or clogged toilets suggest binge–purge episodes.
- Complaints about excessive weight gain or "being fat," prior history of dieting and frequent weight checks or body checks (looking in mirrors, "pinching" self) are consistent with **anorexia nervosa** (**AN**).
- Odd eating behaviors such as cutting food into small pieces, smearing food on the plate, throwing food away or hoarding food are common with **eating disorders** (**ED**).
- Males may experience a decline in libido: inquire about last erection. These become more infrequent as malnutrition results in a decline of testosterone.
- Dysphagia preceeding the weight loss suggests **achalasia**.
- Intense hunger and increasing caloric consumption suggests **hyperthyroidism**.
- History of vomiting *following* weight loss of any origin, or being placed in a lordotic cast suggests **superior mesenteric artery** (**SMA**) **syndrome**.

- Weight loss may be the initial symptoms of pancreatic failure in mild cases of **cystic fibrosis (CF)**, often in teens with a history of asthma.

Menstrual History

- Determine the last menstrual period and previous episodes of amenorrhea.
- A new episode of amenorrhea, persistent emesis and weight loss may indicate **hyperemesis gravidum**.

Past Medical History

- Postpartum weight loss and amenorrhea following a severe intrapartum hemorrhage suggests the panhypopituitarism of **Sheehan's Syndrome**.
- Evaluate for anxiety and depression which may coexist with, precede or follow an ED.
- Investigate suicidal ideations (8% suicide mortality in AN).
- Explore other psychiatric illnesses that can cause weight loss: phobias about eating solids following an episode of choking, obsessive compulsive disorder (OCD) involving food, psychotic fear of poisoning or a major depressive illness.

Social History

- Decline in school performance, things disappearing from home, change of friends and/or increased time spent away from home raise suspicion for stimulant abuse.

Review of Systems

- Complaints of feeling sick or fatigued and worry over the weight loss may indicate **chronic or serious illness**.
- Swallowing difficulty or dysphagia suggests **achalasia**.
- Loose stools suggest **malabsorption** (need to exclude laxative abuse).
- Abdominal pain, diarrhea and rectal bleeding suggest **inflammatory bowel disease (IBD)**.
- Increased appetite, hair loss, fatigue, heat intolerance, palpitations and insomnia suggest **hyperthyroidism**.
- Polyuria, polydipsia and polyphagia suggest **insulin dependent diabetes mellitus**.

- Concomitant headaches and early morning emesis alert to a possible **brain tumor.**
- Fatigue, vomiting, hypotension and bronzed skin characterize **Addison's Disease.**
- Persistent cough, blood in sputum and hemoptysis occur in **tuberculosis.**
- Hematemesis (Mallory Weiss tears) with forceful vomiting can occur with **bulimia.**
- Oral candidiasis and recurrent infections suggests **AIDS wasting syndrome.**

PHYSICAL

Vital Signs

- Low body temperature, bradycardia, hypotension and orthostasis are concerning for severe malnutrition of any cause, most commonly AN.
- Tachycardia and hypertension in a malnourished patient are red flags that suggest intake of stimulants (i.e. cocaine or amphetamines) or hyperthyroidism.

Anthropometric Measurements

- Assess height and weight with patient undressed after emptying bladder and calculate BMI.
- Plot changes over time on a growth curve with the aid of old records.

General Appearance

- Observe for loss of subcutaneous tissue and muscle mass, presence of lanugo (fine downy hair on the trunk and extremities) and acrocyanosis consistent with severe malnutrition.

HEENT

- Ketotic breath is found in semi-starvation and acute diabetic ketoacidosis.
- Parotid hypertrophy can occur with bulimia and AN.
- Oral ulcers raise concern for an underlying autoimmune process.
- Dental enamel erosion can also occur with frequent self-induced vomiting episodes.

Neck

- A goiter and exophthalmos suggest hyperthyroidism.

Cardiac

- Bradycardia can occur with severe malnutrition and may warrant cardiac monitoring.
- Tachycardia and a new onset flow murmur can occur with anemia.
- Cardiac arrhythmia and arrest may be due to hypokalemia secondary to purging.

Abdomen

- A scaphoid or flat abdomen may be noted with weight loss.
- Assess for tenderness which can occur with constipation or underlying IBD.
- Examine for mass/tumor.

Extremities

- Arthritis is seen in granulomatous colitis.

Skin

- Pallor can occur with anemia (poor nutrition or malabsorption from IBD or celiac disease).
- Tanned skin in the winter without tanning treatments suggests Addison's disease ("bronzed" skin).
- Injured and eroded knuckles (Russell's sign) occur with self-induced vomiting.
- "Jaundice" with normal bilirubin, associated with hypercarotinemia, is classically seen in AN.
- Patients with AN may have growth of fine hair across the body, also known as lanugo.
- Scars from "cutting" behaviors can occur in patients with ED who have comorbid psychiatric illnesses.
- Perianal skin tags and mucosal ulcerations can occur with IBD.

Neurologic

- A fine tremor, sometimes detected by placing a sheet of paper over extended fingers, is common in **hyperthyroidism**.

STUDIES

ROUTINE TESTS

Complete Blood Count

- Elevated hemoglobin and hematocrit indicate hemoconcentration.
- Anemia is unusual in ED, and is more characteristic of end stage illness.
- Presence of marked anemia is suspicious for an organic cause, most commonly a granulomatous colitis.
- Hemolytic anemia can occur during refeeding.
- Leukopenia occurs often in malnutrition.
- Blast cells confirm malignancy.

Sedimentation Rate

- An elevated sedimentation rate suggests an inflammatory process, most frequently Crohn's disease (CD) or malignancy.
- This value is very low in patients with AN.

Comprehensive Metabolic Panel

- Liver enzymes may be abnormal due to fatty infiltrate of the liver secondary to malnutrition.
- Liver enzymes can also be elevated in granulomatous colitis.
- BUN may be high due to dehydration while creatinine is normal or even low.
- Cholesterol is often paradoxically elevated in AN.
- Electrolytes, total protein and albumin tend to be normal in patients with AN.
- Albumin tends to be very low in patients with IBD but normal in patients with ED.

- Prealbumin, with a much shorter half life than albumin, is a good marker for very recent fasting or dieting.
- Hyponatremic, hypochloremic alkalosis occurs with purging; hyponatremic acidosis can occur with laxative abuse; and dilutional hyponatremia with low osmolality occurs with water intoxication.
- Hyperkalemia is associated with Addison's Disease.
- Hypoglycemia occurs in AN when the reserve liver glycogen stores have been emptied.
- Alkaline phosphatase may be low due to growth cessation.

Serial Phosphorus and Magnesium

- Monitor for sudden drops in value that can occur with refeeding syndrome in those undergoing intense nutritional rehabilitation (Table 3).

Zinc

- Can be low in AN causing loss of or abnormal taste sensation.

Amylase

- When elevated, it may be a marker for frequent vomiting.

Thyroid Studies

- T3, the active thyroid hormone, declines during malnutrition (adaptive mechanism) while TSH is typically normal even with very low T3.
- High TSH in a depressed patient losing weight because of eating poorly indicates hypothyroidism.

Urinalysis

- Glucosuria and proteinuria suggests insulin dependent diabetes mellitus.
- Proteinuria and microhematuria can occur with intense exercise.
- High specific gravity occurs with dehydration while low specific gravity occurs with "water loading" or isosthenuria.
- Ketones are present following starvation episodes or during an episode of diabetic ketoacidosis.

Pregnancy Test

- Pregnancy is the most common cause of secondary amenorrhea.

Drug Toxicity Screen

- Consider drug screens whenever substance abuse is suspected.

SPECIAL TESTS

Celiac and/or IBD Panel

- Send for all malnourished patients without a classic history for an ED, especially if they are anemic and have other symptoms.

Stool Tests

- Fecal calprotectin and occult blood can be seen in IBD.
- H. Pylori Antigen should be considered if peptic ulcer disease is suspected.
- Fat content (steatorrhea) can be evaluated in cases of malabsorption.

Sweat Test

- Can diagnose cystic fibrosis.

Vitamin D

- This is low in those with severe malnutrition.
- Also consider other vitamin studies depending on history and physical exam findings.

Cortisol

- Low in Addison's disease.
- There is a delayed clearance of cortisol in AN.

HIV Antibody Test

- Routinely recommended for adolescents 13 and older, since history may not be accurate.
- Always test if the patient has a history of child abuse, sexual activity, IV drug use or opportunistic infection.

EKG

- To document bradycardia, rule out arrhythmias and measure the QT interval.

Flat Plate of Abdomen

- Consider if evaluating for constipation: intestines "full of stools" is a common finding in patients with AN.
- If NG tube feeding will be initiated, an x-ray is also indicated post insertion to assess appropriate tube placement.

Upper GI Study

- This can detect the post-stenotic esophageal dilatation of achalasia.
- It can also detect intermittent obstruction or compression of the third portion of duodenum caused by the collapse of the SMA against the aorta (due to loss of omental fat), also known as SMA syndrome.
- Delayed gastric emptying secondary to malnutrition and impaired intestinal motility can also be assessed, but this is usually a clinical diagnosis.

Upper GI Study with Small Bowel Follow Through

- Look for findings suggesting achalasia or granulomatous colitis.

Echocardiogram

- Consider if a patient has abnormal EKG findings other than sinus bradycardia.

Bone Density Test

- A dexa scan with z score may detect low bone density, osteopenia or osteoporosis.
- Consider if there is a high risk of osteopenia, especially if the patient has primary or secondary amenorrhea (older than 15 years, with symptoms lasting more than 6 months).

Endoscopy/Colonoscopy

- Consider if granulomatous colitis or IBD is suspected.

Chest X-Ray

- Order when a patient has a positive tuberculin skin test or whenever weight loss remains unexplained.

Brain Imaging

- This is rarely needed, but should be done if there is a high degree of suspicion for an underlying brain tumor.

DISPOSITION

Patients with ED are best managed with the support of a multidisciplinary team addressing both nutritional and mental health issues.

- Support parents in being firm as they guide their teen towards improved nutrition (Maudsley approach: a family based monitoring and supervision of meals).
- In patients with rapid, severe and uncontrollable weight loss, rescue hospitalization (even against the patient's will) has been proven effective.
- Gradual nutritional rehabilitation is essential to avoid refeeding syndrome (Table 3).

Refer to appropriate subspecialty teams based on exam findings:

- Gastroenterology if underlying achalasia, IBD, celiac or other GI disorder is suspected to perform endoscopy or colonoscopy.
- Endocrinology if diabetes, thyroid disease or Addison's disease are suspected.
- Pulmonary for a patient with cystic fibrosis.
- Infectious Diseases if tuberculosis is confirmed.
- Hematology/Oncology for suspected cases of malignancy.
- Psychiatry should be consulted to co-manage ED, especially when co-morbid psychiatric conditions are suspected. Often, patients undergoing nutritional rehabilitation for an ED subsequently require long-term treatment plans with multi-disciplinary teams, either through outpatient day treatment programs or residential facilities.
- Substance abuse counseling programs for substance abusing teens.

What is unique about weight loss in adolescents?

- ED are the most common cause of weight loss in adolescents.
- Many patients give a false history of eating well and report having menstrual periods when they do not, to avoid detection or hospital admission.
- Parents and/or siblings, and sometimes even classmates are often the ones to raise the alarm that "something is wrong."
- Older adolescents with ED tend to drink lots of water in order to "make weight." This water loading can lead to irritability and seizures.
- Adolescents with ED have a better prognosis than their adult counterparts.
- The incidence of hyperthyroidism in adolescence is similar to that of AN: tachycardia, elevation of blood pressure, a developing goiter and a fine tremor should raise suspicion.
- Males with ED have a decline in the frequency of their erections. These return to normal with nutritional rehabilitation. Males tend to have better prognosis than females.
- Adolescents who lose weight due to an organic disease are very concerned and distressed about their state of malnutrition while those with an ED are not.

TEST YOUR KNOWLEDGE ANSWERS

21. B. SMA syndrome is a condition that arises from the loss of intra-abdominal fatty omentum that normally maintains the open angle formed between the aorta and the SMA that emerges from it. This results in the external compression of the third portion of duodenum which leads to intermittent obstruction and emesis. Any disease that causes weight loss can result in SMA. Patients with AN afflicted by this complication are sometimes unfairly accused of self-induced vomiting. Nutritional rehabilitation via a jejunostomy tube resolves this complication for as nutrition improves, the omentum is reconstituted. Hypophosphatemia (not hyperphosphatemia) is a complication of refeeding. Most patients with AN develop some degree of delayed gastric emptying as malnutrition progresses.
22. E. Some diuretics may change the color of urine (blue). Microhematuria and proteinuria in a patient with an ED strongly suggest "purging"

through compulsive exercise (usually running). Patients with Gilbert's Syndrome have worsening indirect hyperbilirubinemia when fasting. A patient with AN should be suspected of having Gilbert's syndrome if she becomes jaundiced after food restriction. Liver enzymes remain normal in Gilbert's Syndrome and these patients are no more at risk for liver failure than any other patient with an eating disorder (and certainly less than one with persistent elevation of liver enzymes). Abnormal weight loss and malnutrition lead to a compensatory "euthyroid hypothyroidism" which protects the body from acute starvation via a hypometabolic state. Patients with AN suffer a decline in their T3, which is the active metabolic hormone. Elevated cholesterol and carotene are often seen with AN. There is no need for an endocrine consult with these findings; in fact, giving these patients thyroid hormone could worsen their condition.

Table 1. Causes of Abnormal Weight Loss and Malnutrition.

Behavioral or Psychiatric Disorder	Eating Disorders: Anorexia Nervosa, Bulimia or EDNOS Major Depression Psychosis Schizophrenia Substance Abuse (cocaine, amphetamines) Swallowing Phobia (post-choking) Obsessive Compulsive Disorder Dysmorphophobia
Endocrine Disorder	Hyperthyroidism Insulin Dependent Diabetes Mellitus Addison's Disease Hypothalamic Tumors Sheehan's Syndrome
Gastrointestinal Disorder	Achalasia Celiac Disease and other Malabsorption Syndromes Inflammatory Bowel Disease Superior Mesenteric Artery Syndrome
Infectious Disease	Tuberculosis, HIV/AIDS
Malignancy	Brain Tumors and Other Cancers
Other Causes	Hyperemesis Gravidarum, Cystic Fibrosis

Table 2. Eating Disorders.*

Anorexia Nervosa	• Intense fear of gaining weight. • Denial of seriousness of weight loss or body image disturbance. • Refusal to maintain body weight above 85% of ideal body weight. • Amenorrhea (for at least three months). • Two types: restricting and purging.
Bulimia Nervosa	• Recurrent episodes of binging. • Recurrent episodes of inappropriate behavior to prevent weight gain (self induced vomiting, ipecac, appetite suppressants, laxatives or compulsive exercise). • Self-evaluation unduly influenced by weight and body shape. • Binging/purging episodes have taken place on average twice a week for 3 months.
Eating Disorder, NOS	• Does not meet criteria for anorexia nervosa. • Significant eating disorder that does not meet the above criteria.

**Note*: This classification has come under criticism because over time, the same patient may meet criteria for more than one diagnosis. In addition, this classification does not apply as well to younger adolescents and males.

Table 3. Refeeding Syndrome.

Etiology	Occurs in malnourished patients who receive too much food at a rapid rate. Initially described in alcoholic patients receiving total parenteral nutrition, but can also occur in patients with ED.
Mechanism	Extracellular phosphorus rapidly enters the cells now replenished with nutrients. This leads to hypophosphatemia and sometimes hypomagnesemia.
Symptoms	Peripheral edema, tachycardia, cardiac insufficiency, confusion or delirium and bone pain. Death may occur.
Treatment	Regulating food intake, gradual nutritional rehabilitation and providing supplemental phosphorus.

WEB REFERENCES

- American Academy of Pediatrics Publications (www.pediatrics.aappublications.org)
  - Rome, ES et al. (2003) 'Children and Adolescents with Eating Disorders: The State of the Art', Pediatrics 2003; lll(l); e98–el08, Retrieved from http://pediatrics.aappublications.org/Content/lll/l/e98.full?sid=f6cl870b-ef5c-45c7-ab8f-987b9210a294
  - Rosen, DS and the Committee on Adolescence (2010) 'Identification and Management of Eating Disorders in Children and Adolescents', Pediatrics 2010; 126(6); 1240–1253, Retrieved from http://pediatrics.aappublications.org/content/126/6/1240.full?sid=f6c1870b-ef5c-45c7-ab8f-987b9210a294
- Golden NH, et al. (2003) 'Eating disorders in adolescents: position paper of the Society for Adolescent Medicine'. Journal of Adolescent Health, December 2003; 33(6); 496–503, Retrieved from http://www.jahonline.org/article/S1054-139X(03)00326-4/fulltext
- Le Grange D, Lock J, Loeb K, Nicholls D (2010) 'Academy for Eating Disorders Position Paper: The Role of the Family in Eating Disorders', International Journal of Eating Disorders, 2010; 43(l); l–5, Retrieved from http://www.maudsleyparents.org/images/Role_of_Family.pdf
- PubMed Health (February 13, 2012), 'Anorexia Nervosa' Retrieved from http://www.ncbi.nlm.nih.gov/pubmedhealth/PMH0001401/

Additional Clinician and Patient Resources:

- Academy for Eating Disorders, Retrieved from http://www.aedweb.org/AM/Template.cfm?Section=Home
- Eating Disorder Referral and Information Center, Retrieved from www.EDReferral.com
- Families Empowered and Supporting Treatment of Eating Disorders, Retrieved from www.FEAST-ED.org
- The International Association of Eating Disorders Professionals Foundations, Retrieved from http://www.iaedp.com/
- Maudsley Parents, A Site for Parents of Eating Disordered Children, Retrieved from www.maudsleyparents.org
- National Alliance on Mental Illness (www.nami.org)
  - Duckworth K, Freedman JL (January 2013) 'Anorexia Nervosa' Retrieved from http://www.nami.org/Template.cfm?Section=By_Illness&template=/ContentManagement/ContentDisplay.cfm&ContentID=7409
- National Eating Disorders Association, Retrieved from www.edap.org
- Something Fishy, Website on Eating Disorder, retrieved from www.somethingfishy.org

16

BULIMIA

Rosina Pellerano

TEST YOUR KNOWLEDGE

23. Which one of the following statements is true?
    A. Self induced vomiting leads to hypokalemic metabolic acidosis.
    B. Russell's sign is characterized by edema of the lower extremities.
    C. Frequent purging may cause bilateral parotid swelling.
    D. All the above.
    E. None of the above.

24. Which one of the following statements is true?
    A. Constant exposure to gastric secretions can cause pre-cancerous mucosal changes in the esophagus.
    B. A 17 year old male with unexplained hypokalemic metabolic alkalosis probably has renal disease.
    C. Type I diabetics with bulimia may increase their insulin dose to lose weight.
    D. All the above.
    E. None of the above.

Refer to end of chapter for answer on page 189.

"For the past 3 weeks, my daughter has complained of having heartburn and belly pain. I also noticed that she goes to the bathroom immediately after meals at home or in restaurants."

BACKGROUND

- Adolescents rarely present to their doctors because they are distressed by their binge eating or purging. Instead, this problem often comes to a doctor's attention because friends or schools report concerns to parents or because parents catch their teens binge eating or purging.
- Many adolescents experiment with purging. The possibility of their developing bulimia nervosa (BN) is a concern. BN is characterized by:
  - Recurrent episodes of binge eating, stemming from the patient's lack of control.
  - Recurrent compensatory behaviors to avoid weight gain, such as self induced vomiting; use of laxatives, diuretics, ipecac or appetite suppressants; and/or compulsive exercising.
  - Self worth unduly influenced by weight and body shape.
  - Binges and inappropriate compensatory behavior have taken place at least twice a week for a minimum of 3 months.
- BN occurs in both females and males.
- A significant number of patients with BN may have associated problems linked to an impulse disorder, such as substance use, self cutting, shoplifting and sexual promiscuity.
- Gastrointestinal complaints such as nausea and vomiting are common; hence, even if the chief complaint raises suspicion of an eating disorder, other entities should be considered (Table 1).

ASSESSMENT

HISTORY

- Usually a variety of symptoms provide clues to the diagnosis of BN (Table 2).

History of Present Illness

Does the teen report any gastrointestinal complaints or symptoms? If so, what is the duration and frequency of these symptoms?

- Recurrent episodes of abdominal cramps, nausea, weight loss, fever and/or vomiting and diarrhea with or without hematochezia suggests **inflammatory bowel disease (IBD).**
- Epigastric discomfort after meals, nausea, recurrent bouts of vomiting, dysphagia, dark colored stools, bloating and fatigue suggests **peptic ulcer disease (PUD).**
- Nausea, vomiting, upper abdominal pain that worsens after a meal, weight loss and steatorrhea suggests **chronic pancreatitis.**
- Bloating, abdominal cramps, nausea, vomiting, loss of appetite, foul smelling loose stools and fever suggests an **intestinal parasitic infection.**
- Intermittent vomiting (usually after meals), epigastric pain, nausea, weight loss (can be significant) and volume depletion occurs in **gastric outlet syndrome.**
- Hematemesis with or without abdominal pain occur with **Mallory-Weiss** esophageal tears.

Get a detailed history of dietary behaviors and weight changes.

- What has been the teen's highest and lowest weight recorded?
- Does the teen admit to binge eating or purging episodes?
- Has the teen ever felt so full after eating that he/she made him/herself sick?
- After episodes of overeating is there an intense need to get rid of the food and calories?
  - If so, how often does this occur?
  - Is this a daily, weekly or monthly occurrence?
- On what foods does the teen binge?
- Is there a time of day during which the teen chooses to binge?
- Ask if the teen engages in regurgitating food, re-chewing and subsequently swallowing again. This behavior suggests **rumination** and most teens will not disclose unless asked directly.

- How does the teen induce vomiting?
  - Does the teen use fingers, a toothbrush, ipecac syrup or fluids?
  - Other methods such as laxatives, diuretics, enemas or weight loss teas?
- Does the teen skip family meals or eat meals alone?
- What is the teen's exercise pattern?
  - Exercise may be used as a form of purging: does the teen compulsively exercise?
  - How does the teen feel if an exercise session is missed?
- Determine the teen's core beliefs regarding weight, size and body shape.
  - Does the teen have an ideal weight goal that would make him/her happy?
  - Does self esteem and mood depend on weight fluctuations?

Medications

- Inquire if over the counter medications were taken to relieve gastrointestinal symptoms?
- Chronic constipation suggests **atonic** or **cathartic colon** from long term laxative abuse.
- If the teen is a diabetic, determine if they have ever skipped a dose of or overused insulin.
- Determine if the teen has used ipecac, which can cause muscle weakness (myopathy) and arrhythmias (cardiomyopathy).
  - Each bottle contains 32 mg of emetine and frequent exposure has a cumulative effect.
  - A dose of 1,250 mg can lead to cardiac damage over a period of months.

Social History

- Assess a patient's psychological state.
- Have there been any recent problems at school or with peer or family relationships?
- Has the teen experienced any recent changes to friendships, bullying or decline in school performance?
- What is the teen's general mood?

- Does the teen use alcohol such as beer, wine or hard liquor?
  - How often and how much?
  - Does the teen binge drink or drink so much that they experience black outs?
- Is the teen smoking cigarettes or marijuana?
  - Determine quantity and frequency of use.
- Is the teen using any other illicit substance?

Review of Systems

- Severe chest and abdominal pain, dyspnea and upper back pain is an emergency as there may be an esophageal rupture, or **Boerhaave syndrome**, following very forceful vomiting.
- Increased appetite and thirst, fatigue, nausea, vomiting and frequent urination suggests **diabetes.**
- Swollen salivary glands, sore throat, difficulty swallowing, reflux and altered intestinal motility suggests **scleroderma.**
- Coughing after eating, heartburn, difficulty swallowing and halitosis suggests **Zenker's diverticulum.**
- Headaches, early morning vomiting without nausea, weight loss, abnormal gait, seizures, visual field defects and/or changes in mood or memory problems characterize a **brain mass.**
- Hyperphagia, irritability, excessive sleep and behavior problems characterize **Klein Levine Syndrome.**
- Recurrent episodes of nausea with intractable vomiting lasting several days and symptom free intervals of several weeks, indicate **cyclic vomiting syndrome.** This can be due to a variety of causes, ranging from migraines to cannabis abuse.

PHYSICAL

Vital Signs

- Temperature may be normal or low depending on weight.
- Check for orthostatic changes to blood pressure and pulse (from lying to sitting to standing) which can occur with volume depletion and low body weight.

- Orthostatic hypotension with a drop in blood pressure of 20 mm Hg upon standing or an increase in pulse more than 20 beats per minute upon standing needs further evaluation.
- Respiratory rate: dyspnea, severe chest pain and shock suggest **Boerhaave syndrome**, an esophageal rupture leading to mediastinitis.

Anthropometric Measurements

- Weigh the patient with the patient's back to the scale and determine BMI. Plot measurements on a growth chart. Weight may be normal or low for height and age.
  - Laxative and diuretic abusers may experience rapid weight gain whenever they stop using the medication. This is due to the edema of secondary aldosteronism.

HEENT

- Injected ocular conjunctiva, subconjunctival hemorrhage, periorbital edema or facial petechiae can occur from forceful vomiting.
- Assess for hypertrophy of salivary glands.
- Painless bilateral parotid swelling is often the result of frequent purging.
  - In cases of parotid swelling, also consider **parotitis** of viral (i.e. mumps) or bacterial etiology, **obstruction of the salivary duct, poor hygiene** or **Sjögrens Syndrome** if associated with dry mouth (xerostomia) or dry eyes (keratoconjunctivitis sicca).
  - Salivary glands can also be enlarged from **sarcoidosis** (look for uveitis, rash, arthritis and pulmonary infiltrates), **tuberculosis, hypovitaminosis A, cat scratch disease, alcohol abuse, HIV, diabetes, hypothyroidism** or **severe dehydration.**
- Complete a thorough oral exam.
  - Observe for perimolysis, or erosion and discoloration of dental enamel on the lingual surface of the upper teeth.
  - Is there evidence of pyorrhea: friable, sensitive or recessed gums?
  - Is there notable dental caries which may increase due to purging?
  - Does the teen have cheilosis, or painful fissures in the corners of the mouth, also related to frequent purging episodes?

Lungs

- Shortness of breath and rales may indicate aspiration.

Heart

- Auscultate for irregular rhythm. Arrhythmia may be due to **electrolyte imbalances** and/or **ipecac use**.
- A mid-systolic click is associated with **mitral valve prolapse** in low weight teens.

Abdomen

- Right upper quadrant tenderness along with weight loss may indicate **gallstones.**
- A nontender mass palpated in the lower quadrants may be stool.

Neurologic

- Examine optic fundi for papilledema to rule out vomiting due to increased intracranial pressure from a **brain tumor**.

Skin

- Calluses or scars on the dorsal surface of the hands, also known as "Russell's sign," occur when vomiting is induced with fingers that are repeatedly rubbed against upper incisors.
- Circular or linear scars on inner thighs, abdomen or arms, caused by cigarette burns or sharp metal objects, indicates **dermatitis artefacta**, caused by self harm (i.e. cutting).
- Clubbing of fingers may be seen with laxative abuse.
- Edema of lower extremities, also known as **Pseudo-Bartter's Syndrome**, occurs when frequent purging produces volume depletion and hyperaldosteronism.

STUDIES

Complete Blood Count

- Anemia and a low red blood cell count may indicate blood loss due to IBD, intestinal infection, PUD or Sjögren's syndrome.

- An elevated WBC suggests inflammation and may be elevated in gastrointestinal illness.
- A low WBC is seen with malnutrition.

Comprehensive Metabolic Panel

- Hypokalemia and metabolic alkalosis can result from purging.
  - Hypokalemia less than 3.6 mmol/L can cause fatigue, muscle weakness, constipation and palpitations.
  - Hypokalemia less than 2.5 mmol/L can cause cardiac arrythmias, heart failure and sudden death.
  - Metabolic alkalosis is common in patients with BN and bicarbonate levels range from 30–40 mEq/L (normal: 22–28 mEq/L).
- Consider checking potassium on a spot urine sample:
  - Urinary potassium less than 10 mmol/liter suggests a gastrointestinal cause for the potassium loss.
- Hypomagnesemia suggests diuretic abuse.
- Hyperchloremic metabolic acidosis may occur with diarrhea or laxative abuse.
- Elevated BUN and creatinine may occur from dehydration (purging) or gastric outlet obstruction.
- Elevated fasting blood sugar of 126 mg/dl or higher suggests diabetes.

Serum Amylase and Lipase

- Elevated amylase and lipase suggests pancreatitis.
- Elevated amylase with a normal lipase suggests salivary origin of hyperamylasemia. This is seen with significant, repeated self-induced vomiting.
- Fractionation of serum amylase will also confirm a salivary gland origin.

SPECIAL TESTS

EKG

- Can show changes due to hypokalemia such as ST segment depression, T wave flattening or inversion and U waves.
- Hypocalcemia and hypomagnesemia can cause prolonged QT interval and T-wave changes.

Chest X-ray

- Unilateral pulmonary effusion (more often on the left side) or pneumomediastinum in a rapidly deteriorating patient suggests Boerhaave syndrome.

Thyroid Studies

- TSH and T4 are usually normal in BN and T3 is low with malnutrition.

Antinuclear Antibody (ANA) and Rheumatoid Factor (RF)

- Positive tests suggest underlying autoimmune etiology such as Sjögren's disease.
- Immunoglobulins would also be elevated in autoimmune processes.

Urinalysis

- A high specific gravity indicates volume depletion.
- A comprehensive urine laxative screen can be positive up to 24 hours and can be ordered if laxative abuse is suspected.

Stool Tests

- For travelers, consider stool culture, stool for ova and parasites and parasite specific IgG serum tests to rule out parasitic intestinal infection.
- May also send stool for occult blood and calprotectin if IBD is suspected.

GI Studies

- An upper GI with small bowel follow through can be helpful to diagnose IBD.
- An upper endoscopy would identify bleeding sites in cases of suspected Mallory-Weiss esophageal tears.
- An esophagogastroduodenoscopy and abdominal CT would diagnose a gastric outlet obstruction.
- A barium swallow would be helpful in suspected cases of Zenker's diverticulum.
- An abdominal CT and ultrasound should be ordered if chronic pancreatitis is suspected.

Salivary Gland Biopsy

- Would diagnose Sjögren's syndrome.
- In addition, a sialogram helps to determine salivary flow while the Shirmer test measures tear duct production in Sjögren's.

MRI of Brain

- Consider if a brain mass is suspected.

DISPOSITION

Ideally the treatment of BN should include a multidisciplinary team approach with professionals who have experience treating eating disorders.

- The team should consist of a psychologist, nutritionist, clinician and consulting psychiatrist.
- The level of care recommended should be discussed between the team and family.
- The primary care clinician and medical team should also educate the patient and family on medical complications and negative outcomes that can occur from engaging in unhealthy compensatory behaviors.
- The team's goal is to help the teen move away from an unhealthy preoccupation with body weight and shape. With ongoing therapy, compensatory thoughts and behaviors can remit, leading to a healthy and productive life.

The medical management of a teen diagnosed with BN will depend on their presenting signs and symptoms:

- Patients with ongoing purging behaviors require frequent outpatient follow up for repeat laboratory studies (screening for hypokalemia) and oral potassium supplementation.
- Patients with hypokalemia (below 2.5 mEq/L) and metabolic alkalosis should be hospitalized and treated with IV hydration as well as potassium repletion.

- Clinicians can initiate pharmacotherapy.
  - Fluoxetine, a selective serotonin reuptake inhibitor (SSRI), dosed up to 80 mg/day (gradually increased as tolerated) may help.

- Psychiatric consult/referral is required when patients present with comorbid psychiatric conditions (Table 3) and/or are suicidal.
- Long-term purging behaviors can lead to significant oral hygiene issues and tooth decay. Teens should be advised to rinse their mouth with a mixture of baking soda and water after purging episodes to help prevent enamel erosion, gum disease and dental caries.
- A dental referral needs to include information about the self-induced vomiting.

What is unique about BN in adolescents?

- Some adolescents deal with painful emotions or inner turmoil through unhealthy behaviors that eventually culminate in the development of BN.
- BN carries the stigma of a shameful, secretive illness that adolescents do not want their parents to discover.
- Impulse disorder (i.e., alcohol intoxication, shoplifting, social acting out or cutting) may be a presenting symptom that upon further inquiry, leads to the discovery of BN.
- Through acceptance and a nonjudgemental approach to care, an alliance can be built between health care providers and teens.
- A combination of empathy and gentle firmness can lead a reluctant teen to accept medical and psychological care.
- Early treatment in adolescence leads to a better prognosis.

TEST YOUR KNOWLEDGE ANSWERS

23. C. Bilateral parotid swelling (sialoadenosis) is painless and persists even after purging has ceased. The glands become hypertrophied due to overstimulation: frequent contact with gastric contents produces increased stimulation of the cholinergic nerve. It improves with sucking on lemons or sour candies, warm compresses and cessation of purging. Pedal edema may be found in laxative and diuretic abusers. Hypokalemic metabolic alkalosis first develops due to a loss of sodium chloride, producing volume contraction which leads to the secretion of aldosterone from the adrenal glands. Subsequent salt and bicarbonate absorption occur. There is also

loss of acid from vomiting. Russell's signs are small scars on the dorsum of the hand formed from contact with teeth to induce vomiting.

24. A. Barrett's esophagus is a precancerous transformation that develops from repeated exposure to stomach acid. Patients may complain of heartburn or be asymptomatic. Males may also present with BN. Other causes of metabolic alkalosis include: diuretic and laxative abuse (though this can also manifest as acidosis), villous adenoma and excessive licorice intake. Type I diabetics may choose to miss an insulin dose to lose weight through ketoacidosis. They may increase their insulin dose to cover binge episodes.

Table 1. Differential Diagnosis of Bulimia Nervosa.

Inflammatory Bowel Disease
Peptic Ulcer Disease
Pancreatitis
Diabetes
Scleroderma
Intestinal Infections: Parasitic
Zenker Diverticulum
Gastric Outlet Syndrome
Malignancy: Hypothalamic or Brain Tumor
Klein-Levin Syndrome
Recurrent Cyclic Vomiting

Table 2. Clinical Clues that a Patient may have Bulimia Nervosa.

- Fatigue
- Swollen face or "chipmunk cheeks"
- Sore throat with or without esophageal irritation
- Teeth are sensitive to hot or cold foods or liquids
- Palpitations that can be due to dehydration, hypokalemia, hypomagnesemia or occur after purging (sinus tachycardia)
- Complaints of bloating
- Swelling of hands, abdomen and/or feet
- Diarrhea or constipation
- Diffuse abdominal pain
- Anxiety
- Feelings of sadness, or signs of depression
- Irregular menses
- Reports of blood in vomitus which suggests a Mallory-Weiss tear
- Unexplained hypokalemia or bouts of dehydration requiring emergency room visits
- Family reports vomiting with no concomitant illness
- Family reports evidence of excessive amounts of food disappearing or evidence of laxative use

Table 3. Comorbid Psychiatric Conditions.*

- Mood disorders
- Anxiety disorders
- Attention deficit hyperactivity disorder
- Drug or alcohol abuse
- Personality disorder: cluster B traits presenting with lack of impulse control and mood instability

*These may precede, coexist with or follow the eating disorder.

WEB REFERENCES

- Cleveland Clinic: Center for Continuing Education, Publications (www.clevelandclinicmeded.com/medicalpubs):
  - Franco, K, 'Eating Disorders', Retrieved from http://www.clevelandclinicmeded.com/medicalpubs/diseasemanagement/psychiatry-psychology/eating-disorders/

- PubMed Health (February 13, 2012), 'Bulimia' Retrieved from http://www.ncbi.nlm.nih.gov/pubmedhealth/PMHOOO1381/
- Rosen DS, and the Committee on Adolescence (2010) 'Clinical Report: Identification and Management of Eating Disorders in Children and Adolescents', Pediatrics November 2010;126(6);1240–1253, Retrieved from http://pediatrics.aappublications.org/content/126/6/1240.full?sid=8a937852 9d68-4f58-a842-900eea2ff096

Additional Clinician and Patient Resources:

- Academy for Eating Disorders, Retrieved from http://www.aedweb.org/AM/Template.cfm?Section=Home
- Eating Disorders, Resources for Recovery Since 1980: http://www.bulimia.com/index.cfm
- National Alliance on Mental Illness (www.nami.org)
  - Duckworth K, Freedman JL (January 2013) 'Bulimia Nervosa' Retrieved from http://www.nami.org/Template.cfm?Section=By_Illness&Template=/ContentManagement/ContentDisplay.cfm& ContentID=149448
- National Eating Disorders Association: http://www.edap.org/

17

ANEMIA

*Carleen Townsend-Akpan**

TEST YOUR KNOWLEDGE

25. A 15 year old African-American girl with a history of heavy menses comes to your office for evaluation of fatigue and pallor. Her hemoglobin is 7.2, MCV 55, Retic 0.5%, WBC 7.5 (with normal differential), and platelet count 555 K. The smear shows marked microcytosis and occasional basophilic stippling. What is the *MOST* likely diagnosis?

    A. Acute Leukemia
    B. Autoimmune Hemolytic Anemia
    C. Iron Deficiency Anemia (IDA)
    D. Beta Thalassemia Trait
    E. Alpha Thalassemia Trait

26. A 15 year old Chinese-American boy consults for evaluation of fatigue and pallor. His hemoglobin is 7.2, MCV 55, Retic 1.5%, WBC 7.5 (normal differential), and platelet count 255 K. The smear shows marked microcytosis and 2+ target cells. Ferritin, TIBC and iron level were normal. You obtain a hemoglobin electrophoresis that shows 98.4% Hgb A, 1.5% Hgb A2, and 0.1% Hgb F. Mom reports that she has

Refer to end of chapter for answers on page 202.

*We thank Dr. Helge Hartung for providing chapter questions and answers.

been "iron deficient" for many years, despite good adherence to oral iron supplementation. What is the *MOST* likely diagnosis?

A. Acute Leukemia
B. Autoimmune Hemolytic Anemia
C. Iron Deficiency Anemia (IDA)
D. Beta Thalassemia Trait
E. Alpha Thalassemia Trait

A 14-year-old female presents for routine physical. She is in excellent health and was doing well at school, until her grades recently started slipping. She seems more tired and her grandmother is concerned that she eats erratically and skips breakfast. On exam, she has pale conjunctiva and is mildly tachycardic, with a grade I/VI systolic murmur.

BACKGROUND

- Anemia is defined as a reduction of red blood cells or concentration of hemoglobin.
- Iron deficiency anemia (IDA) is the most common cause of anemia in adolescent females and will therefore be prominently addressed in this chapter.
- Iron deficiency can cause physical, cognitive, and social impairments.
- In IDA, there are decreased red blood cells due to low iron resulting in abnormally small red blood cells (microcytic) and a decreased amount of hemoglobin (hypochromic).
- Adolescence is a time of rapid growth during which 20% of final adult height and 50% of adult weight are attained. Teens have increased iron needs due to increases in blood volume and muscle mass.
- Males usually regain adequate iron status at the end of their growth spurt while females are more likely to remain deficient due to increased iron requirements from menses, poor diet, and in some cases, pregnancy and lactation.
- The causes of iron deficiency include:
  - Blood loss (including loss from heavy menstrual flow).
  - Poor dietary intake of iron.
  - The Centers for Disease Prevention (CDC) estimates that among adolescents, 75% of females and 17% of males do not get enough iron in their diet.
  - Poor iron absorption.
  - Less common causes of anemia include hemolytic anemias, hemoglobinopathies, chronic illness, blood loss and malignancies.

ASSESSMENT

HISTORY

History of Present Illness

- Fatigue, decrease in appetite, poor physical performance, and/or dropping school grades may be presenting complaints.
- Rarely, teens may experience "**pica**," which is a persistent and compulsive craving to eat nonfood items such as dirt, cornstarch, or ice chips. One of many causes of pica may be a lack of iron in the diet.
- Assess menstrual history. Females with **menorrhagia** and/or **metrorrhagia** (heavy menses greater than 80 ml/month or frequent bleeding, respectively) are at higher risk.
- Patients may report melena or hematochezia and these symptoms should raise the concern for **peptic ulcer disease, Meckle's diverticulum**, and **NSAID** or **aspirin** use.

Past Medical History

- Has there been IDA in the past and if so, did the teen respond to treatment?
- Teens living with chronic illness are more likely to be anemic than healthy teens.
- Certain inherited conditions, such as **glucose-6-phosphate dehydrogenase deficiency (G6PD)** can exhibit non-immune hemolytic anemia. Males are much more likely to have this disorder than females.
- Consider a patient's ethnic background in your evaluation. **Sickle cell disease** is more common in African-Americans and **thalassemia** can be seen across several ethnic groups.

Family History

- Questions about prior transfusions in family members, gallstone disease or splenomegaly may uncover an inheritable form of hemolytic anemia or hemoglobinopathy.

Diet History

- A diet that lacks sufficient iron, vitamin B12 and folic acid can lead to anemia.
- This is more likely to occur in teens who follow strict vegetarian or vegan diets or have low intake of meat, fish, poultry or iron-fortified foods.
- IDA occurs more frequently in those who have a low intake of vitamin C rich foods.
- Also consider IDA in teens who frequently diet, restrict eating or skip meals or suffer chronic or significant weight loss (i.e. those with **eating disorders**).

Medications

- Some **antibiotics, anti-inflammatory drugs** and **anticonvulsants** can cause suppression of the bone marrow and subsequent hemolytic anemia.

Social History

- IDA is more common in those who abuse substances (usually correlates with poor diet).
- Recent teen immigrants from developing countries may experience higher rates of IDA from poor nutrition and/or parasitosis (i.e. **ancylostoma duodenale**).

Review of Systems

- Does the patient have signs or symptoms of an infection? **Hepatitis** and **parvovirus** can suppress the bone marrow whereas **Epstein-Barr virus, cytomegalovirus** and **mycoplasma pneumonia** can all cause a hemolytic anemia.
- Teens may complain of dizziness or lightheadedness, headaches, shortness of breath or taste disturbance.

PHYSICAL

- Anemia may be mild to severe; even those with mild anemia can present with symptoms of weakness and fatigue.

Vital Signs

- Tachycardia may occur with mild to severe anemia.

Anthropometric Measurements

- Measure weight and height.
- Patients who are underweight (BMI $<$5th percentile) or obese (BMI $>$95th percentile) likely have poor diets placing them at higher risk of IDA.

HEENT

- Observe for pale conjunctiva and/or gums, blue hue of the sclera or angular stomatitis.

Cardiac

- A flow murmur may be heard on exam.

Skin

- Pallor
- May also notice spooning of the nails.

STUDIES

- Recent guidelines (CDC, Bright Futures) recommend anemia screening in females one year post menarche and every 5 years thereafter, unless risk factors indicate annual screening.
- Screening is not indicated in males unless there are risk factors. Males participate in endurance sports at an early age and 17% of adolescent males do not get enough iron in their diet: a single screening during the early stage of adolescent development (12–14 year) can be considered.

Hemoglobin

- An iron-containing protein found in red blood cells that is a more sensitive and direct indicator of anemia than the hematocrit.
- A venous sample is more reliable than a finger stick.

- Presumptive diagnosis of IDA can be made if the hemoglobin is low and there is response to iron therapy after 1 month.
- Hemoglobin levels usually rise after 2–3 weeks on iron therapy. If it does not improve, inquire about non-adherence.
- If adherent to treatment and there is no rise in hemoglobin, further testing is indicated to rule out other causes of anemia such as thalassemia minor.

Mean Corpuscular Volume (MCV)

- A measure of red blood cell size that indicates IDA or thalassemia when less than the lower limit of normal (microcytic).
- The Mentzer index can be used to differentiate IDA from beta-thalassemia.
  - If the MCV divided by the red blood cell (RBC) count is greater than 13, a diagnosis of IDA is supported.
  - If the MCV divided by RBC value is less than 13, a diagnosis of beta-thalassemia is supported.

Red Blood Cell Distribution Width (RDW)

- Used to determine the cause of anemia and compares red blood cell size in a blood sample.
- A low MCV and RDW support the diagnosis of IDA.

Reticulocyte Count

- Measures the rate of new red blood cell (reticulocyte) production by the bone marrow and subsequent release into the bloodstream.
- Reticulocytes are in the blood for about 2 days before developing into mature red blood cells. Normally, about 1% to 2% of the red blood cells in the blood are reticulocytes.
- The reticulocyte count rises when there is significant blood loss or in disease states where red blood cells are destroyed prematurely.
- Conversely, a low reticulocyte count in the face of anemia suggests decreased production or release of red blood cells, as may be seen in IDA.
- In the case of IDA, a reticulocyte count is ordered to measure the response to iron therapy treatment. Reticulocyte counts rise after a few days of supplement use.

White Blood Cells and Platelets

- If these indices are low, consider aplastic anemia.
- Thrombocytosis can sometimes be seen with IDA as well as inflammatory processes.
- Thrombocytopenia can be seen with systemic illnesses such as lupus.

Ferritin

- Is a measure of iron stored in the body. Low ferritin and hemoglobin levels confirms the diagnosis of IDA.
- High levels indicate an inflammatory process.

Total Iron Binding Capacity

- Measures the ability of blood to bind with iron via transferrin, and is elevated with IDA.

Iron Level

- If normal, it rules out IDA and other causes of anemia need to be investigated.
- Low levels confirm a diagnosis of IDA.

Sickle Cell Prep and Hemoglobin Electrophoresis

- Consider if a hemoglobinopathy is suspected.

Coomb's Test and Haptoglobin

- May detect hemolytic anemias.

G6PD

- To determine risk of hemolysis with medication.

Peripheral Blood Smear

- Small cell size and hypopigmentation (hypochromia) suggests IDA or a hemoglobinopathy.
- Macrocytosis suggests vitamin B deficiency.

- Anisocytosis and poikilocytosis suggests hemolysis.
- Blasts indicate an underlying malignancy.

C-Reactive Protein and Sedimentation Rate

- May indicate inflammation or infection; however, a high sedimentation rate is usually a non-specific finding with any type of anemia.

Complete Metabolic Panel

- In cases where chronic illness is suspected.

SPECIAL TEST

Bone Marrow Biopsy

- When either malignancy or aplastic anemia is suspected.

DISPOSITION

- Replenishing iron stores and raising the hemoglobin level is the goal of IDA therapy. Treatment involves iron supplements (ferrous sulfate) and dietary education to include foods rich in iron and vitamin C (aids iron absorption).
- Iron supplements are indicated when diet alone cannot replenish iron stores to normal.
- Supplemental iron is available in 2 forms: ferric and ferrous.
  - Ferrous iron salts (i.e. ferrous sulfate, ferrous fumarate and ferrous gluconate) are better absorbed forms of iron.
  - Elemental iron is the amount of iron in a supplement that is available for absorption.
  - Ferrous fumerate contains 33% of elemental iron, ferrous sulfate 20% and ferrous gluconate 12%.
  - The CDC recommends 50–60 mg of oral elemental iron (found in one 300 mg ferrous sulfate tablet), twice daily for three months for the therapeutic treatment of IDA.
  - In very rare situations, IM or IV iron may be warranted.
- To increase adherence with iron therapy, it is important to educate the adolescent on the following factors:

  - Constipation and dark stools are common side effects.
  - Iron is best absorbed if taken on an empty stomach.
  - Iron pills maintain potency stored away from heat and humidity (<u>not</u> in the bathroom).
  - To prevent poisoning, keep away from young children and pets.
  - Antacids and milk can interfere with iron absorption.
  - It is important to follow-up with a physician to monitor the success of treatment.

- Dietary sources of iron are found in both animal (heme iron) and plant (nonheme) sources, and heme iron is much better absorbed than non-heme.
  - Animal sources include red meats, fish and poultry.
  - Plant sources include lentils and beans, as well as non-heme iron added to fortify foods.
- For other causes of anemia, consider a hematology consult.

What is unique about anemia in adolescents?

- Adolescents are at higher risk for IDA due to increased iron needs during puberty, menstrual losses, poor dietary intake of iron and poor dietary habits.
- Adolescent females are 10 times more likely than boys to be deficient in iron.
- A diet rich in iron is essential to maintain adequate iron stores.
- IDA can be prevented by discouraging meal-skipping and dieting and encouraging the key recommendations established by "2010 Dietary Guidelines for Americans," jointly issued and updated every 5 years by the Department of Agriculture (USDA) and the Department of Health and Human Services (HHS).

TEST YOUR KNOWLEDGE ANSWERS

25. C. This teen has microcytic anemia confirmed on smear review. The differential diagnosis for microcytic hypochromic anemia includes IDA, thalassemia trait (alpha and beta), as well as lead poisoning. Given the history of heavy menses, low reticulocyte count and slightly elevated platelet count, IDA is the most likely diagnosis. Autoimmune hemolytic

anemias are typically normocytic and characterized by a high reticulocyte count. Acute leukemias are important to consider whenever more than one cell lineage is affected-in this case, the anemia is isolated. Thalassemia trait is a possibility, and should be considered if the patient does not respond to oral iron supplementation. A full iron panel including ferritin, TIBC and serum iron should distinguish IDA from thalassemia, as these tests are normal in thalassemia patients. A hemoglobin electrophoresis can identify and confirm any hemoglobinopathy.

26. E. In this case, the normal iron panel argues against IDA. Furthermore, smear findings of homogeneously small cells with prominent targeting, are classic for thalassemia. The history of IDA resistant to oral iron therapy is classic for undiagnosed thalassemia trait (alpha or beta). Beta thalassemia trait always demonstrates a high Hgb A2 on electrophoresis, which is low normal in our case. Furthermore, alpha thalassemia is more common in patients of Southeast Asian heritage.

WEB REFERENCES

- American Academy of Family Physicians (www.aafp.org):
  - Killip S, Bennett JM, Chambers MD (2007) 'Iron Deficiency Anemia' American Family Physician. 2007;75(5);671–678, Retrieved from http://www.aafp.org/afp/2007/0301/p671.html
- Centers for Disease Control and Prevention (http://www.cdc.gov)
  - Iron and Iron Deficiency Anemia (February 23, 2011), Retrieved from http://www.cdc.gov/nutrition/every one/basics/vitamins/iron.html
  - Recommendations and Reports: Recommendations to Prevent and Control Iron Deficiency in the United States. MMWR. 1998;47(RR-3); 1–36, Retrieved from http://www.cdc.gov/mmwr/preview/mmwrhtml/00051880.htm
- Stang J, Story M. eds. Guidelines for adolescent nutrition services. Minneapolis, MN: Center for Leadership, Education and Training in Maternal and Child Nutrition, Division of Epidemiology and Community Health, School of Public Health, University of Minnesota; 2005: Chapter: Iron Deficiency Anemia by Irene Alton: http://www.epi.umn.edu/let/pubs/img/adol_ch9.pdf

Additional Clinician and Patient Resources:

- American Society of Hematology: 'Iron Deficiency Anemia' (2011), Retrieved from http://www.hematology.org/Patients/Blood-Disorders/Anemia/5263.aspx
- Cafasso, J (2012) 'Iron Deficiency Anemia', Retrieved from http://www.healthline.com/health/iron-deficiency-anemia

- eHow Health: The Signs and Symptoms of Anemia in Teens, Retrieved from http://www.ehow.com/about5218572_signs-symptoms-anemia-teens.html#ixzzlAZpGMknN
- MedlinePlus, NIH. Iron deficiency anemia-children, Retrieved from www.nlm.nih.gov/medlineplus/ency/article/007134.htm
- Office of Dietary Supplements, NIH. Dietary supplement fact sheet. Available online: http://ods.od.nih.gov/factsheets/Iron-HealthProfessional/
- USDA: Center for Nutrition Policy and Promotion: http://www.cnpp.usda.gov
- US National Library of Medicine, NIH. Iron deficiency anemia, http://www.nhlbi.nih.gov/health/health-topics/topics/ida/

18

HEADACHES: COMMON, CHRONIC AND RECURRENT

Stephanie Addison

TEST YOUR KNOWLEDGE

27. A 15 year old male presents to the office because of persistent unilateral pulsating frontal headache that is worsened with bright lights and sound. He refuses examination with the ophthalmoscope. There are no focal neurological findings on physical exam. What is the next *BEST* step in evaluation of his headache?

    A. Laboratory studies to rule out temporal arteritis.
    B. Lumbar puncture to measure cerebrospinal fluid pressure.
    C. Brain Imaging.
    D. First C, then B.
    E. No further evaluation is warranted and he may begin symptomatic treatment.

28. A 13 year old female presents to your office with her mother who is very concerned because there has been a change in the pattern of her daughter's usual migraine headaches. According to her mother, the patient developed a fever, headache, fatigue and seems to be moving in and out of her usual consciousness. A few days prior to presentation she had mild cold symptoms. On physical exam you notice patient has an altered mental

Refer to end of chapter for answers on page 213.

status and abnormal exam. What is the next *BEST* step in evaluation of this patient?

A. Send the patient to the lab for a complete blood count and viral panel and then home with supportive care instructions.
B. Obtain a lumbar puncture in your office.
C. Send the patient to Emergency Department for laboratory studies, head CT and further management.
D. Obtain an MRI as an outpatient.
E. None of the above.

"My head hurts all the time and I can't even study. What should I do?"

BACKGROUND

- Headaches become increasingly prevalent in adolescence and are a frequent chief complaint.
- By mid-adolescence, a higher ratio of females suffer from chronic and recurrent headaches.
- Chronic headaches are defined as headaches that occur more than 15 days per month for at least 3 months.
- Headaches are categorized as either primary or secondary.
  - Primary headaches (i.e. migraines, tension and cluster headaches) have no underlying demonstrable pathology.
  - Secondary headaches are related to an underlying cause such as head and/or neck trauma, intracranial pathology, infection (i.e. meningitis) or use or withdrawal of medications.
- For isolated, acute severe headaches, refer to Chapter 59.

ASSESSMENT

HISTORY

History of Present Illness

Pain characteristics:

Timing

- How often do headaches occur and how long do they last? **Primary headaches** have a variable time course with some migraines lasting up to 72 hours.
- When do the headaches occur? Early morning headaches or headaches that wake the teen up at night are concerning for **intracranial pathology.**
- What is the acuity of the headache? **Cluster headaches** occur suddenly while **migraine** and **tension headaches** have gradual onset or a waxing and waning course.

Quality

- What is the quality of the headache? Is it sharp, stabbing, pulsating, dull or achy?
- A pulsating headache may be a sign of a **migraine headache without aura.**

Severity

- A change in pattern or sudden onset of a very severe headache warrants immediate evaluation to rule out **subarachnoid hemorrhage**.

Location

- Where is the pain located and does it radiate? **Cluster headaches** are usually unilateral whereas **tension headaches** may be bilateral and often have a band like distribution around the head. **Migraines** can present either unilaterally (hemicrania), bilaterally or they may switch sides on different occasions.
- Are there any relieving or aggravating factors? Patients may complain of phonophobia, photophobia or report that their headaches improve with rest.
- Trimenical neuralgia, or tic douloureux, is associated with pain concentrated in the facial region.

- What symptoms are associated with the headache?
  - Associated nausea, vomiting, blurry vision, or weakness may distinguish **migraines** from **tension or cluster headaches.**
  - Morning emesis without nausea may be a sign of more serious etiology such as **intracranial mass.**
- Does that patient know when the headache is going to occur?
  - Do menses herald the headaches?
  - Are there any warning signs? An aura (flickering lights) may be a sign of an imminent **migraine with aura.**
- Poor sleep habits (i.e. going to bed late and waking early for school) can trigger headaches.
- Poor dietary habits (i.e. skipping meals) and poor hydration can also trigger headaches.

Past Medical History

- A thorough history is essential in the work up of chronic and recurrent headaches.
- Viral upper respiratory infections (URIs) may be associated with fevers and headache.
- A history of poorly controlled hypertension could signal a hypertensive crisis.
- A history of allergic rhinitis could herald sinusitis with headaches.
- Does the patient have a history of hydrocephalus and/or VP shunt placement? A headache could indicate shunt failure.
- A history of HIV or cancer may suggest underlying infection or malignancy.
- Rapid weight gain or morbid obesity may lead to **pseudotumor cerebri.**

Medications

- Obtain a complete list of medications, supplements or herbal medications that the patient has used: overuse or withdrawal may be a precipitating factor.
- Be aware that the prolonged use of anlagesics can cause or prolong headaches.
- Headaches could also occur as a medication side effect (e.g. Fluoxetine and other SSRIs).
- A number of medications including but not limited to oral contraceptives, isotretinoin, minocycline, tetracycline, nitrofurantoin, phenytoin, steroids and sulfa drugs can induce **pseudotumor cerebri,** an increased intracranial pressure.

Social

- Are there any school or life related stressors?
- Illicit substance use, including marijuana and other street drugs, could cause headaches.
- Teens recovering from an alcohol or drug binge may experience headaches when "hungover."

Review of Systems

- Itchy eyes, nasal congestion, rhinorrhea, post nasal drip and itchy throat are all characteristic features of **allergic rhinitis**, that if poorly controlled, could manifest as sinus pressure and headache.
- Purulent nasal discharge, nasal obstruction or frontal maxillary pain could signal an underlying **sinus infection.**
- Patients who report difficulty seeing the blackboard or blurry vision may have poor vision with headaches occurring at the end of the school day because of frequent eye straining.
- Reports of blurred vision, diplopia or vision loss, tinnitus, dizziness and/or nausea with symptoms that get worse during physical activity suggests **pseudotumor cerebri.** Untreated, this can lead to blindness.
- Early morning projectile emesis without nausea can signal a **brain tumor.**

PHYSICAL

Vital Signs

- Fever suggests an underlying infection.
- Assess for elevations in blood pressure.

HEENT

- Vision screening when a patient reports blurry vision or changes to visual acuity. Patients with headaches require fundoscopic evaluation to rule out papilledema.
- Inflammed or boggy turbinates and/or frontal-maxillary tenderness can occur with URIs, allergic rhinitis or sinus congestion.
- Fluid noted behind the tympanic membranes could indicate inflammation along the eustachian tube that can occur with allergic rhinitis or acute URIs. Evaluate for signs of otitis media or externa which could also trigger headaches.

Neurological Exam

A complete neurological evaluation is always warranted.

- Assess baseline mental status, as altered sensorium may require more urgent evaluation.

- Assess for nuchal rigidity or other meningeal signs.
- Complete a fundoscopic exam to assess optic disc margins for signs of papilledema, a hallmark of increased intracranial pressure.
- Assess for localizing neurological deficits.

STUDIES

- Laboratory studies, lumbar puncture and EEG are *not* considered routine studies in the evaluation of headaches.

CT or MRI Study

- Consider if exam findings include neurological deficits.
- If a brain tumor or pseudotumor cerebri is suspected, neuroimaging should be obtained PRIOR to doing a lumbar puncture to measure CNS fluid pressure.
- Consider in cases of suspected trauma (as teens may hide having been in a fight or accident) or when more serious pathology is suspected such as malignancy or subarachnoid hemorrhage.

TREATMENT

- A variety of treatment approaches, both non-pharmacologic and pharmacologic, can help manage headaches.

Non-Pharmacologic Treatment Strategies

- A headache diary can be a useful tool to define headache characteristics, identify triggers or aggravating factors and help educate teens about headache prevention strategies.
  - For example, a teen may discover that their headaches are worse after a poor night's rest. They can then work to improve sleep habits to prevent future headaches.
- Improve sleep hygiene, physical activity and fluid intake.
- Encourage eating three healthy, well balanced meals per day.
- Consider dietary changes when there is a link between certain foods and onset of headache:

- Monosodium glutamate (MSG) is found in many food products and may exacerbate headaches, especially migraines, and should be avoided.
- Caffeine may also exacerbate migraines.

- Decrease and/or gradually discontinue use of products with caffeine including teas, sodas, coffees and chocolate to avoid caffeine withdrawal headaches.
- Biofeedback therapy has been proven beneficial.
- Some advocate massage, acupuncture and homeopathy, with less evidence.

Pharmacologic Treatment

- The first line of treatment for headaches are over the counter analgesics such as acetaminophen or NSAIDs.
- There are a number of abortive and preventive prescription drugs available to treat headaches (Table 1).

DISPOSITION

- If there are no concerning findings on history or physical exam, primary headaches are likely to be the underlying etiology of chronic headaches.
- Treatment should include a combined approach with non-pharmacological modalities such as lifestyle changes and pharmacologic treatment if warranted.
- If the patient is not responsive to appropriate medical intervention or if the clinician is not comfortable prescribing preventive medications, consultation with a neurologist is warranted.

What is unique about headaches in adolescents?

- Teens may *overuse* over the counter headache medications, often exacerbating headaches.
- Teens on oral contraceptives may need to switch to a different form of contraception if their migraine headaches worsen.
- Menstruating females can experience headaches before and during menses secondary to hormonal influence.
- More commonly, adolescents are obtaining higher doses of caffeine from energy, sports, soda and coffee drinks that may exacerbate headaches.

- Obese teens with rapid weight gain and those on medications such as birth control pills, may develop pseudotumor cerebri.
- Teens, especially competitive athletes, may not share a history of head trauma. Post-concussion headaches should be considered, especially if school performance deteriorates or there are reports of problems with memory.
- Adolescents may have co-existing conditions such as hypertension or diabetes which may alter a clinician's choice of medication.

TEST YOUR KNOWLEDGE ANSWERS

27. E. A patient presenting with a history concerning for migraines and normal neurological exam does not require further studies.
28. C. This patient has a very concerning history: a change in the usual pattern of headaches is always alarming. She has altered mental status, a headache and fever, which should make the provider suspicious for encephalitis. She warrants further evaluation as there are many etiologies for meningo-encephalitis. A head CT should be obtained prior to lumbar puncture as she may have increased intracranial pressure due to a yet undiagnosed intracranial pathology.

Table 1. Pharmacologic Therapies to Treat Headaches.

Abortive Therapies	Acetaminophen Ibuprofen Naproxen Sodium Ergotamine Tartrate 5-HT Agonists
Preventive Therapies	Cyproheptadine Topiramate Valproic Acid Gabapentin Amitriptyline Nortiptyline Naproxen Sodium Verapamil Propanolol
Alternative and Complementary Medicine	Vitamin B2 Calcium Magnesium Essential Fatty Acids Butterbur Feverfew 5- Hydroxytryptophan Coenzyme Q10

WEB REFERENCES

- Kabbouche MA, Gilman DK. 'Management of migraine in adolescents', Neuropsychiatric Disease and Treatment. 2008 June;4(3);535–548, retrieved from http://www.ncbi.nlm.nih.gov/pmc/articles/PMC2526375/
- Lewis, DW. 'Headaches in Children and Adolescents', American Family Physician. 2002 Feb 15;65(4);625–633, Retrieved from http://www.aafp.org/afp/2002/0215/p625.html
- Shah UH, Kalra V. 'Review Article: Pediatric Migraine', International Journal of Pediatrics. 2009, retrieved from http://www.hindawi.com/journals/ijped/2009/424192/
- Tkachuk GA, et al. 'Factors Associated With Migraine-Related Quality of Life and Disability in Adolescents: A Preliminary Investigation', Headache. 2003 October;43(9):950–955, retrieved from http://www.ncbi.nlm.nih.gov/pmc/articles/PMC2128716/

Additional Clinician and Patient Resources:

- HealthyChildren.org, Teenagers and headaches: When It's Cause for Concern (last updated 11/19/2012), retrieved from http://www.healthychildren.org/English/health-issues/conditions/head-neck-nervous-system/pages/Teenagers-and-Headaches-When-Its-Cause-for-Concern.aspxnfstatus=401&nftoken=00000000-0000-0000-0000-000000000000&nfstatusdescription=ERROR%3 a+No+local+token
- Migraine Headache Guide, retrieved from http://www.webmd.com/migraines-headaches/guide/migraines-headaches-overview
- National Headache Foundation (2013), retrieved from http://www.headaches.org/
- Teenagers and Headaches: When It's Cause for Concern (last updated 11/19/2012), retrieved from http://www.healthychildren.org/English/health-issues/conditions/head-neck-nervous-system/pages/Teenagers-and-Headaches-When-Its-Cause-for-Concern.aspx
- Teens Health from Nemours: Migraine Headaches, retrieved from http://kidshealth.org/teen/diseases conditions/brain nervous/migraines.html

19

BELL'S PALSY (7th NERVE OR FACIAL NERVE PALSY)

Jonathan Fanburg

TEST YOUR KNOWLEDGE

29. A 15 year old female, presenting with sudden right facial palsy with both the top and bottom part of the face involved, is mortified by her appearance. What is the next step?
    A. Give prednisone for a week followed by a week of tapering.
    B. Give anti-viral medication for a week.
    C. Obtain an EMG at 3 weeks to determine prognosis.
    D. Counsel her that her findings are likely to go away within 3 weeks.
    E. All the above.
30. Every patient who presents with a facial palsy should have the following:
    A. An MRI of the nerve to rule out tumor.
    B. An EMG of the nerve to determine prognosis.
    C. A Lyme titer to rule out Lyme disease.
    D. An otoscope exam to look for cholesteotoma.
    E. Ibuprofen to decrease inflammation.

Refer to end of chapter for answers on page 221.

A 15 year old female comes into the urgent care clinic with a 1 day history of being unable to move the right side of her face. She is very upset about her appearance and is crying.

BACKGROUND

- Most teens with unilateral facial paralysis will have Bell's Palsy.
- Symptoms that make the diagnosis more likely include unilateral involvement of both the upper and lower parts of the face.
- Use of steroids improves prognosis, but most cases resolve without intervention.

ASSESSMENT

HISTORY

- History is only marginally contributory to the diagnosis.

History of Present Illness

- Upper respiratory illness precedes the palsy.
- Ear tingling or pain commonly precede exam findings by 1–2 days.
- Palsy has a rapid onset (1–2 days).

Past Medical History

- Critical history can exclude other causes of facial palsies:
  - History of tick bite, antecedent skin rash, heart block, arthritis, vertigo, hearing loss, or swelling/erythema of the face preceding palsy suggest **Lyme disease.**
  - The patient is NOT likely to have lyme disease if coexisting findings are not present before or at the time of the palsy.
  - Multiple asymptomatic viruses/bacteria are possible causes which may or may not have exam findings, but won't change the management: **herpes zoster, cytomegalovirus, Epstein Barr virus, adenovirus, rubella, mumps, influenza B, coxsackievirus, chicken pox, mycoplasma, cat-scratch, and rickettsial infection.**

PHYSICAL

HEENT

- Exam reveals **absent nerve function in the upper and lower face *only* on the affected side.**
- Typical symptoms appear unilaterally and can include:
  - Inability to create forehead wrinkles or raise eyebrow.
  - Inability to fully close eye.
  - Loss of nasolabial fold.
  - Inability to raise corner of mouth with possible drooping of involved corner.
  - Loss of taste in the anterior 2/3 of the tongue.
- Critical exam findings will exclude other causes of facial palsies.
  - Bilateral facial involvement is more likely to be seen with **Guillain-Barré syndrome** (also has diminished lower extremity reflexes) or **sarcoidosis** (rare in teens).
  - Voice changes and difficulty with oral secretions are found with **Guillain-Barré syndrome, poliomyelitis,** and **brain stem gliomas.**
  - Prolonged onset of palsy symptoms or palsy not recovering to normal after 3–4 months is reason to work up for **tumor.**
  - The ability to wrinkle the forehead or move the orbital muscle suggests that the palsy is solely in the lower part of the face. This type of palsy suggests a central upper motor neuron facial palsy or supranuclear lesion (like **brainstem glioma**) on the contralateral side.
  - Preceding facial twitch or spasm suggests irritation from a **tumor.**
  - Exam of the ear is warranted: **bacterial infection** of the inner ear as well as **cholesteatomas** can cause a palsy.
  - Patients with a fissured tongue, facial swelling and facial paralysis may have the rare triad seen in adolescents called **Melkersson Rosenthal Syndrome,** a syndrome that doesn't have a known cause or treatment.

STUDIES

Laboratory tests are not indicated unless the exam is not fully consistent with the diagnosis.

Lyme Titer

- May be useful in endemic areas but titer testing should not be done unless there are coexisting symptoms.
- IgM may be falsely negative in the first 3–6 weeks.

CT and MRI

- Useful if tumor or malignancy is suspected.

EMG

- Used to predict resolution of symptoms but only consider after at least 3 weeks of palsy.

DISPOSITION

- Most patients (85–99%) recover from Bell's Palsy without any treatment within 3 weeks but symptoms can persist upto 6 months. It is important to reassure your teen patient.
- Steroids can improve the prognosis if initiated in the first 2 weeks of symptoms (1–2 mg/kg/day, max 60 mg/day) for 7 days, followed by a 1 week taper. Maximal efficacy is seen if initiated within 1 day of symptoms.
- Antiviral medications have no benefit alone, yet may have some benefit when combined with steroids in cases where herpes virus is the cause. Current recommendations are to take antivirals for 1 week as data is conflicting.
- Protection of the eye surface with lubricants, tears, sunglasses, and/or a patch is indicated.
- Prognosis is better when facial nerve involvement is limited and when there are signs of recovery in the first 3 weeks.
- The obvious psychosocial implications of a palsy in adolescents need to be addressed.

What is unique about Bell's Palsy in adolescents?

- An adolescent's sense of time can make it very difficult for him or her to comprehend that it could take several weeks for a full recovery to be made. Self-image can be so threatened that teens may become desperate.

- Adolescent girls may be specifically afflicted as so much of their social life is infused with ideas of personal beauty. Depressive episodes, withdrawal and even suicidal ideations may complicate Bell's Palsy recovery.
- It is important to provide reassurance to the teen patient as well as close follow up to ensure uncomplicated recovery.

TEST YOUR KNOWLEDGE ANSWERS

29. E. There are limited interventions effective at treating Bell's Palsy; fortunately, most cases resolve without intervention. Steroids have some limited benefit. Antivirals may have benefit when used with steroids (no benefit alone) and are recommended. EMG is indicated after 3+ weeks if the patient has continued symptoms. Early initiation of steroids and less severe palsy are associated with better prognosis. Improvement in the first 3 weeks versus later, has a better likelihood of recovery.
30. D. Unlike many diseases in which the history is the most important part of the diagnosis, an exam is the most important component when evaluating an adolescent with Bell's Palsy. In addition to determining the unilateral involvement of facial nerves in both the upper and lower part of the face, it is important to rule out other diagnoses. In particular, examine patients carefully for other nerve palsies in the face, otitis media and cholesteatoma, rash and decreased distal reflexes. MRI is only indicated if the patient doesn't have classic Bell's Palsy exam findings and has a slower onset of symptoms. Lyme titers are only indicated if the patient has other Lyme disease findings or lives in an endemic region. EMG is only indicated if resolution does not occur after 3+ weeks. Ibuprofen is not used for treating Bell's Palsy, but one may use steroids and anti-viral medications.

WEB REFERENCES

- Anderson, P. 'New AAN Guideline on Bell's Palsy', Neurology. 2012;79;l–5, retrieved from http://www.medscape.com/viewarticle/774056
- Gronseth GS, Paduga R. 'Evidence-based guideline update: Steroids and antivirals for Bell palsy: Report of the Guideline Subcommittee of the American Academy of

Neurology', Neurology. 2012. Retrieved from http://www.neurology.org/content/early/2012/11/07/WNL.0b013e318275978c.full.pdf

- Murthy JMK, Saxena AB. 'Bell's palsy: Treatment guidelines', Annals of Indian Academy of Neurology. 2011 July;14(supplel);S70–S72, retrieved from http://www.ncbi.nlm.nih.gov/pmc/articles/PMC3152161/
- PubMed Health: Bell's Palsy (last reviewed May 12, 2012), retrieved from http://www.ncbi.nlm.nih.gov/pubmedhealth/PMH0001777/

Additional Clinician and Patient Resources:

- Bells Palsy Association: www.bellspalsy.org.uk
- Bell's Palsy Information Site: www.bellspalsy.ws
- National Institute of Neurological Disorders and Strokes (last updated September 4, 2012), retrieved from www.ninds.nih.gov/disorders/bells/bells.htm
- TeensHealth from Nemours: Bell's Palsy, retrieved from http://kidshealth.org/teen/diseases_conditions/brain_nervous/bells_palsy.html

20

ASTHMA, EXERCISE INDUCED BRONCHOSPASM (EIB) AND VOCAL CORD DYSFUNCTION (VCD)

Anthony P. Acquavella

TEST YOUR KNOWLEDGE

31. An adolescent seen frequently for poorly controlled asthma, including 2 prior ICU admissions, should be evaluated for vocal cord dysfunction if complaining of:

    A. Stridor
    B. Hoarseness
    C. Throat tightness
    D. Symptoms associated with stress or anxiety
    E. All the above

32. All the following will improve control of exercise induced bronchospasm (EIB) *EXCEPT*:

    A. Pretreatment with an inhaled short-acting $beta_2$ agonist.
    B. Adequate warm up period before engaging in sports.
    C. Covering the nose and mouth during cold weather.
    D. Participating in sports later in the day.
    E. Pretreatment with an inhaled long-acting $beta_2$ agonist.

Refer to end of chapter for answer on page 230.

"My 16 year old son has been having trouble breathing and is now using his sister's inhaler." This patient recently began having episodes of shortness of breath with exercise.

BACKGROUND

- Reactive airway disease and exercise induced bronchospasm (EIB) are usually a manifestation of asthma while marked dyspnea with inspiratory stridor may be due to vocal cord dysfunction.
- Wheezing is common in adolescence while stridor is not.

ASSESSMENT

HISTORY

History of Present Illness

- Assess for any current symptoms such as shortness of breath with activities or at rest.
- Assess rescue inhaler use. How often is the teen using their rescue inhaler?
- Review medication compliance and if there is a need for prescription refills. Is the teen using daily controller medications as prescribed?
- Do symptoms occur at night?

Past Medical History

- Did the patient experience wheezing, respiratory infections and/or difficulty breathing in infancy or childhood?
- Is there a history of recurrent pneumonias or bronchopulmonary dysplasia that could predispose the patient to lung damage.
- Determine severity of asthma course. Is there a history of emergency department visits and/or hospitalizations requiring intensive care admission or intubation?

Family History

- Determine if there is a family history of asthma, allergies, eczema or nasal polyps.

Review of Systems

- Ascertain current symptoms including recurrent episodes of wheezing, nighttime cough, EIB, wheezing associated with exposures to airborne allergens, and/or upper respiratory infections which "settle in the chest" and take up to one week to resolve.
- Assess for prodromal symptoms, rapidity of onset, and symptom duration and frequency.
- Determine limitations to activity due to recurrent symptoms. Estimate the number of exacerbations in the past 6–12 months and calculate missed days from school or work.
- Clarify the degree of EIB, wheezing or coughing during exercise or up to 15–20 minutes thereafter.
- Obtain a list of triggers:
  - Primary or secondary smoke exposure.
  - Indoor allergens such as dust mites, animals and molds.
  - Outdoor allergens such as pollens, trees, grasses and/or seasonal variations.
  - Weather changes including cold weather.
  - Exercise.
  - Upper respiratory infections.
  - Rarely food allergies can cause wheezing or bronchospasm.
- Unusual symptoms such as stridor, hoarseness, throat tightness or symptoms associated with stress or anxiety suggest **vocal cord dysfunction** (VCD). Consider in patients who are difficult to treat or unresponsive to routine medications.

Medications

- Determine current and past medication use including inhaled or oral steroids.
- Have symptoms responded to medications in the past?
- Determine if the teen uses medications appropriately:
  - Does the teen correctly use a spacer with inhalers?
  - Does the teen know how to use a peak flow meter?

- Is the teen overusing medications due to anxiety or inability to understand symptoms?
- Assess current level of symptom control (Table 1).
- Determine the teen's and/or parents' knowledge of asthma, its chronicity as well as their beliefs regarding medication use.

PHYSICAL

Anthropometric Measurements

- Patients should have their height and weight assessed using standard growth charts.
- **Chronic lung disease** may cause a growth delay.

HEENT

- Assess the upper airway for nasal secretions, abnormal turbinates, nasal polyps or enlarged tonsils.

Chest

- Observe for hyperexpansion of the chest or chest wall deformities and auscultate for wheezing, prolonged inspiratory or expiratory phases, and stridor.
- Signs of non-pulmonary causes for shortness of breath such as abnormal heart murmurs, pulmonary or peripheral edema, hepatosplenomegaly or ascites are consistent with **right-sided heart failure**.
- Stridor is typical of **VCD**.

Skin

- Look for atopic dermatitis, eczema or clubbing.

STUDIES

Consider Peak Flow Assessment

- Obtain peak flow meter readings at each office visit.
- Review proper peak flow meter use. Advise patients to:

- Record peak flow readings twice daily for 2–3 weeks *when well* to determine personal best values.
- Record a peak flow reading before and after short-acting $beta_2$ agonist use.
- Use a peak flow meter to determine worsening asthma control and then follow the individualized asthma action plan.
- Optimal peak flow is determined by the patient's height percentile.

Chest Radiograph

- Only when needed to exclude other etiologies or complications such as pneumothorax, pneumonia and middle lobe syndrome.

SPECIAL TESTS

Pulmonary Function Testing (PFT)

- The gold standard for diagnosis and more accurate and reliable than peak flow testing, but requires pulmonary or allergy referral.
- Can be performed with methacholine, histamine, cold air or exercise challenge as needed.
- Expect flattening of the inspiratory curve in patients with VCD.

Allergy Testing

- Consider referral to an allergist for full testing if the patient has significant allergic triggers.

Direct Laryngoscopy

- Refer to an otolaryngologist for direct laryngoscopy if considering VCD.

DISPOSITION

Medical Treatment

- Follow a stepwise approach as detailed below (Table 2):
  - **Step 1** Short-acting $beta_2$ agonist.
  - **Step 2** Low dose inhaled corticosteroid (alternative: leukotriene modifier/ 5-lipoxygenase inhibitor).

- **Step 3** Low dose inhaled corticosteroid plus long-acting $beta_2$ agonist or medium dose inhaled corticosteroid. (Alternative: low dose inhaled corticosteroid plus leukotriene modifier/5-lipoxygenase inhibitor.)
- **Step 4** Medium dose inhaled corticosteroid plus long-acting $beta_2$ agonist. (Alternative: medium dose inhaled corticosteroid plus leukotriene modifier/5 lipoxygenase inhibitor.)
- **Step 5** High dose inhaled corticosteroid plus long-acting $beta_2$ agonist and consider immunomodulator.
- **Step 6** High dose inhaled corticosteroid plus long-acting $beta_2$ agonist plus oral corticosteroid and consider immunomodulator.

- Treat comorbid conditions that may affect the course of asthma (Table 3).

Asthma Action Plan

Teach patients how to:

- Recognize early symptoms of worsening asthma.
- Use a peak flow meter to monitor changes in asthma control.
    - 80–100% of personal best peak flow values: no change in medications.
    - 60–80% of personal best values: adjust medications.
    - Less than 60% of personal best values: seek medical care.
- Develop a plan to adjust medications to treat worsening asthma.
- Develop a plan to monitor response to changes in medication and know when to seek medical care.

Prevention is an Essential Component of Treatment

Take steps to reduce exposure to known triggers for asthma.

- Encourage the teen/family to quit smoking and prohibit smoking in the home or car.
- Reduce exposure to dust mites.
- Encase the mattress and pillows in dust mite proof covers.
- Reduce indoor humidity to below 60% via an air conditioner or dehumidifier.
- Remove carpets if possible.
- Reduce exposure to pet dander by either removing pets with fur from the home or at least from the patient's bedroom.
- Control cockroach exposure.

- Frequent vacuuming by someone else twice weekly or dust mask use when vacuuming.
- Minimize household molds by preventing free standing water from leaky plumbing or wet basements.
- Use air conditioning or air filters to minimize exposure to outdoor pollens.
- Limit exposure to wood burning stoves, kerosene heaters or fireplaces.
- Refrain from eating foods with sulfites if they are a trigger.
- Keep nose and mouth covered in very cold weather.

Exercise Induced Bronchospasm (EIB)

- Determine the degree of EIB, wheezing or cough during exercise or up to 15-20 minutes after.
- Warm up for a significant period of time before beginning any sports activity.
- Check peak flows before beginning activity to assure adequate asthma control.
- Consider pre-sports treatment with a short-acting $beta_2$ agonist.
- Keep nose and mouth covered in very cold weather.

Vocal Cord Dysfunction

- Refer patients to speech therapy and mental health services if needed.

What is unique about caring for adolescents with asthma?

Teens may not know the true severity of their illness or understand that asthma can be life threatening. Review their understanding of the disease including its pathophysiology.

- As teens become more independent, with parents managing their symptoms less, it is important to review their understanding of the need and use of chronic medications.
- Teens should demonstrate the correct use of a metered dose inhaler during an office visit.
- Develop the simplest treatment plan possible.
- Determine barriers that prevent compliance with treatments, such as using medicines at school.

- Explain that peak flow readings indicate times of both good and poor asthma control. This is reassuring to families, especially during times of mild upper respiratory infections.
- Achieving a personal best peak flow allows the adolescent to prove that he/she is well enough to participate in activities such as sports.
- Smoking, often initiated during adolescence, should be considered as a potential trigger for asthma exacerbation.
- The annual flu vaccine is recommended for all asthmatics as they tend to have more severe complications when diagnosed with influenza. The flumist nasal vaccine is contraindicated in asthmatics.
- Adolescents should have frequent scheduled follow-up medical visits to assure a good understanding of the treatment plan, to ensure compliance and to address problems early.
- Anxious adolescents, who may or may not suffer from asthma, can have sudden acute dyspnea and diminished air entry. They may be treated inappropriately either repeatedly or in an intensive care unit, when what they require is outpatient therapy for vocal cord dysfunction.

TEST YOUR KNOWLEDGE ANSWERS

31. E. Many adolescents carry an erroneous diagnosis of asthma when what they actually have is vocal cord dysfunction (VCD). They usually have a history of repeated emergency room visits and are labeled as either non-compliant or in poor control. They are then given repeated courses of oral steroids with no improvement. "Asthmatic" patients with symptoms associated with anxiety or stress not only need an evaluation for an anxiety disorder but also for VCD. A referral to an otolaryngologist for direct laryngoscopy is needed to make the diagnosis.
32. D. Pretreatment with inhaled short-acting $beta_2$ agonists before activity may help for up to 3 hours. Long-acting $beta_2$ agonists (LABA) are also helpful up to 12 hours but have a decreased duration of effect if used daily. Frequent use of a LABA as pretreatment may also disguise poorly controlled asthma. For these reasons a LABA is not recommended for the treatment of EIB. Nedocromil and Cromolyn have been shown to be effective but not as effective as inhaled short-acting $beta_2$ agonists.

An adequate pre-activity warm up is also helpful in decreasing EIB as is covering the nose and mouth.

Table 1. Assessment of Asthma Control.

	Controlled	Partial Control	Not Controlled
Symptoms	≤Twice a week	≥Twice a week	Daily
Nighttime Awakenings	≤Twice a month	1–3 Times a week	≥4 Times a week
Limited Activity	None	Some	Regularly
Beta2 Agonist Use	≤Twice a week	>Twice a week	Several times a week

Table 2. Classes of Medications.

Short-acting Beta2 Agonist	Albuterol
	Levabuterol
	Pirbuterol
Inhaled Corticosteroids	Beclomethasone
	Budesonide
	Flunisolide
	Fluticasone
	Mometasone
	Tramicinolone acetonide
Long-acting Beta2 Agonist	Salmeterol
	Formoterol
Leukotriene Modifiers	Montelukast
	Zafirlukast
	Zileuton (5-lipoxygenase inhibitor)
Immunomodulator	Omalizumab
Combined Inhalers	Fluticasone and Salmeterol
	Budesonide and Formoterol
Other Medications:	
Anticholinergics	Ipratropium bromide
Mast Cell Stabilizers	Cromolyn, Nedocromil
Methylxanthines	Theophyline

Table 3. Comorbid Conditions that May Affect Ashtma Management.

Gastroesophageal Reflux Disease (GERD)	Treating GERD may help control asthma symptoms especially in teens with frequent nighttime symptoms.
Allergic Bronchopulmonary Aspergillosis	Consider in teens with pulmonary infiltrates.
Obesity	Weight reduction may improve overall asthma control.
Obstructive Sleep Apnea (OSA)	Undiagnosed OSA may be a cause of poor asthma control.
Chronic Sinusitis and Rhinitis	Control of upper airway symptoms will improve asthma control.
Depression and Stress	Helping the teen deal with these issues, as well as coping with a chronic disease, could help improve teen's overall health.

WEB REFERENCES

- Akinbami, LJ, Office of Analysis and Epidemiology. 'The State of Childhood Asthma, United States, 1980–2005', 2006 December;381, retrieved from http://www.cdc.gov/nchs/data/ad/ad381.pdf
- Couriel, J. 'Asthma in Adolescence', Pediatric Respiratory Reviews. 2003 March;4(l);47–54, retrieved from http://www.prrjournal.com/article/Sl526-0542(02)00309-3/fulltext
- The Global Initiative for Asthma (GINA) (http://www.ginasthma.com/)
  - Pocket Guide for Asthma Management and Prevention (for adults and children older than 5 years). Updated 2012. Retrieved from http://www.ginasthma.org/local/uploads/files/GINA_Pocket_Guide_2012_wms.pdf
- Lougheed MD, et al. 'Canadian Thoracic Society Asthma Management Continuum — 2010 Consensus Summary for children six years of age and over, and adults'. Canadian Respiratory Journal. 2010 Jan;17(l);15–24 retrieved from http://www.respiratoryguidelines.ca/sites/all/ files/cts_asthma_consensus_summary_2010.pdf
- National Heart, Lung, and Blood Institute
  - Guidelines for the Diagnosis and Management of Asthma, US Department of Health and Human Services (2007), retrieved from http://www.nhlbi.nih.gov/guidelines/asthma/index.htm
  - National Asthma Education and Prevention Program: http://www.nhlbi.nih.gov/about/naepp/naep_pd.htm

Additional Clinician and Patient Resources:

- Canadian Thoracic Society Guidelines (2010), http://www.respiratoryguidelines.ca/guideline/asthma
- Centers for Disease Control (CDC): Asthma and Schools (February 13, 2013), retrieved from http ://www. cdc.gov/HealthyYouth/asthma/
- The Global Initiative for Asthma (GINA) http://www.ginasthma.com/
  - Instructions for Inhaler and Spacer use: http://www.ginasthma.org/documents/ll
- National Heart, Lung, and Blood Institute
  - Patient Education: http://www.nhlbi.nih.gov/health/dci/Diseases/Asthma/Asthma_WhatIs.html
  - Publications for Health Professionals: Asthma, retrieved from http://www.nhlbi.nih.gov/about/naepp/naep_pd.htm

21

GYNECOMASTIA

Amy L. Weiss

TEST YOUR KNOWLEDGE

33. A 14 year old male confides that he feels embarrassed changing clothes in the school locker room because he has breasts. He is otherwise healthy, takes no medicines, and denies illicit drug use. On exam, you note bilateral, firm, rubbery masses under his nipples, measuring about 3 cm each. He is Tanner stage 3 for genital maturation. What is the next *BEST* step in your evaluation?

    A. Obtain an ultrasound of his breasts.
    B. Perform a urine drug screen.
    C. Reassure him that this is a common, benign condition that should resolve on its own.
    D. Check thyroid function as well as testosterone and DHEAS hormone levels.
    E. None of the above.

Refer to end of chapter for answer on page 239.

A 13 year old male presents for his annual physical and his mom reports concern that he has breasts. When addressed, the boy shrugs his shoulders.

BACKGROUND

- Gynecomastia is a benign proliferation of glandular breast tissue in males and is common in adolescence.
- It is thought to be caused by an increased estrogen to androgen ratio, which induces development and maturation of ductal breast tissue. This can result from decreased androgen production or circulating androgens, or increased estrogen or estrogen precursors.
- Typically physiologic, it can also be caused by drugs (Table 1), endocrinopathies or other systemic diseases.

ASSESSMENT

HISTORY

History of Present Illness

- Assess duration of symptoms. How long has the breast tissue been enlarged?
- Is breast enlargement unilateral or bilateral? Gynecomastia often starts unilateral and then is typically bilateral.
- Is there use of marijuana or other illicit drugs (can induce gynecomastia)?

Past Medical History

- Are there any underlying medical problems? Endocrinopathies, liver and kidney diseases can be associated with enlarged breast tissue.
- Inquire about renal disease and symptoms of renal insufficiency such as edema, fatigue, change in urinary habits, and decreased appetite.
- Lack of progression through puberty (delayed maturation of the genitals, no deepening of the voice, no body hair growth, and/or scant muscle mass development) is consistent with hypogonadism (e.g. **Klinefelter's Syndrome**).

Medications

- What medicines is the patient taking? Ask about over-the-counter drugs, supplements, and homeopathic or herbal therapies (Table 1).
- Marked muscular development, severe acne, mood changes and testicular atrophy suggest the use of **anabolic steroids**.

Review of Systems

- Symptoms of weight loss, insomnia, palpitations, hair loss and heat intolerance suggest **hyperthyroidism**.
- Jaundice, itching, easy bruising or bleeding, edema and ascites suggest **cirrhosis**.

PHYSICAL

General

- Look for signs of drug abuse such as injected conjunctiva, altered sensorium, pupillary dilation and needle tracks.

Neck

- Examine the thyroid for the presence of a goiter.

Breasts

- Examine the chest for a firm, rubbery mass, extending concentrically from the nipple. A mass of tissue measuring greater than 0.5 cm in diameter is considered gynecomastia.
- Fat deposition without glandular breast tissue is called **pseudogynecomastia** and can be seen in overweight or obese young men. A ridge of glandular tissue should be felt to confirm true gynecomastia.
- Assess if enlarged tissue is present unilaterally or bilaterally. Breast cancer is extremely rare in men but typically presents unilaterally and is *not* centered on the nipple.

Abdomen

- Examine the abdomen for liver span and ascites.

Genital

- Perform a genital exam for Tanner staging and to look for testicular tumors or atrophy.

STUDIES

- Laboratory tests are unnecessary when certain of the diagnosis.
- Consider thyroid function tests if hypothyroidism is suspected.
- Consider gonadotropin screen for Klinefelter's Syndrome. If elevated, obtain a chromosomal study (XYY).
- Check renal and liver functions if either renal insufficiency or cirrhosis, are suspected, respectively.
- Check serum human chorionic gonadotropin (HCG) if a testicular tumor is suspected.
- Ultrasound is the best modality to evaluate breast tissue in adolescents but is not indicated to evaluate gynecomastia.

DISPOSITION

- Reassure parents and teens that 85–90% of gynecomastia resolves within 6 months to 2 years, but typically by 18 months after presentation.
- Gynecomastia rarely persists beyond the age of 17 years.
- Observe with regular (every 6 months) follow-up until resolved.
- Discontinue any medications that may be causing the gynecomastia.
- Treatment with androgens, selective estrogen receptor modulators, aromatase inhibitors or surgery is rarely required.

What is unique about gynecomastia in adolescents?

- The prevalence of gynecomastia is as high as 69% in teens.
- Gynecomastia can have an onset as early as 10–12 years, with typical peak between 13–14 years.
- Gynecomastia is most commonly seen in boys who are Tanner stage 3.
- Adolescents may be upset about their gynecomastia but may not relay their concerns. Some are teased and bullied and may become withdrawn while

younger adolescents may develop concerns such as "Am I turning into a woman?"

TEST YOUR KNOWLEDGE ANSWER

33. C. Gynecomastia is extremely common in adolescence, typically presenting at age 14 or Tanner stage 3. It is a bilateral enlargement of the glandular breast tissue though it often begins unilateral. If the history and physical exam are consistent with gynecomastia, no further evaluation is needed. Reassure the patient, and follow regularly to ensure resolution.

Table 1. Medications and Drugs that can cause Gynecomastia.

Antiandrogens	Cyproterone acetate Flutamide, Bicalutamide, Nilutamide Finasteride, dutasteride Spironolactone Ketoconazole PC-SPECS (OTC herbal) Lavender oil Tea tree oil
Antibiotics	Ethionamide Isoniazid Ketoconazole Metronidazole
Hormones	Androgens Anabolic steroids Chorionic gonadotropin Estrogens Growth hormone
Chemotherapeutic Drugs	Alkylating agents Methotrexate Vinca alkaloids Combination chemotherapy Imatinib
Cardiovascular Drugs	ACE inhibitors: Captopril, Enalapril Amiodarone

(*Continued*)

Table 1. (*Continued*)

	Calcium channel blockers: Diltiazem, Nifedipine Digitoxin Methyldopa Reserpine
Drugs of Abuse	Alcohol Amphetamines Heroin Marijuana Methadone
Antiulcer Drugs	Cimetidine Ranitidine Omeprazole
Psychoactive Drugs	Diazepam Haloperidol Phenothiazines Tricyclic antidepressants
Miscellaneous	Auranofin Diethylproprion Domperidone Etretinate HAART therapy Metoclopramide Phenytoin Penicillamine Sulindac Theophylline

WEB REFERENCES

- Bembo SA, Carlson HE. 'Gynecomastia: Its features, and when and how to treat it', Cleveland Clinic Journal of Medicine. June 2004;71(6);511–517, retrieved from http://www.ccjm.org/content/71/6/511.full.pdf+html
- Carlson, HE. 'Approach to the Patient with Gynecomastia', The Journal of Clinical Endocrinology & Metabolism', January 2001;96(l);15–21, retrieved from http://jcem.endojournals.org/content/96/l/15.full

- Goldman, RD. 'Drug-induced gynecomastia in children and adolescents', Canadian Family Physician. April 2010;56(4);344–345, retrieved from http://www.cfp.ca/content/56/4/344.full.pdf+html
- Laituri CA, et al. 'Treatment of adolescent gynecomastia', Journal of Pediatric Surgery. 2010;45;650–654, retrieved from http://www.clsnyder.com/Publications/20223338.pdf

Additional Clinician and Patient Resources:

- Emedicine from WebMD, Gynecomastia (updated April 16, 2012), http://emedicine.medscape.com/article/120858-overview
- Teens Health from Nemours: I'm a Guy... So How Come I'm Developing Breasts?: http://kidshealth.org/teen/sexual_health/guys/boybrst.html
- Young Men's Health, Children's Hospital Boston, Gynecomastia: http://www.voungmenshealthsite.org/gynecomastia.html

22

RECURRENT OR CHRONIC ABDOMINAL PAIN

Oscar Taube

TEST YOUR KNOWLEDGE

34. Which of the following statements is true?
    A. Weight loss is a common finding in adolescents with functional abdominal pain.
    B. Adolescents and their families do best with an approach to abdominal pain that strictly separates the pain into organic and stress related causes.
    C. Parents don't believe that chronic abdominal pain in their teens is related to stress.
    D. Irritable bowel syndrome (IBS) is *not* associated with changes in bowel frequency or form.
    E. All the above.
    F. None of the above.

Refer to end of chapter for answer on page 249.

A 17 year old female with several months of sharp, stabbing abdominal pain presents to clinic. She has seen several sub-specialists with an extensive negative diagnostic work up. She and her mother are frustrated: "What's wrong with me! I just want to get better!"

BACKGROUND

- There are a wide range of conditions that can cause chronic or recurrent abdominal pain in adolescents (Table 1).
- Many teens may have functional gastrointestinal disorders (Table 2).
- Clinicians must be alert to "red flag" findings that point to an organic diagnosis (Table 3).
- Stress or psychogenic causes require positive history findings and should not be considered a diagnosis of exclusion.

ASSESSMENT

HISTORY

History of Present Illness

Pain Characteristics

- Night-time pain, awakening from sleep, or pain relieved by food ingestion suggests **peptic ulcer disease (PUD)**. Pain on weekdays (causing school absence) but not on weekends or vacations suggests a **functional/ psychogenic** cause.
- Pain location can help narrow the focus of the differential:
  - Right upper quadrant pain suggests **hepatitis** or **cholecystitis.**
  - Right upper quadrant pain, exacerbated by fatty food intake (especially in an overweight female) suggests **biliary tract disease (cholecystitis, cholelithiasis).**
  - Recurrent right lower quadrant pain suggests **inflammatory bowel disease (IBD)**, sequelae of **pelvic inflammatory disease (PID)** and/or an indolent **tubo-ovarian abscess (TOA).**

  - Epigastric pain suggests **gastritis, PUD, pancreatitis** (especially if the pain is sharp and radiates to back) or **pericarditis.**
  - Periumbilical pain suggests **functional pain, gastroenteritis** or **parasitosis.**
- Recurrent abdominal pain that improves with defecation and is associated with changes in stool frequency or form suggests **irritable bowel syndrome (IBS).**
- Infrequent bowel movements that are hard and painful to pass suggests **constipation.**

A multitude of findings strongly indicate a psychogenic/somatoform disorder (Table 4).

Menstrual History

- Pain occurring with menses suggests primary **dysmenorrhea** or **endometriosis.**
- Recurrent lower abdominal pain in a female who has had PID/TOA suggests **adhesions.**
- Amenorrhea, nausea and weight gain with a history of unprotected sexual intercourse raises concern for **pregnancy** (distention of the broad ligaments can be quite uncomfortable).

Past Medical History

- Prior surgery or diagnosis of PID/TOA increase the risk of painful **adhesions.**

Family History

- A family history of IBD or celiac disease suggests **IBD** or **celiac disease,** respectively.
- The presence of family members with chronic pain or somatoform disorders suggests **psychogenic/functional pain.**

Social History

- Assess psychosocial functioning: HEEADDSSS questions, GAPS questionnaire, Youth Symptom Checklist, and Beck Depression Inventory are good screens for diagnosing psychosocial dysfunction; positive findings suggest a **psychogenic** etiology.
- Alcohol abuse is a marker for psychological stress, and it can cause **gastritis** with associated abdominal pain.

Review of Systems

- Fever, weight loss, bloody stool, joint symptoms, rash, chronic diarrhea, oral ulcers, and growth or pubertal delay suggests **IBD.**

PHYSICAL

Anthropometric Measurements

- Weight, height and BMI calculations are important.
- A low BMI, poor growth and malnutrition suggest an organic diagnosis.

General

- Oral ulcers (aphthous stomatitis) as well as other systemic findings such as peripheral arthritis, episcleritis, uveitis, erythema nodosum or pyoderma gangrenosum suggest **IBD.**

Abdomen

- Check for guarding, rebound tenderness, psoas or obdurater signs and hepatosplenomegaly.

Genital

- Assess Tanner stage as pubertal delay may suggest an organic diagnosis.
- Pelvic exam may be clinically indicated to rule out an indolent **TOA.**

Anal

- Observe for perianal pathology and consider a rectal exam to evaluate the rectal vault.

STUDIES

- Unless the history and physical exam point toward a particular disease process that indicates otherwise, only a *limited* number of tests are appropriate including:

Complete Blood Count (CBC)

- Consider infectious etiology with elevated white count.
- Consider **IBD** with anemia.

ESR or CRP

- Elevations suggest underlying inflammatory condition such as **IBD.**

Urinalysis/Urine Culture

- Consider if a **urinary tract infection** is suspected.

SPECIAL TESTS

Amylase and Lipase

- May uncover recurrent **pancreatitis.**

Liver Enzymes, Bilirubin and Alkaline Phosphatase

- May be elevated with **cholelithiasis.**

Stool Studies

- Occult blood in stools may occur with **IBD** and **PUD.**
- Calprotectin is positive with **granulomatous colitis.**
- H. pylori antigen in stools is positive with **PUD.**

TREATMENT

- Supportive treatment is recommended for functional bowel disease:
- If diagnosed with functional dyspepsia:
  - Discontinue dyspepsia causing medications (i.e. ibuprofen) and foods.
  - Trial H_2 receptor antagonists or proton pump inhibitors.
  - Trial low-dose tricylic antidepressants.
- If diagnosed with IBS and:
  - Diarrhea is the featured symptom, recommend dietary modifications including reduced intake of sorbital, fructose and gas forming vegetables.
  - Constipation is the featured symptom, increase water intake and consider a stool softener.
  - Rifaximin (oral antibiotic) may be therapeutic in severe IBS without constipation.

DISPOSITION

- The clinician's primary goal for an adolescent with abdominal pain is to restore the teen to normal function in family and society. Frequent follow up visits are often necessary.
- If a specific disease is suspected, further diagnostic tests and treatment may be indicated.
- Early in the evaluation, bring up the idea that you are searching both for organic diagnoses AND for stress related diagnoses. If you first mention stress related causes of abdominal pain AFTER your "organic work up" is negative, the patient and family will assume that you are diagnosing a stress related disease "because you can't find anything wrong."
- Avoid the "mind-body split," the idea that organic diagnoses have nothing to do with psychological issues and vice versa.
  - An example is the presentation of red facial flushing that can occur with embarrassment. The trigger is stressful feelings (embarrassment), but a physiologic change occurs (dilation of facial blood vessels).
  - The teen should understand that the gastrointestinal tract is very prone to altered functioning in the presence of stress ("the gut flushes").
- Ask the teen/parents about their theories and worries regarding the cause of pain.

- Urge consolidation of care: limit the number of new consultations and encourage one primary care team to follow up.
- Encourage the use of self-monitoring techniques such as progressive muscle relaxation, yoga and maintenance of a diary.
- Patients with a history of recurrent abdominal pain are not immune to conditions that can cause acute abdominal pain.
  - For instance, an adolescent suffering from IBS can experience an ectopic pregnancy.
  - A change in the nature of pain should alert the clinician to such possibilities.
- Treat co-morbid psychiatric disease and gain the family's permission to have ongoing contact with mental health providers.

What is unique about recurrent or chronic abdominal pain in adolescents?

- It is very common: Approximately 13% of middle school teens experience abdominal pain at least weekly; 32% experience pain more than 5 times per year; 24% have abdominal pain that is severe enough to affect activities. The findings are similar for high school students.
- A careful and thorough history and physical exam is valuable as a diagnostic tool and communicates to the family that you are not dismissing the adolescent's pain.
- Although much of the pain can be functional or psychogenic, adolescents engage in lifestyle choices (e.g. alcohol use, unprotected sexual intercourse) that can place them at risk for significant abdominal problems.
- IBD, a significant gastrointestinal disease with long-term implications often first presents during adolescence.

TEST YOUR KNOWLEDGE ANSWERS

34. F. Central to the definition of IBS is that the pain IS associated with changes in bowel frequency or form. Adolescents, their families and clinicians would do best to recognize functional, stress related, psychogenic and organic diagnoses as existing along a continuum. Acknowledging this continuum will help the clinician to more accurately diagnose the problem

and win the confidence of the teen and their family. Parents frequently acknowledge "stress" as a causative factor; therefore, asking the teen and parents to contribute their ideas regarding etiology is always a good idea. Weight loss in a teen with abdominal pain should alert the clinician to the possibility of a serious condition such as IBD.

Table 1. Causes of Chronic Abdominal/Pelvic Pain in Adolescents.

Disorders	**Differential Diagnosis**
Functional Bowel Disorders	Functional Dyspepsia
	Irritable Bowel Syndrome (IBS)
	Childhood Functional Abdominal Pain Syndrome
	Constipation
Organic GI Disorders	Gastritis (e.g. alcohol related)
	Gastroesophageal reflux
	Peptic Ulcer Disease (PUD)
	Biliary Tract Obstruction/Biliary Colic
	Pancreatitis
	Gastroparesis
	Lactose Intolerance
	Inflammatory Bowel Disease (IBD)
	Celiac Disease
	Chronic Infection (e.g. Giardiasis)
	Eosinophilic Esophagitis/Gastritis
Genitourinary Conditions	Adhesions following Pelvic Inflammatory Disease (PID)
	Tubo-Ovarian Abscess (TOA)
	Mittelschmerz (pain with ovulation)
	Dysmenorrhea
	Endometriosis
	Ovarian Mass with Episodes of Torsion
	Urinary Tract Infections (UTI)
	Pregnancy

Table 2. Definitions of Functional Abdominal Pain Disorders.

Disorder	**Definition**
Functional Dyspepsia	Persistent, recurrent abdominal pain centered in upper abdomen above the umbilicus. Pain not relieved by defecation, nor associated with onset of changes in stool frequency or form. No evidence of inflammatory, anatomic, or neoplastic process to otherwise explain symptoms. Must be present at least once a week for at least 2 months.
Irritable Bowel Syndrome (IBS)	Recurrent abdominal pain or discomfort at least 3 days a month for the past 3 months. There is no evidence of an inflammatory, anatomic or neoplastic process. The pain is associated with 2 or more of the following: 1) improvement with defecation, 2) onset associated with change in stool frequency; and 3) onset associated with change in stool form.
Childhood Functional Abdominal Pain Syndrome	Episodic or continuous abdominal pain must be present at least once a week for 2 months. Insufficient criteria for other functional gastrointestinal disorders and no evidence of an inflammatory, anatomic or neoplastic process. Pain is accompanied by some loss of daily activity, and/or additional somatic symptoms such as headache, limb pain or difficulty sleeping.

Table 3. Red Flags: Findings on History and/or Physical which Suggest Organic Disease.

	Findings
History	Weight loss
	Unexplained fevers
	Pain radiating to the back
	Abdominal pain distant from umbilicus
	Bilious emesis
	Hematemesis
	Chronic diarrhea (>2 weeks)
	Gastrointestinal blood loss
	Dysphagia
	Nocturnal symptoms
	Dysuria, urinary urgency and/or frequency
	Arthritis
	Family history IBD/Celiac Disease/PUD
Physical	Delayed puberty/deceleration of linear growth velocity
	Anemia/Pallor
	Oral ulcers
	Unexplained rashes
	Hepatosplenomegaly
	Perianal abnormalities such as tags or fissures

Table 4. Findings on History which Suggest Psychogenic or Somatoform Disorders.

History of multiple somatic complaints (e.g. headache, abdominal pain, backache, fatigue).
History of multiple primary care physician visits for these problems.*
History of multiple specialty consultations for these problems.*
History of extensive diagnostic testing for these problems.*
Family members with chronic and recurrent symptoms.
Pain causing dysfunction in the primary areas of life: family/school/peers/activities.

*Consultations have not resulted in a diagnosis.

WEB REFERENCES

- American College of Gastroenterology, Clinical Guidelines: http://gi.org/clinical-guidelines/clinical-guidelines-sortable-list/
- Campo JV, et al. 'Adult Outcomes of Pediatric Recurrent Abdominal Pain: Do They Just Grow Out of It?', Pediatrics. 2001;108(l);el, retrieved from http://www.pediatricsdigest.mobi/content/108/l/el.full
- Chiou E, Nurko S. 'Management of Functional Abdominal Pain and Irritable Bowel Syndrome in Children and Adolescents', Expert Reviews Gastroenterology & Hepatology. 2010;4(3); 293–304, retrieved from http://www.medscape.com/viewarticle/723605
- Francavilla R, et al. 'A Randomized Controlled Trial of Lactobacillus GG in Children With Functional Abdominal Pain', Pediatrics. 2010 Nov;126(6);el445–el452, retrieved from http://pediatrics.aappublications.org/content/126/6/e1445.full?sid=fb68937b-6f7c-46ea-8d0b-3651a4ac4096
- Rome Foundation (www.romecriteria.org)
  - Rome III Diagnostic Criteria for Functional Gastrointestinal Disorders, retrieved from http://www.romecriteria.Org/assets/pdf/l9_RomeIII_apA_885-898.pdf
- Subcommittee on Chronic Abdominal Pain. 'Chronic Abdominal Pain in Children', Pediatrics. 2005;115(3);812–815, retrieved from http://pediatrics.aappublications.org/content/115/3/812.full
- Thompson WG, et al. 'Functional bowel disorders and functional abdominal pain', Gut. 1999;45(Suppl II);II43–II47, retrieved from http://www.ncbi.nlm.nih.gov/pmc/articles/PMC1766683/pdf/v045p0II43.pdf
- Wedert JA, Ball TM, Davis MF 'Systematic Review of Treatments for Recurrent Abdominal Pain', Pediatrics. 2003;lll;el, retrieved from http://pediatrics.aappublications.org/content/lll/l/el.full.pdf+html?sid=fb68937b-6f7c-46ea-8d0b-3651a4ac4096

Additonal Clinician and Patient Resources:

- American College of Gastroenterology, Patient's section on Abdominal pain: http://patients.gi.org/topics/abdominal-pain/
- Center for Young Women's Health, "Health Guides A to Z" for discussions on irritable bowel syndrome, lactose intolerance and constipation: www.youngwomenshealth.org
- Chacko, MR. 'Patient Information: Chronic abdominal pain in children and adolescents (Beyond the Basics)', Up To Date (last updated December 16, 2011), retrieved from

http://www.uptodate.com/contents/chronic-abdominal-pain-in-children-and-adolescents-beyond-the-basics

- GastroKids (Help & Hope for Children with Digestive Disorders): www.gastrokids.org
- Young Mens Health, "Health Guides A to Z" for discussions on irritable bowel syndrome, lactose intolerance and constipation: http://www.youngmenshealthsite.org/

23

CONSTIPATION AND ENCOPRESIS

Promise Ahlstrom

TEST YOUR KNOWLEDGE

35. All the following contribute to constipation in teens *EXCEPT*:
    - A. Irritable Bowel Syndrome
    - B. Hypothyroidism
    - C. Compulsive water drinking
    - D. Stool holding
    - E. Use of iron tablets

Refer to end of chapter for answer on page 260.

A 14 year old boy complains of intermittent abdominal pain with no other symptoms. On exam, hard stools are detected on palpation.

BACKGROUND

- Constipation is caused by the increased absorption of water from stool during a long transit in the colon.
- It is more likely due to the delayed passage of stool. Withholding and the subsequent delay in stool transit can lead to harder stools, anal pain and rectal bleeding.
- Stools may be small and pebbly or huge and hard.
- Hard stool in the rectum causes dilation of the rectum, decreased sensation of the urge to defecate and can progress to fecal impaction.
- Encopresis is the overflow of stool, often diarrhea, around the hard stool in the rectum. It often originates in childhood as an intentional, willful withholding, sometimes stemming from an acute episode of painful passage of stool.

RISK FACTORS

Teen Behaviors

- Rushed morning routine and frequent skipping of breakfast prevent taking advantage of the gastro-colonic reflex active upon arising in the morning.
- Avoidance of public bathrooms for reasons of privacy, cleanliness or harassment at school.

Poor Dietary Habits

- Low fiber diet: teens usually have low intake of fruits, vegetables and whole grains.
- Lower water intake.
- High intake of caffeine-containing drinks which have a mild diuretic effect and may contribute to constipation.
- Late onset cow's milk allergy.

Medications

- Opiates (prescribed by a doctor or illicit), iron and calcium supplements, anticholinergics and some psychiatric medications may contribute to constipation.
- Complication of laxative or enema abuse.

ASSESSMENT

HISTORY

History of Present Illness

- Assess the size, frequency and consistency of stools. Abnormal stools are often hard and either pebbly or large in diameter.
- Determine if there is soiling of the undergarments as this suggests impacted stools.
- Determine if there is frequent urination, enuresis or urinary tract infections as these are often linked to impacted stools.
- Ask about symptoms between bowel movements. Pain, bloating and malaise suggest **irritable bowel syndrome (IBS).**

Medications

- Ascertain if medicines are being used that could change stools such as laxatives or enemas.

Review of Systems

- Complaints of cold intolerance, fatigue, weakness, coarse hair or depression suggests **hypothyroidism**.

PHYSICAL

Anthropometric Measurements

- Measure height and weight.
- Growth delays may be the first signs of an underlying systemic illness.
- Low weight or significant weight loss may occur with insufficient caloric intake as with **eating disorders.**

Abdomen

- Look for distention and palpate for stool masses or tenderness.
- If the patient is ill-appearing, vomiting, has acute abdominal pain or tender abdomen with guarding or rebound, consider obstruction: **volvulus** or **Hirschprung's disease.**

Back

- A sacral dimple or tuft of hair suggests **tethered cord syndrome**.

Rectal

- Adolescents are often uncomfortable with the idea of rectal exams: be prepared to provide an unrushed explanation.
- Observe for hemorrhoids, anal fissures, or bleeding.
- Can hard stool be felt? Is the rectal tone normal?
- A dilated, low tone rectum is associated with chronic constipation.

STUDIES

No lab tests are required if the history and physical are normal.

Abdominal X-ray (KUB)

- Shows the amount of stool and degree of fecal impaction.

SPECIAL TESTS

Basic Metabolic Panel

- Electrolyte levels can be disrupted in cases of laxative or enema abuse.

TSH/T4

- Consider if the patient has cold intolerance, myxedema and/or hoarseness.

TREATMENT

Effective treatment strategies include:

- Dietary modifications:
  - Increase fluid intake. Prune, pear, and apple juices are high in sorbitol which is a hyperosmotic laxative promoting increased fluid absorption by stool.
  - Decrease intake of caffeine-containing drinks which have a mild diuretic effect and can contribute to relative dehydration.
  - Increase fiber rich food products such as high fiber cereals or breads, and fiber rich fruits and vegetables.
  - Assess for constipating effects of excess milk intake in some individuals.
- Behavioral modifications:
  - Establish a bowel routine. Make time for a relaxed bathroom routine, preferably after meals or in the a.m., when the gastrocolic reflex is strong.
  - Discourage holding of stool to prevent chronic problems.
- Maintenance medications:
  - Stool softeners should be used with goal of soft, painless stools every one to two days. Individuals often stop medicines too early; medicines are often needed for 6 months or longer. If the therapy is ended too early in encopresis, rectal tone will not have a chance to return to normal.
  - Polyethylene glycol is preferred due to its lack of taste, high efficacy and lack of systemic absorption. Typical dose is 17 gm, or one capful, in 8 ounces of clear liquid to be used daily. Dose can be titrated as needed. Diarrhea, gas or cramping are side effects if too large a dose is administered.
  - Docusate sodium tablets promote water and fat absorption into stool for softer passage and are generally taken as 1–3 doses per day.
  - Magnesium hydroxide (Milk of Magnesia) works as an osmotic laxative, increasing fluids into colon up to 30–60 ml daily.
  - Laxatives should be used only temporarily until bowel habits return to normal.
  - Senna stimulates peristalsis and is available in tablet form (Senakot, senna tabs), chew tablets (Ex-Lax chocolate squares), or film strips and can be used as needed to promote daily or every other day stools.
  - Bisacodyl (Ducolax) tablets also stimulate peristalsis.

- Disimpaction may be necessary if fecal impaction is detected on abdominal or rectal exam or on abdominal x-ray:
  - Oral medications are more likely to be tolerated by teens; however, with severe constipation, an enema may be necessary to provide colonic disimpaction.
  - Magnesium citrate solution: 150–300 ml use once.
  - Polyethylene glycol powder (MiraLax) in a high dose: 1.5 gm/kg/day.
  - Polyethylene glycol (GoLYTELY) is available as a prescription-only product. A flavored electrolyte solution designed for colonic clean-out.

What is unique about constipation and encopresis in adolescence?

- Many teens don't like to talk about stools or bowel habits and even serious constipation may go unreported.
- Teens may be embarrassed to have this problem or may try to hide it.
- Constipation presents in adolescence secondary to teen behaviors such as limited time for relaxed bathroom use, poor eating habits and scant fluid intake.

TEST YOUR KNOWLEDGE ANSWER

35. C. A common contributor to constipation is mild dehydration due to insufficient fluid intake. IBS can present with constipation and tenesmus alternating with loose stools. Constipation, cold intolerance and fatigue are common signs of hypothyroidism. Stool holding, or the desire to delay defecation because of school fears or dislike of public restrooms, can compound the problem. Finally, iron commonly causes constipation. Compulsive water drinking induces polyuria but not constipation.

WEB REFERENCES

- Furuta GT, et al. "Management of Constipation in Children and Adolescents With Autism Spectrum Disorders', Pediatrics. 2012;130(Suppl 2);S98–S105, retrieved from http://pediatrics.aappublications.org/content/130/Supplement_2/S98.full.pdf+html?sid=116b3afc-afb8-45f9-a525-98fb98e4dfd5

- National Collaborating Centre for Women's and Children's Health. 'Constipation in Children and Young People: Diagnosis and Management of Idiopathic Childhood Constipation in Primary and Secondary Care', NICE Clinical Guidelines. 2010;99, retrieved from http://www.ncbi.nlm.nih.gov/pubmedhealth/PMH0033416/
- Rasquin A, et al. 'Childhood Functional Gastrointestinal Disorders: Child/Adolescent', Gastroenterology. April 2006;130(5);1527–1537, retrieved from http://www.gastrojournal.org/article/S0016-5085(06)00518-X/fulltext#section42
- Tabers MM, et al. 'Nonpharmacologic Treatments for Childhood Constipation: Systematic Review', Pediatrics. 2011;128(4);753–761, retrieved from http://pediatrics.aappublications.org/content/128/4/753.full.pdf+html?sid=116b3afc-afb8-45f9-a525-98fb98e4dfd5

Additional Clinician and Patient Resources:

- American Academy of Pediatrics (AAP) Healthy Children, Constipation (last updated 7/30/2012), retrieved from http://www.healthychildren.org/English/health-issues/conditions/abdominal/Pages/Constipation.aspx
- Center for Young Women's Health, Constipation http://www.youngwomenshealth.org/constipation.html
- International Foundation for Functional Gastrointestinal Disorders:
  - About Constipation (last modified March 4, 2013), retrieved from www.aboutconstipation.org
  - About Kids and Teens GI Health: http://www.aboutkidsgi.org/
- National Institutes of Health, Constipation : http://vsearch.nlm.nih.gov/vivisimo/cgi-bin/query-meta?query=constipation&v%3Aproject=nlm-main-website
- GI Kids, Constipation search: http://www.gikids.org/content/94/en/
- PubMed Health, Encopresis (last reviewed August 1, 2012), retrieved from http://www.ncbi.nlm.nih.gov/pubmedhealth/PMH0002537/
- Teenshealth from Nemours, Constipation, retrieved from http://kidshealth.org/teen/diseases_conditions/digestive/constipation.html
- Young Men's Health, Constipation, retrieved from http://www.youngmenshealthsite.org/constipation.html

24

ENURESIS

Promise Ahlstrom

TEST YOUR KNOWLEDGE

36. Which one of the following statements is true:

    A. Most individuals diagnosed with childhood enuresis continue to have problems well into their teen years.
    B. Desmopressin (DDAVP) cures enuresis.
    C. There is usually a strong family history of enuresis in enuretic males.
    D. The alarm treatment for enuresis is risky because of electrical discharges.
    E. Enuresis is usually not a big concern for affected teens.

Refer to end of chapter for answer on page 268.

"My 12 year old son still wets his bed almost every day! He is so lazy!"

BACKGROUND

- Enuresis in adolescents is most often nocturnal and is more common in males.
- Teens who have never established urinary continence have primary enuresis while those who have had at least 6 months of continence have secondary enuresis. Diurnal enuresis is very unusual and occurs day and night.
- Nocturnal enuresis (NE) usually resolves during adolescence.
  - By age 5, 15% of children have NE and by age 10, only 5% suffer from NE.
  - Approximately 15% of children spontaneously outgrow their incontinence each year thereafter. By adolescence, only about 1% of teens have NE.
- Primary NE has 3 components: nocturnal polyuria (high urine volume due to immaturity in the release of antidiuretic hormone), overactive bladder (small functional bladder capacity), and poor night time arousability (deep sleepers).
- Secondary NE can be caused by urinary tract infection (UTI), constipation, encopresis, diabetes mellitus or stress.
- Consider co-morbid conditions that could cause or exacerbate enuresis (Table 1).

ASSESSMENT

HISTORY

History of Present Illness

- Determine duration of symptoms. How old was patient at onset?
- Do symptoms occur during the day, night or both? Daytime dribbling in females suggests **urologic malformations** such as the ureter entering the vagina instead of bladder.
- Does the patient ever experience a dry period?

- Is there a history of normal daytime urination? Does the patient experience dribbling or stress incontinence? Is the urinary stream normal?
- Does the patient have symptoms of polydipsia or polyuria suggesting **diabetes mellitus?**
- Is there a history of **constipation?** This can lead to urinary tract obstruction and hydronephrosis.

Past Medical History

- Have there been past interventions, medicines or enuresis alarms used?

Family History

- Is often positive for enuresis in family members.

Review of Systems

- Assess for sleep disorders. Overweight or obese teens who snore may have **obstructive sleep apnea.**
- Determine if the patient has any urogenital complaints. Vaginal discharge or irritation may indicate an underlying **vulvovaginitis.**

PHYSICAL

Vitals Signs

- If the patient presents with fever, consider an infectious etiology such as UTI or cystitis.

Abdomen

- Examine for masses or palpable stool which could compress the bladder or urethra.
- Assess for tenderness that may occur with a mass or stool.

Back

- A sacral dimple or tuft of hair suggests **tethered cord syndrome.**

Genital

- Observe for **vaginal adhesions, vulvovaginitis or foreign bodies.**

Rectal

- Perform if necessary to rule out rectal impaction.

STUDIES

ROUTINE TESTS

Urinalysis

- The presence of white blood cells, leukocyte esterase or nitrates suggests infection.
- Protein spilling into the urine may indicate a renal problem.
- The presence of glucose and ketones spilling into the urine suggest diabetes mellitus.
- A urine specific gravity greater than 1.015, makes the diagnosis of diabetes insipidus unlikely.

Urine culture

- Can rule out urinary tract infections.

SPECIAL TESTS

Sleep Study

- Consider in patients who snore, have enlarged tonsils, are obese or are resistant to treatment.

Urologic Work Up

- Is usually unnecessary unless daytime voiding dysfunction accompanies nocturnal enuresis.
- However, measurement of bladder capacity may be of interest if the bladder capacity exceeds the amount of nighttime urine production.

EEG

- Consider in patients with suspected serizures.

TREATMENT

- In cases of secondary enuresis, first treat the cause (i.e. UTI or constipation).
- In cases of primary enuresis, effective therapeutic strategies include:

Behavioral modification

- Establish bedtime voiding habits and consider setting an alarm to wake up during the night for voiding purposes in patients with small bladder capacities.
- Limit caffeine intake, especially later in the day.
- Limit fluid intake at bedtime. Excessive evening fluid intake can lead to hyponatremia and seizures if the patient is on DDAVP.

Enuresis alarm

- Is very effective yet requires motivation and parental supervision. Can be bought online for under $100.
- Waterproof the bed and encourage nightly use of an alarm. Urinating completes the electric circuit sounding the alarm: teen wakes up, removes the alarm, and finishes voiding in the bathroom. The alarm is replaced and the teen goes back to sleep.
- Parents supervise to ensure that the teen is waking up fully and voiding in the bathroom.
- Used nightly until successfully dry for 14 days and often takes less than 2–3 months.

Desmopressin (DDAVP)

- DDAVP is the synthetic analogue of vasopressin (anti-diuretic hormone) and works by reducing urine production.
- Available in tablet form (0.1 and 0.2 mg doses), usual dose 0.2–0.6 mg given 1 hour before bedtime. Also available as a nasal spray but the FDA contraindicates its use for enuresis.
- DDAVP therapy is easier, requires less motivation and parental involvement, and yet is only effective while the medicine is being used. There is a high relapse rate with discontinuation of the medicine.
- Advantage: can be used temporarily for camp and sleep-overs.
- DDAVP has substituted imipramine and despramine, both once used to treat enuresis but no longer recommended because of their anticholinergic effects and high rates of toxicity.

DISPOSITION

Close outpatient follow up is crucial to ensure interest and compliance with the enuresis alarm. Schedule phone contact at weekly intervals until success is achieved.

- Patients with normal bladder capacities but nocturnal polyuria may try DDAVP first.
- Patients with a small bladder capacity, normal urine production and a poor response to DDAVP usually show a good response to the enuresis alarm.

Referral to a Urologist may be necessary for:

- Daytime bladder symptoms and treatment resistant individuals to assess urinary tract, urinary flow, functional bladder capacity, and post-void residual urine volume.
- Adolescent females who have both day and night enuresis, as they can be found to have an anomalous insertion of the urethra into the vagina that warrants surgical correction.

What is unique about enuresis in adolescents?

- NE can be a difficult experience for adolescents, both socially and psychologically and yet they are reluctant to talk about it.
- Adolescents are likely to avoid overnight stays with friends or summer camps secondary to potential embarrassment related to NE.
- If parents have reacted to NE in a punishing or critical way, it can affect self-esteem and teens may present with depressive symptoms.
- An unusual triad of enuresis, cruelty to animals and fire setting has been described.

TEST YOUR KNOWLEDGE ANSWER

36. C. By adolescence, most individuals have outgrown enuresis. However, teens still suffering from enuresis need treatment because bedwetting is very upsetting for them, even if they are reluctant to discuss this. Alarm results are long-lasting and do not have any associated risks. DDAVP does not cure enuresis; nevertheless, it works by causing the kidney to produce less urine during the night via its antidiuretic effect. Since enuresis often

resolves with age, any "cure" that results from DDAVP use is due to maturation of the system that releases antidiuretic hormone.

Table 1. Co-morbid Conditions.

- Constipation and fecal impaction which can then cause pressure or obstruction of the bladder.
- Neuro-psychiatric conditions such as ADHD, autism, developmental delay, or neurologic dysfunction such as seizures.
- Upper airway obstruction and obstructive sleep apnea, especially in overweight teens with NE who fail to respond to standard treatment.
- Diabetes
- Emotional stress
- Compulsive water drinking.
- Females with day and night wetting may have an anomalous urethral insertion in their vaginas.

WEB REFERENCES

- Lawless MR and McElderry DH. 'Nocturnal Enuresis: Current Concepts', Pediatrics in Review. December 2001. 22(12);399–407, retrieved from http://www.fmed.ulaval.ca/pediatrie/fileadmin/docs/serveur_pediatrie/Acces_reserve/Medecins/Articles_scientifiques/recueil/Enuresis.pdf
- National Institute for Health and Clinical Excellence. 'Nocturnal enuresis: The management of bedwetting in children and young people', NICE Clinical Guideline lll;October 2010, retrieved from http://www.nice.org.uk/nicemedia/live/13246/51367/51367.pdf
- 'Practice Parameter for the Assessment and Treatment of Children and Adolescents with Enuresis' Journal American Academy of Child Adolescent Psychiatry. 2004;43(12):1540–1550, retrieved from http://www.aacap.org/galleries/PracticeParameters/Enuresis.pdf
- Robson WLM. 'Enuresis Treatment & Management' (last updated April 30, 2012), retrieved from http://emedicine.medscape.com/article/1014762-treatment

Additional Clinician and Patient Resources:

- American Academy of Pediatrics (AAP) Healthy Children, Nocturnal Enuresis in Teens (last updated 2/27/2013) retrieved from http://www.healthychildren.org/English/health-issues/conditions/genitourinary-tract/Pages/Nocturnal-Enuresis-in-Teens.aspx
- Center for Young Women's Health, Ask Us: I wet the bed every night and ear diapers. How can I stop?, retrieved from http://www.youngwomenshealth.org/askus/nocturnal_enuresis.html

- National Kidney Foundation, Bed-Wetting in the Young Adult, retrieved from http://www.kidney.org/patients/bw/BWyoungadults.cfm
- Schmitt BD. 'Bed-Wetting (Enuresis): Teen Version' Pediatric Advisor 2012.2 published by Relay Health (last reviewed 6/6/2011), retrieved from http://www.cpnonline.org/CRS/CRS/patnbedwethhg.htm
- Teenshealth from Nemours, What is Enuresis, retrieved from: http://kidshealth.org/teen/diseasesconditions/urinarv/enuresis.html

25

DYSURIA, URINARY TRACT INFECTIONS AND PYELONEPHRITIS

Amy E. Klamberg

TEST YOUR KNOWLEDGE

37. A diabetic adolescent develops a urinary tract infection (UTI). Which of the following is *MOST* likely to be true?

    A. She has begun having sexual intercourse.
    B. She should be treated with an antibiotic for 3 days.
    C. Because she is a diabetic, she should have a voiding cystourethrogram (VCUG).
    D. All the above.
    E. None of the above.

Refer to end of chapter for answer on page 278.

"It hurts and burns when I have to pee and I'm running to the bathroom every 10–15 minutes!"

BACKGROUND

- Urinary tract infections (UTI), or uncomplicated cystitis, are common in female adolescents and are often markers for sexual intercourse ("honeymoon cystitis").
- For most patients who are treated for a UTI there are no serious long-term complications.
  - Females with urologic abnormalities are usually diagnosed during childhood.
  - Males with UTI often have underlying urologic abnormalities.
- E. coli is the most common cause of uncomplicated UTI in young women, followed by Staphylococcus saprophyticus and other gram-negative organisms.
- Klebsiella, enterococci, pseudomonas and proteus species are more common causes of chronic or recurrent infections.
- Gram negative bacilli account for 75% of UTIs in males, but trichomonas and Gardnerella can also cause infection and pyuria in males.
- Dysuria mimicking UTI is often caused by urethritis secondary to a sexually transmitted infection (STI).
- Patients with frequent or untreated UTIs can develop more serious complications of an upper-UTI or pyelonephritis.
- Renal scarring, hypertension, and end-stage renal disease are uncommon but more serious consequences of pyelonephritis.

ASSESSMENT

HISTORY

History of Present Illness

- Ascertain the onset, severity and duration of dysuria. Acute onset suggests **cystitis** while gradual onset with mild symptoms suggests **urethritis.**

- Timing of the dysuria is important. With **urethritis**, pain is often worse with initiation of urine stream; terminal pain is often associated with **cystitis.**
- Determine if there is frequency or urgency associated with urination. Lack of frequency and urgency suggests **vaginitis or urethritis.**
- The presence of vaginal discharge can result in abnormal urinalysis and raises concern for a **STI, bacterial vaginosis,** or **yeast infection.**
- Ask about a patient's bowel habits. Frequent stool retention and constipation are risk factors for UTIs.
- Have there been any recent chemical exposures or trauma to the perineum? Frequent bubble baths, scented panty liners and use of thong underwear may contribute to irritation, dysuria and erythema of the urethra.

Past Medical History

- Has the patient had a UTI in the past or recurrent UTIs?
- A history of neurogenic bladder or bladder dysfunction may cause a patient to be more susceptible to recurrent UTIs due to prolonged urinary stasis.
- A history of vesicoureteral reflux (VUR) can predispose to renal complications.
- Did the patient have a recent upper respiratory infection? **Adenovirus cystitis** should be considered in adolescents with hemorrhagic cystitis.
- Ask if the patient has recently been hospitalized. Catheter associated UTIs and cystitis are the most common nosocomial infections reported to the National Nosocomial Infection Surveillance (NNIS).

Social History

- Detailed sexual activity, including condom use at last sexual activity, can guide assessment.
- Sexually active females have a higher likelihood of developing UTIs than those who are not and are also at higher risk of developing STIs.
- Ask about recent travel as parasites are a common cause of cystitis in certain parts of the world. ***Schistosoma hematobium*** may be a cause of cystitis and hematuria in Africa and the Middle East.

Review of Systems

- Are there associated symptoms such as fever, chills or malaise?
- Is there associated fever, back or flank pain? This suggests progression to **pyelonephritis.**

PHYSICAL

Vital Signs

- Document temperature, pulse and blood pressure to assess for underlying infectious process and hemodynamic stability.

General Appearance

- Is the patient comfortable or in acute distress?

Abdomen

- Assess for abdominal, pelvic or suprapubic pain.

Back

- Assess for CVA or flank tenderness to percussion.

Genital

- In females, assess for vaginal discharge or other signs of vulvovaginitis.
- In males, assess for meatal irritation, urethral discharge or signs of epididymitis.
- Genital ulcers or lesions may also have associated dysuria.

Pelvic with Bimanual

- May sometimes be necessary in a sexually active teen suspected of having concurrent PID.

Lymph Nodes

- Check for inguinal lymphadenopathy.

STUDIES

Urine Dipstick and/or Urinalysis

- White blood cells (WBC) and/or nitrites indicate a UTI; however, WBCs alone suggest an STI as a cause of dysuria. For females, a clean catch specimen is more accurate.

Urine Culture

- Uncomplicated UTIs can be treated empirically and urine cultures are not required. Consider in cases of recurrent UTI's to ascertain the antibiotic susceptibility panel.

Gonorrhea/Chlamydia Testing

- Urine nucleic acid amplification tests or cervical cultures should be considered in a sexually active teen.

Wet Prep Specimen

- Allows for visualization of trichomonads, WBCs, clue cells and yeast as sources of dysuria.

Urine Pregnancy Test

- Can help guide treatment plan. Some antibiotics are contraindicated during pregnancy.

SPECIAL TESTS

ESR and *C-Reactive Protein*

- Can be useful as markers for inflammation.

Blood Cultures

- Consider if there is concern for sepsis related to pyelonephritis.

Renal Ultrasound and *Voiding Cystourethrogram (VCUG)*

- Are not routinely recommended for female teens with uncomplicated UTI/cystitis who respond well to antibiotic therapy in the first 48–72 hours of treatment.
- Adolescent males with a first UTI should have these studies to rule out renal abscess, calculi, anatomic abnormalities or other causes of obstruction.

Technetium-99m-labeled Dimercaptosuccinic Acid (DMSA) Scans

- This is a sensitive method to assess for acute changes in the kidneys associated with pyelonephritis.
- May be an important investigative tool in evaluating teens with febrile UTIs for acute pyelonephritis.

TREATMENT

- Treatment will depend on whether the diagnosis is uncomplicated UTI, uncomplicated pyelonephritis, or complicated UTI/pyelonephritis.

Uncomplicated UTI or Cystitis

- Teens diagnosed with uncomplicated UTI or cystitis based on their clinical symptoms and urine dipstick findings, may be treated empirically without further work up.
- Antibiotic treatment is recommended and there are many available options:
  - First line treatment: Sulfamethoxazole/Trimethoprim, although urinary pathogens are showing increased drug resistance to this antibiotic and alternative treatment options should be considered.
  - Second or third generation cephalosporins, such as Ceftin or Cefpodoxime may be considered.
  - Fluoroquinolones, such as Ciprofloxacin and Ofloxacin are recommended in older adolescents and young adults, but are not approved for teens under 16 years.
  - A 3 day course of treatment for uncomplicated UTI is sufficient.

- For teens with symptoms over 1 week or with a concomittant chronic illness such as diabetes mellitus or sickle cell disease, treatment should be extended to 7 days.
- Uncomplicated UTI in pregnancy should be treated for 7 days. Sulfamethoxazole/trimethoprim and fluoroquinolones are not recommended during pregnancy while cefuroxime is pregnancy category B and is considered safe during pregnancy.
- Treatment drug of choice should be based on resistance patterns in the community.
- With recurrences, check urine culture and sensitivities as the patient may be resistant to the initially prescribed antibiotic.

Uncomplicated Pyelonephritis

- If there is pyelonephritis but no nausea or vomiting, outpatient oral antibiotic therapy for 10–14 days is recommended. Administer a loading dose of ceftriaxone 500 mg.
- A teen treated as an outpatient for uncomplicated pyelonephritis should be followed-up within 48 hours for response to therapy.

Complicated UTI or Pyelonephritis

- For severe cases of pyelonephritis where the patient is unable to tolerate oral medications or has a chronic illness, hospitalize and treat with parenteral antibiotics.
- Hospitalization is also recommended for pregnant teens with pyelonephritis.
- Third and fourth generation cephalosporins (ceftriaxone, cefotaxime) and aminoglycosides are appropriate parenteral therapy for pyelonephritis.
- Post coital prophylaxis may be considered for adolescent females with recurrent UTIs.
- Continuous prophylaxis of daily antibiotics has been recommended for individuals with recurrent UTIs (>3 per year) but there is no supportive evidence base and the development of resistance may be a concern.

What is unique about UTIs and pyelonephritis in adolescents?

- UTIs can be a manifestation of the initiation of sexual intercourse in females and should prompt a reproductive health evaluation.
- Female adolescents are often reluctant to follow the advice of emptying their bladder before sexual intercourse because it "interrupts the moment;" however, they need to be reminded. An empty bladder allows for the epithelial cells to secret IgA to protect against an infection while a full bladder is an ideal culture medium for bacteria to grow. If they forget, or are reluctant, postcoital voiding may offer some protection.
- Young adolescent females may not be aware that the vaginal vestibule can be colonized with intestinal bacteria if they wipe themselves back to front post bowel movement.
- Many adolescents suffer from constipation and this can predispose to UTIs. Routinely counsel on good dietary habits including adequate daily fiber intake and appropriate intake of water.
- UTIs are very uncommon in otherwise healthy adolescent males so this diagnosis warrants further urologic work-up.

TEST YOUR KNOWLEDGE ANSWER

37. A. Like any other teen, a diabetic patient who develops a UTI may have had her infection following sexual debut. While an uncomplicated UTI only requires 3 days of antibiotic treatment, a patient with a chronic illness such as diabetes requires a seven day course of antibiotics. There is no indication for a VCUG study in a diabetic patient with a UTI.

WEB REFERENCES

- Clausius, I. 'Dysuria in adolescents', Western Journal of Medicine. 2000 March; 172(3); 201–205, retrieved from http://www.ncbi.nlm.nih.gov/pmc/articles/PMC1070807/
- Colgan R and Williams M. 'Diagnosis and Treatment of Acute Uncomplicated Cystitis', American Family Physician. 2011 October; 84(7); 771–776, retrieved from http://www.aafp.org/afp/2011/10017p771.html
- Kodner CM and Gupton EKT. 'Recurrent Urinary Tract Infections in Women: Diagnosis and Management', American Family Physician. 2010 September 15; 82(6); 638–643, retrieved from http://www.aafp.org/afp/2010/0915/p638.html

- Nguyen H and Weir M. 'Urinary Tract Infection as a Possible Marker for Teenage Sex', Southern Medical Journal. 2002; 95(8), retrieved from http://www.medscape.com/viewarticle/444325
- Raz R, Chazan B, Dan M. 'Cranberry Juice and Urinary Tract Infection', Clinical Infectious Diseases. 2004. 38(10); 1413–1419, retrieved from http://cid.oxfordjournals.org/content/38/10/1413.1ong
- Stamm We and Norrby SR. 'Urinary Tract Infections: Disease Panorama and Challenges', The Journal of Infectious Diseases. 2001; 183(Suppl 1); S1–S4, retrieved from http://jid.oxfordjournals.org/content/183/Supplement_l/Sl.full.pdf+html

Additional Clinician and Patient Resources:

- American Family Physician, Educational Resources on Urinary Tract Infections/Dysuria, retrieved from http://www.aafp.org/afp/topicModules/viewTopicModule.htm?topicModuleId=30
- Center for Young Women's Health, Urinary Tract Infections (Last updated 11/15/2012), retrieved from http://www.youngwomenshealth.org/uti.html
- Emedicine Health, Urinary Tract Infections in Teens and Adults, retrieved from http://www.emedicinehealth.com/urinary_tract_infections_in_teens_and_adults-health/article_em.htm
- Hooton TM. 'Patient Information: Urinary tract infections in adolescents and adults (Beyond the Basics)', Up To Date. Last Updated May 2, 2012, retrieved from http://www.uptodate.com/contents/urinary-tract-infections-in-adolescents-and-adults-beyond-the-basics
- Mayo Clinic, Kidney Infection (Aug 9, 2011), retrieved from http://www.mayoclinic.com/health/kidney-infection/DS00593
- National Institute of Diabetes and Digestive and Kidney Diseases, Pyelonephritisi: Kidney Infection (last updated June 11, 2012) retrieved from http://kidney.niddk.nih.gov/KUDiseases/pubs/pyelonephritis/index.aspx
- National Kidney Foundation, Patient handout on Urinary Tract Infections, retrieved from http://www.kidney.org/atoz/pdf/uti.pdf
- National Kidney and Urologic Diseases Information Clearinghouse, Patient handouts on Urinary Tract Infections, retrieved from http://www.kidney.niddk.nih.gov/KUDiseases/topics/uti.aspx

26

PROTEINURIA

Lawrence J. D'Angelo

TEST YOUR KNOWLEDGE

38. The *MOST* common cause of proteinuria in adolescents is
    A. Poststreptococcal glomerulonephrits
    B. Systemic Lupus Erythematosus
    C. Orthostatic Proteinuria
    D. Alport's Syndrome
    E. Heart Failure

Refer to end of chapter for answer on page 287.

A 17 year old male patient presents for STI screening. A urine dipstick is done to check for leukocytes. The test is negative but 3 + protein is found incidentally.

BACKGROUND

- Asymptomatic proteinuria is proteinuria not associated with other physical (i.e. hypertension, rash, etc.) or urine findings (i.e. hematuria, pyuria, etc.).
- It is a common finding on a screening urinalysis in adolescents.
- Screening for proteinuria is not cost-effective: minor abnormalities may lead to unnecessary and expensive work up. Nevertheless, urinalysis is a fairly common test and that is how proteinuria is often identified.
- For the majority of teens with proteinuria, no significant renal disease is present and the long-term prognosis is excellent.
- The presence of proteinuria may lead to difficulties in acceptance for employment, insurance, or the armed services.
- Clinicians need to determine the degree and significance of proteinuria when it exists (Table 1).
- The leading causes are "benign persistent proteinuria" and orthostatic proteinuria.
- Functional proteinuria can also occur with exercise, fever and congestive heart failure.
- Other etiologies are more ominous as they involve more significant renal disease (Table 2).

ASSESSMENT

HISTORY

History of Present Illness

- Does the patient report a recent upper respiratory tract or skin infection that suggests **streptococcal infection?**

Past Medical History

- Has the patient been diagnosed with diabetes mellitus? Ten to fourteen years of diabetes is usually required before clinical detection of proteinuria; detection of microalbuminuria is possible at earlier stages of disease.

- Does the patient have any known history of allergic reactions to drugs or bee stings?
- Does the patient have a history of drug intoxication?

Family History

- Is there a family history of **systemic lupus erythematosus** (SLE), **diabetes mellitus** or other renal disease?

Review of Systems

- Skin rashes, arthralgias or photosensitivity may indicate an underlying autoimmune process such as **SLE.**
- Flank pain, fever, and prior urinary tract infection suggests **pyelonephritis.**
- Does the patient report hearing loss or joint pain?

PHYSICAL

- Vision and hearing screens should be considered if **hereditary nephritis** is a diagnostic consideration.

Vital Signs

- A fever would indicate underlying infection while abnormalities in blood pressure may indicate **renal pathology**.

Anthropometric Measurements

- Height and weight percentiles should be calculated. Growth delays may indicate chronic disease.
- **Obesity** can be complicated by proteinuria.

Heart Exam

- Assess for any signs of **congestive heart failure** or other **cardiac abnormalities.**

Abdomen

- Assess for the presence of an abdominal mass.

Musculoskeletal

- Are there any abnormalities on the joint exam? Patients who complain of joint pain should be assessed for tenderness or swelling.

Skin

- Careful skin exam is warranted as autoimmune processes such as **SLE** may present with rashes.
- Assess for the presence of edema, most likely in the lower extremities.

STUDIES

Urine Dipstick

- The qualitative dipstick test for protein can detect protein levels as low as 10 to 30 mg/dL.
- An initial positive test result should be confirmed with two subsequent tests because many individuals have transient initial proteinuria with negative findings on subsequent testing.
- False-positive test results can be seen with highly concentrated urine, gross hematuria, or with antiseptic contamination.

Sulfosalicyclic Acid Test

- If proteinuria is confirmed on repeated dipstick testing, the next diagnostic step is a protein precipitation test such as the sulfosalicyclic acid test on a first morning void sample.
- If this confirms findings, laboratory work up is indicated to rule out significant disease.

Urinalysis

- Proteinuria refers to the urinary excretion of more than 150 mg of protein per day.
- Small amounts of protein in the urine are normal. Most individuals excrete 30 to 130 mg of protein per day.
- Completely healthy adolescents may excrete up to 300 mg/day without any evidence of renal disease.

- Up to 10% to 19% of healthy adolescents have protein in their urine on a dipstick test of a random urine sample.
- This prevalence falls with repeated testing.
- The diagnosis of persistent proteinuria should be based on three separate urine tests.
- Prevalence peaks at about 16 years of age.

Urine Protein/Creatinine Ratio

- The most practical method of estimating total urinary protein excretion is a spot urine protein/creatinine ratio.
  - A random urine sample is analyzed for protein and creatinine.
  - When both are expressed in milligram amounts, a ratio of less than 0.2 is normal and a ratio greater than 1.0 signifies nephrotic-range proteinuria.
- The urine protein/creatinine ratio closely correlates with the daily excretion of protein in $g/1.73m^2$. This is based on the fact that the average daily excretion of creatinine is approximately 1000 mg/24 hours/1.73 m^2.
- If the urine protein/creatinine ratio is >0.5, then further evaluation is indicated.
- A spot urine protein/creatinine ratio of >1.0 suggests that a 24-hour protein concentration will be greater than 1,000 mg.
- Timed urine collection (ideally over 24 hours) is another option, but adherence to instructions is often suboptimal.

Complete Blood Cell (CBC) Count

- Can identify anemia.

Serum BUN and Creatinine

- Can detect loss of kidney function.

SPECIAL TESTS

- Not all tests need to be done at once. Clinical history and physical exam findings should direct the order and extent of testing.

Antistreptolysin O titer

- Consider testing in a patient with recent upper respiratory or skin infection as these findings in the context of proteinuria suggests post-streptococcal glomerulonephritis.

Complement Levels

- Should be considered when the adolescent has symptoms that suggest nephrotic syndrome.

Ultrasonography or CT Scan

- These tests may yield useful information, such as the number of kidneys present (1 in every 1,000 people is born with a single kidney), the size of the kidneys (small kidney size reflects chronic disease), and "echogenicity" suggestive of "medical renal disease" that may require further evaluation.

Renal Biopsy

- Common lesions can be diagnosed by history, physical exam and laboratory findings; therefore, the indications for a renal biopsy are limited.
- A biopsy may be needed to define the severity of the lesion and determine disease prognosis.
- The final diagnostic step in evaluating patients with severe, persistent proteinuria is a renal biopsy.

DISPOSITION

- The approach to proteinuria is best established by determining the severity, if any, of the underlying condition. Underlying etiology will dictate treatment course.
- Table 1 lists etiologies most likely to cause proteinuria.
- When the clinician feels that a biopsy may be necessary, referral to a nephrologist for further evaluation is appropriate.
- Factors that may influence this decision include:
  - An unclear diagnosis, particularly when significant disease is suspected in cases of proteinuria, hematuria, hypertension or renal insufficiency.
  - Nephrotic range proteinuria is present, particularly if there is no response to a therapeutic trial of corticosteroids for "minimal change disease."
  - Renal function is deteriorating.
  - The patient and/or family express the need for prognostic information.

What is unique about proteinuria in adolescents?

- Most adolescents with proteinuria are healthy, have a functional cause such as fever or exercise or at most have a benign persistent proteinuria or orthostatic proteinuria. These patient's proteinuria is often discovered incidentally.
- Orthostatic (postural) proteinuria occurs when a patient is upright but not while recumbent. It is common in adolescents.
- The etiology of orthostatic proteinuria is unclear, although exaggerated hemodynamic response to the upright position and functional compromise of the left renal vein have been postulated as two possible causes.
- Orthostatic proteinuria of adolescence is characterized by:
  - Onset between 10 to 20 years of age.
  - The absence of physical or laboratory signs of other disease.
  - Urine dipstick findings limited to 1+ to 3+ protein.
  - Significantly less protein detected in a urine specimen obtained immediately after patient arises in the morning.
  - Negative findings on evaluating the urine sediment.
  - Normal renal function and no evidence of hypoalbuminemia or hyperlipidemia.
- A minority of adolescents who do not fulfill criteria for functional or orthostatic proteinuria may have conditions outlined in Table 1 and will require referral or consultation with a nephrologist.

TEST YOUR KNOWLEDGE ANSWER

38. C. The most common cause of proteinuria in adolescents is orthostatic proteinuria. The other entities are much less common. Post-streptococcal glomerulonephritis can be a complication of impetigo. Alport's syndrome is a hereditary nephritis associated with hearing loss. Though proteinuria is present in both post-streptococcal glomerulonephritis and Alport's syndrome, hematuria is usually a more prominent symptom. Heart failure can indeed cause proteinuria but it is rare in adolescents.

Table 1. Causes of Proteinuria (by Protein Excretion Rates).

Mild Asymptomatic Proteinuria Expected excretion of protein: less than 500 mg/m^2 in 24 hours.	Benign persistent proteinuria Orthostatic or postural proteinuria (proved with split 24-hour urine collection) Functional: Fever or exercise Pyelonephritis (usually with fever and pyuria) Renal tubular disorders Chronic interstitial nephritis Congenital dysplastic lesions Congestive heart failure (severe)
Moderate Proteinuria Expected excretion of protein: 500 to 2,000 mg/m^2 in 24 hours.	Acute poststreptococcal glomerulonephritis (PSGN) Primary glomerulonephritis Hereditary chronic nephritis (Alport syndrome) Systemic diseases: SLE
Severe Proteinuria Expected excretion of protein: more than 2,000 mg/m^2 in 24 hours; usually more than 3.5 g	Typically associated with edema, hypoalbuminemia and hypercholesterolemia (nephrotic syndrome) Idiopathic glomerulonephritis • Minimal change disease • Focal sclerosis • Membranous or membranoproliferative glomerulonephritis Systemic disease • SLE • Amyloidosis (in setting of chronic inflammatory disease or familial Mediterranean fever) Less common • Infections: Bacterial endocarditis, hepatitis, malaria, human immunodeficiency virus • Toxins: Mercury, heroin, gold, penicillamine Uncommon • Allergens: Bee stings • Mechanical: Pericarditis, renal vein thrombosis • Cancer: Hodgkin disease, lymphoma • Pregnancy • Congenital: Fabry disease and Alport syndrome

Table 2. Renal Diseases.

Disease	Pathophysiology
Primary Glomerulopathies IgA Nephropathy Minimal Change Disease Membranous Nephropathy **Secondary Glomerulopathies** Diabetes Mellitus Systemic Lupus Erythematosus (SLE)	Increased glomerular permeability
Monoclonal Gammopathies	Increased production of abnormal proteins
Fanconi Syndrome Aminoglycoside Nephrotoxicity Chronic Interstitial Nephritis	Decreased tubular reabsorption of proteins, as in tubular disease

WEB REFERENCES

- Gattineni, J. 'Review Article: Highlights for the Management of a Child with Proteinuria and Hematuria', International Journal of Pediatrics. 2012, retrieved from http://www.hindawi.com/journals/ijped/2012/768142/
- Hogg, RJ. 'Adolescents With Proteinuria and/or Nephrotic Syndrome', February 2015, retrieved from http://www.redorbit.com/news/health/127735/adolescents_with_proteinuria_andor_the_nephrotic_syndrome/
- Hogg RJ, et al. 'Evaluation and Management of Proteinuria and Nephrotic Syndrome in Children: Recommendations From a Pediatric Nephrology Panel Established at the National Kidney Foundation Conference on Proteinuria, Albuminuria, Risk, Assessment, Detection, and Elimination', Pediatrics. 2000. 105(6); 1242-1249, retrieved from http://pediatrics.aappublications.org/content/105/6/1242.abstract
- Loghman-Adham, M. 'Evaluating Proteinuria in Children', American Family Physician. 1998 Oct 1;58(5); 1145–1152, retrieved from http://www.aafp.org/afp/1998/1001/pll45.html
- Naderi ASA and Reilly RF. 'Primary Care Approach to Proteinuria', Journal of the American Board of Family Medicine. Novemeber-December 2008. 21(6); 569–574, retrieved from http://www.jabfm.org/content/21/6/569.full

Additional Clinician and Patient Resources:

- HealthyChildren.org from the American Academy of Pediatrics, 'Proteinuria' (last updated 1/9/2012), retrieved from http://www.healthychildren.org/English/health-issues/conditions/genitourinary-tract/pages/Proteinuria.aspx?nfstatus=401&nftoken=00000000-0000-0000-0000-000000000000&nfstatusdescription=ERROR%3a+No+local+token

- Kallen RJ. 'Pediatric Proteinuria: Orthostatic Proteinuria' (last updated November 28, 2011), retrieved from http://emedicine.medscape.com/article/984289-overviewtfaw2aab6b4
- National Kidney & Urologic Disease Information Clearinghouse (NKUDIC):, Proteinuria (March 2009, last updated Sept 2, 2010), retrieved from http://kidney.niddk.nih.gov/kudiseases/pubs/proteinuria

27

HEMATURIA

Lawrence J. D'Angelo

TEST YOUR KNOWLEDGE

39. A 17 year old female comes in complaining that her urine has changed color. She is a basketball player and sometimes, after practice, her urine turns a brown color, taking days to clear. She has no other associated complaints such as back pain or dysuria. There is no family history of kidney disease. Her physical exam is unremarkable with a normal blood pressure and no flank discomfort. Urinalysis reveals 1+ protein and microscopic hematuria but no evidence of white cells. What is the *MOST* likely causes of this teen's problem?

    A. Small kidney stones (gravel) displaced by exercise.
    B. Early onset nephrotic syndrome.
    C. Asymptomatic urinary tract infection.
    D. Exercise induced urinary changes.
    E. Typical findings of chronic dehydration.

Refer to end of chapter for answer on page 297.

An 18 year old adolescent was recently started on oral contraceptives. She begins to complain about groin pain and develops gross hematuria.

BACKGROUND

- Hematuria is defined by the presence of red blood cells (RBCs) in the urine. As little as 1 ml of blood per liter of urine can change its color, so relatively small amounts of blood can bring patients to consult a health care provider.
- Diagnosis is based on finding more than 4 erythrocytes per high-power field (HPF) on a urine sediment specimen. Less than 3% of healthy individuals excrete more than 3 RBCs/HPF.
- Most cases are detected by the reaction of a reagent strip impregnated with ortho-toluidine. This may correlate with as few as 2 to 5 RBCs/HPF in the urine.
- Hematuria in adolescents is usually asymptomatic; however, when symptoms are present, they often point to the etiology.
- The differential diagnosis of hematuria is extensive; however, the common conditions that occur in adolescents are far fewer (Table 1).
- Hematuria can be caused by renal glomerular or non-glomerual diseases (Table 2).
- Rarely, hematuria may be due to systemic coagulation disturbances such as thrombocytopenia or by anti-coagulation medications.
- False hematuria must always be considered in the differential.

ASSESSMENT

HISTORY

History of Present Illness

- Is the hematuria macroscopic (visible to the naked eye)?
- A history of normal urine preceding exercise, followed by hematuria after heavy exercise suggests **marathon runner's (athlete's) hematuria.**
- Recurrent bouts of hematuria following upper respiratory tract infections suggests **immunoglobulin A nephropathy (Berger disease).**

- Is the patient sexually active? **Gonococcal urethritis** can present with macrohematuria.

Past Medical History

- Does the patient report a history of hearing loss? This occurs in **Alport's syndrome.**
- Patients with a history of **nephrolithiasis** can present with recurrences.

Family History

- Is there a family history of hematuria, deafness or known kidney disease?
- Are any relatives currently on dialysis treatment for chronic renal failure?

Medications

- Is the patient currently using oral contraceptives or anticoagulants? **Loin pain hematuria syndrome** can occur in young women on oral contraceptives.

Review of Systems

- Dysuria and frequency suggest **lower urinary tract infections,** while fever and flank pain suggest **upper tract infections.**
- **Renal stones** are accompanied by severe colicky back and flank pain often radiating to the abdomen and/or testicles, whereas **loin pain hematuria** is characterized by episodic unilateral or bilateral loin pain.
- Does the patient report rash, joint pain or bleeding tendencies? Rash and joint pain often accompany **systemic lupus erythematosus (SLE).**
- Early onset renal insufficiency accompanied by abnormalities of the lens and retina as well as high-frequency hearing loss characterize **hereditary nephritis (Alport syndrome).**

PHYSICAL

- Decreased hearing or vision may indicate the presence of familial nephritis.

Vital Signs

- Chronic kidney diseases are often accompanied by elevations in blood pressure.

Abdomen

- Assess for tenderness and abdominal masses.

Skin

- Examine the skin carefully for rashes, ecchymoses or purpura.
- Edema, usually in the lower extremities, suggests chronic kidney disease.
- Abdominal pain and "palpable purpura" suggest **Henoch-Schönlein disease.**

STUDIES

First determine if the hematuria is "true" or "false."

- "True" hematuria
  - A positive dipstick finding is confirmed by the presence of RBCs in a spun urine pellet while spun urine itself is clear.
- "False" hematuria
  - Red blood cell lysis can lead to hemoglobinuria with a positive dipstick finding, negative microscopic examination, red spun urine, and pink spun serum.
  - Muscle breakdown can cause myoglobinuria with a positive dipstick finding, negative microscopic examination, orange-red or brown spun urine and clear spun serum.
  - Menstrual bleeding can easily contaminate urine.
  - Certain foods and drugs have also been known to cause pigmenturia that can mimic hematuria. The dipstick is negative.

Urinalysis

- Hematuria should be confirmed on repeated urinalyses before an extensive evaluation.

- Determine the presence or absence of RBC casts and/or proteinuria.
- RBC casts and greater than 10% dysmorphic RBCs suggest a renal parenchymal origin, usually either glomerulonephritis or interstitial nephritis.
- Significant proteinuria suggests a glomerular cause; however, blood in the urine can cause some proteinuria, even heavy bleeding usually results in less than 1 g/24 hour.
- Idiopathic hypercalciuria is recognized as an important cause of microscopic hematuria and it can be useful to obtain a random urine calcium/creatinine ratio. A ratio of less than 0.2 is normal. With a ratio greater than 0.2, hypercalciuria is likely to be the cause of the hematuria and no further evaluation is required.

Urine Culture

- With signs or symptoms suggestive of infection, obtain a urine culture.

Complete Blood Cell (CBC) Count

- Anemia is common in chronic renal disease.
- Thrombocytopenia can occur with SLE.

Basic Metabolic Panel

- Serum BUN and creatinine are elevated with acute renal failure.
- Electrolyte disturbances may be seen with chronic renal disease.

SPECIAL TESTS

Antinuclear Antigen (ANA), Anti-DNA Antibody, Third and Fourth Components of Complement (C3 and C4), Antistreptolysin O Titer (ASO), Serum Albumin, Cholesterol, Quantitative Urinary Protein, and Creatinine Clearance

- These tests should be considered in adolescents with signs and symptoms suggestive of connective tissue disease or proteinuria and RBC casts.

Prothrombin Time, Partial Thromboplastin Time, Platelet Count, and Bleeding Time

- Consider these tests if a coagulopathy is suspected.

Sickle Cell Screening or Hemoglobin Electrophoresis

- Screen in African-American patients to evaluate for sickle cell trait or disease.

Renal Ultrasound

- If the diagnosis is unclear and hematuria is persistent or recurrent, a renal sonogram may find structural causes of hematuria such as cysts or hydronephrosis.

Cystoscopy

- Consider if the patient has lower tract symptoms of dysuria or urgency and the RBC morphological features are normal.

Renal Biopsy

- Indicated if there is significant proteinuria and RBC casts are present.
- Consider if hypertension accompanies either of these two symptoms.
- Without this history, almost all individuals will have either normal biopsy findings or no significant pathological change.

Renal Angiography

- Consider if gross hematuria persists without an obvious cause or if vascular causes are suspected.

Hearing Test

- Consider if the patient reports hearing loss.

Urine of First-Degree Relatives

- The presence of hematuria in a parent, sibling, or child of an adolescent may indicate either benign familial hematuria (if family members are well) or hereditary nephritis (if family members have renal disease).

DISPOSITION

The management of hematuria in adolescents depends on the diagnosis:

- Marathon runner's hematuria, benign familial hematuria and loin pain hematuria all have a favorable outcome and can be followed by the primary care physician.
- Infectious causes of hematuria such as pyelonephritis, gonorrhea and hemorrhagic cystitis can also be managed by the primary care physician, usually on an outpatient basis.
- For severe infections such as complicated pyelonephritis, inpatient antibiotic therapy may be warranted.
- More complex illnesses such as polycystic disease of the kidneys, hereditary nephritis and immunoglobulin A nephropathy require referral to a nephrologist.

What is unique about hematuria in adolescents?

- This is an age of intensive physical activity and sports participation; hence, the frequency of "Marathon Runner's Hematuria."
- It is also often when oral contraceptive are initiated; hence, the occurrence of "loin pain syndrome."
- Trauma during sports and sometimes during fights may occur due to impulsivity or inexperience.
- Familial conditions often do not manifest until the second decade of life (i.e., IgA Nephropathy, Alport's Syndrome, and Familial Hematuria).
- Adolescent initiation of sexual activity may lead to "honeymoon" cystitis and/or gonococcal urethritis.

TEST YOUR KNOWLEDGE ANSWER

39. D. Gross or microscopic hematuria is associated with many forms of exercise, including baseball, track, football, etc. Nephrotic syndrome is characterized by marked proteinuria and edema. Nephrolithiasis is extremely painful. Asymptomatic urinary tract infection may be associated with leukocyturia and positive nitrates but not hematuria. Severe dehydration indeed has a very abnormal urinalysis but this patient did

not report thirst, oliguria, lightheadedness nor any other symptoms of dehydration.

Table 1. Common Causes of Hematuria in Adolescents.

Marathon Runner's (Athlete's) Hematuria	• Gross or microscopic hematuria associated with many forms of exercise, including baseball, track, football, hockey, boxing, cross-country skiing, swimming, crew, lacrosse, rugby and basic military training. • Normal urine before exercise, with hematuria on the first specimen voided after exercise, lasting up to 24 to 48 hours. • Possibly associated with dysuria and suprapubic discomfort. • Unclear etiology, unrelated to the duration of sustained activity. • Possible causes: decrease in renal plasma flow, local trauma to the bladder, or leakage of blood from spiral vessels in the adventitia of minor calyces. • The prognosis is excellent unless another renal problem is the cause.
Loin-Pain Hematuria Syndrome	• Mainly occurs in young females receiving oral contraceptives. • Recurrent bouts of gross or microscopic hematuria with or without dysuria but often with unilateral or bilateral loin pain. • Blood pressure and renal function are normal. • NSAIDs and calcium channel blockers may be useful. • Oral contraceptives should be discontinued.
Immunoglobulin A Nephropathy (Berger Disease)	• Relatively common cause of gross hematuria in young adults. Associated with IgA and IgG deposits in the mesangium. • 80% of patients are between 16 and 35 years of age. • Male-female ratio is 6:1. • Recurrent bouts of gross hematuria after upper respiratory tract infections. • May have dysuria and flank pain.

(*Continued*)

Table 1. (*Continued*)

	• Renal function is usually normal, but 40% of individuals may progress to renal insufficiency. • Poor prognostic signs include hypertension, renal insufficiency, and persistent proteinuria (protein excretion greater than 1 g/day). • Serum IgA levels are elevated in 50% of patients. • Diagnosis is made by characteristic history or renal biopsy. • No treatment is available.
Hereditary Nephritis (Alport Syndrome) and Polycystic Kidney Disease (PCKD)	• Adult form of PCKD usually manifests in the second or third decade of life with hematuria and hypertension. • Autosomal dominant. • Familial nephritis in males often causes an early onset of renal insufficiency. • Renal disease often accompanied by abnormalities of the lens and retina and high-frequency hearing loss.
Benign Familial Hematuria	• Glomerular hematuria (RBC casts), nonprogressive renal disease, and normal renal function in affected family members. • Associated with thinning of the glomerular basement membrane. • Autosomal dominant. • Diagnosis suggested by (a) hemoglobin or RBC casts in the urine of adolescent and parent or sibling, (b) absence of renal insufficiency, and (c) no history of renal failure or auditory abnormalities in the affected family members. • More common in females.

Table 2. Renal Parenchymal Diseases.

Glomerular Diseases	Primary	IgA nephropathy (Berger disease), membranous or membranoproliferative glomerulonephritis, focal glomerulonephritis or glomerulosclerosis.
	Secondary	Glomerulonephritis associated with connective tissue diseases, hemolytic uremic syndrome, or Henoch-Schönlein purpura. Glomerulonephritis associated with infections such as streptococcal infection, shunt infections, or infective endocarditis.
	Hereditary	Alport syndrome, polycystic kidney disease, medullary sponge kidney.
	Benign familial hematuria	Primary renal hematuria with thin basement membrane.
Nonglomerular Diseases	Vascular diseases	Malignant hypertension, loin-pain hematuria syndrome, arteriovenous malformation, renal arterial emboli.
	Papillary necrosis	Sickle cell disease, diabetes mellitus, alcoholism and analgesic abuse.
	Trauma	Usually significant trauma, as from motor vehicle accidents or contusions from contact sports.
	Acute pyelonephritis	Related to cystitis, malformations, reflux or prostatitis.
	Neoplasms	Kidney or bladder.
	Renal calculi	Hypercalcemia.

WEB REFERENCES

- Gattineni, J. 'Review Article: Highlights for the Management of a Child with Proteinuria and Hematuria', International Journal of Pediatrics. 2012, retrieved from http://www.hindawi.com/journals/ijped/2012/768142/

Additional Clinician and Patient Resources:

- Gulati, S. 'Hematuria', Medscape Reference (updated Jun 19,2012), retrieved from http://emedicine.medscape.com/article/981898-overview
- HealthyChildren.org from the American Academy of Pediatrics, 'Blood in Urine (Hematuria) (last updated 1/9/2012), retrieved from http://www.healthychildren.org/English/health-issues/conditions/genitourinary-tract/pages/Blood-in-Urine-Hematuria.aspx
- National Kidney and Urologic Disease Information Clearinghouse (NKUDIC)
  - 'Hematuria: Blood in Urine', March 2012, retrieved from http://kidney.niddk.nih.gov/kudiseases/pubs/hematuria/
  - Patient handout, "Hematuria: Blood in Urine', retrieved from http://kidney.niddk.nih.gov/KUDiseases/pubs/hematuria/Hematuria_Blood_in_the_Urine_508.pdf

28

LOW BACK PAIN

Alan Morrison

TEST YOUR KNOWLEDGE

40. A 16 year old healthy cheerleader presents with low back pain of 3 weeks duration. Her routines consist of acrobatics including back hand springs. Which of the following radiographic views of the lumbar spine is *MOST* likely to diagnose her condition?

    A. Anteroposterior (AP)
    B. Lateral
    C. Supine
    D. Oblique
    E. None. This teen does not require imaging.

Refer to end of chapter for answer on page 309.

A 16 year old gymnast presents with 3 weeks of lower back pain that has been getting worse over the past few days.

BACKGROUND

- Active teens are prone to back pain. This is commonly due to muscular strain; however, there are many other reasons for back pain (Table 1).
- Spondilolysis and spondylolisthesis tend to occur with activities involving repeated hyperextension.
- Inflammatory and infectious conditions can present with back pain.
- Renal or gastrointestinal problems may present as pain referred to the back.
- Scoliosis is usually not a cause of back pain in adolescents.

ASSESSMENT

HISTORY

History of Present Illness

- Assess Pain Characteristics
  - Location: Upper back pain is characterstic of **Sheurmann's disease**, while mid-lower back pain is often associated with **muscle strain.**
  - Severity: Severe pain that wakes the teen suggests **tumor** or **infection.**
  - Onset and Duration: Pain at rest also raises concern for an underlying **tumor** or **infection.**
- What are some of the triggers and exacerbating factors for pain?
- Does the patient report any recent trauma or injury? Ask the teen about any activities such as sports, work or any heavy lifting.
- Is the patient involved in activities which require frequent hyperextension such as cheerleading or gymnastics? Repeated hyperextension places the teen at risk for **spondilolysis**.
- What type of shoes does the teen regularly wear? Are they on their feet for a large portion of the day?
- Determine the size and type of the teen's back pack. Are they frequently carrying a heavy load? Do they use a one-sided shoulder bag? Do the shoulder straps on their backpack have additional padding for support?

- Is the patient sitting for long periods of time and do they self-report good or poor posture? If they use a laptop, do they generally sit at a desk or table or are they frequently using the laptop on a bed or in their lap?
- Does the patient sleep on an older mattress or sofa? Soft bedding can lead to back pain.
- If the teen has macromastia, does she use an appropriately supportive bra?

Past Medical History

- Does the patient report previous back pain or injury?
- Has the patient been diagnosed with cancer in the past, raising concern for recurrence?
- Is the patient immunocompromised from either a chronic medical condition such as HIV or because of long term steroid therapy?

Social History

- Do patients report IV drug use? If yes, this places them at increased risk of infection.

Review of Systems

- Have there been any changes to bowel or bladder habits?
- Fever, joint pain (arthritis), difficulty urinating (urethritis) or eye problems (iritis) suggest an underlying inflammatory condition such as **ankylosing spondylitis.**
- Recent unexplained fevers, chills or adenopathy suggest an infection.
- Bladder dysfunction including symptoms of retention, frequency or overflow incontinence are consistent with **cauda equina compression,** which can result in progressive neurologic deficits in the lower extremities.

PHYSICAL EXAM

Vital Signs

- Fever suggests an infectious etiology.

Back

- Inspect for asymmetry, kyphosis, lordosis or midline hypertrichosis. Observe for any obvious deformity or signs of trauma.
- Assess patient's range of motion. Is the teen able to flex, extend, rotate and sidebend without pain or difficulty?
- Palpate for any point tenderness over the vertebra, specifically assessing for pain on the spinous or transverse processes.
- Complete maneuvers to elicit source of back pain (Table 2).

Muscle

- Observe the back for any signs of muscle atrophy.
- Does the back feel cool or hot or do the muscles feel tense?

Lower Extremity

- Evaluate gait.
- Examine for leg length discrepancies and assess the feet without shoes for **pes planus.**

Neurologic Exam

- Check reflexes.
  - Diminished patellar reflexes suggests a problem at the L4 level.
  - Diminished ankle jerk suggests a S1 level problem.
  - Presence of the Babinski reflex suggests an upper motor lesion and could represent a demyelinating process.
- Assess muscle strength.
  - Difficulty squatting or rising from a squat suggests a problem at the L4 spinal level.

- Inability to heel walk suggests a problem at the L5 level.
- Difficulty with toe walking suggests a problem at the S1 level.

- Complete sensory testing of the lower extremity.
  - Deficits medially suggests a problem at the L4 level; dorsally, at the L5 level' and laterally; at the S1 level.

Skin

- Note any nevi, cafe au lait spots or other skin changes.
- Assess for any soft tissue masses.

STUDIES

Routine tests are generally not needed for evaluation of a teen with back pain and the decision to obtain laboratory or radiologic studies should be based on the clinical history and physical exam findings.

CBC with Differential, CRP and ESR and Urinalysis

- Consider if the teen is febrile, has red flags suggestive of an infectious or oncologic etiology or has had pain for greater than 3 months.

Imaging studies should be considered when the history and exam findings suggest an underlying pathology such as spondylolysis, spondylolisthesis or ankylosing spondylitis.

Back X-Ray

- Obtain a scoliosis series if curvature is noted on the back exam.
  - Radiologists will calculate the Cobb angle based on the series of x-rays to determine severity of curvature, as well as Risser staging to determine stage of bone growth and development.
- An oblique x-ray should be obtained if spondylolysis or spondylolisthesis is suspected.
  - Classic "scotty dog" can be seen on this view and a break in the neck of the "dog" corresponds to a fracture of the pars interarticularis, which is specific for spondylolysis.

- Spondylolisthesis occurs when there is a bilateral pars defect, leading to slippage of a vertebra over another.

CT Scan

- This study is useful if disc disease or herniation are suspected.
- Is sensitive for detecting spondylolysis, which can be missed on radiograph.

DISPOSITION

- Treatment of back pain should be based on etiology.
- If the teen has experienced a muscular strain, treat supportively.
  - NSAID's can be used to lessen the severity of pain. For acute strains, consider ice therapy for 2–3 days and then switch to moist heat.
  - The patient should be counseled on proper posture when standing and sitting; appropriate shoes with good arch support, especially if found to have pes planus; proper techniques when lifting heavy objects such as bending at the knee and using thigh muscles to assist with lifting versus back muscles; use of bras with appropriate support if large breasted; and use of good mattress for proper back support when sleeping.
  - Physical therapy should be initiated as soon as physically possible.
  - Patients should be advised on back strengthening exercises and should engage in low impact activities such as low-stress aerobics, stationary bike riding or swimming.
  - With more persistent pain, physical therapy consultation should be considered.

- Chronic, or functional back pain may occur and it is important for the patient to maintain their level of activity to prevent further deterioration or dysfunction. Encourage back strengthening exercises and consider physical therapy. Follow up in the office is necessary to determine response to therapy.
- Consider orthopedic consultation if back pain is severe, unremitting or if a more serious condition is suspected.
  - A teen diagnosed with spondylolisthesis should decrease physical activity and start NSAID's for pain relief. If severe, this condition can cause spinal root compression, requiring surgery.

- In cases of disc herniation, recommend analgesics and physical therapy. Steroid treatment and surgery may also be required.
- If an osteomyelitis of the back is diagnosed, the patient will likely require hospitalization and intravenous antibiotics.

What is unique about back pain in adolescents?

- The growth spurt of puberty also involves the spine and this increases the risk of scoliosis in teens; however, this is usually *not* a cause of back pain.
- Athletes who frequently hyperextend their backs, such as cheerleaders and gymnasts, are at greater risk for spondylolysis and spondylolisthesis.
- Older children and younger adolescents (ages 9–15) diagnosed with spondylolisthesis have an increased chance of progressive slippage.
- Back strengthening exercises can prevent recurrence of back pain episodes.

TEST YOUR KNOWLEDGE ANSWERS

40. D. This patient has a history of repeated hyperextension which raises the question of spondylolysis. Of the proposed views, an oblique view of the lumbar spine will show spondylolysis. While AP and lateral views can be helpful they may not show spondylolysis.

Table 1. Differential Diagnosis of Back Pain in Adolescents.

System	Diagnostic Considerations
Musculoskeletal	Muscle strain Trauma Scoliosis Congenital abnormalities Herniated disc Sheurmann's disease (juvenile kyphosis) Spondylolysis (fibrous defect in the pars interarticularis) Spondylolisthesis (spondylolysis with forward displacement of a vertebral segment and most common L5-S1) Pes Planus

(*Continued*)

Table 1. (*Continued*)

System	Diagnostic Considerations
Inflammatory	Reactive arthritis (Reiter's syndrome) Ankylosing spondylitis Discitis
Infectious	Viral syndrome Urinary tract infection Endocarditis Osteomyelitis
Gastointestinal	Cholecystitis Pancreatitis Ulcers
Renal	Pyelonephritis Renal stones Perinephric abscess
Metabolic	Cushing's disease Acromegaly Hyerparathyroidism Osteomalacia
Gynecologic	Endometritis
Functional	Stress
Oncologic	Osteoid osteoma Spinal cord tumor Cauda equina compression from mass effect Leukemia

Table 2. Evaluating a Teen with Back Pain: Physical Exam Maneuvers.

Straight Leg Raising	With the patient lying supine, the examiner lifts the patient's leg while the knee is straight. Pain in the sciatic nerve distribution, when the leg is between 30 and 70 degrees is considered a positive test.
Braggard's Test	After the patient has straightened their legs, passively dorsiflex the ankles by pushing up on the balls of the feet. This test is positive if it produces pain in the spine.
Patrick's Test	With the patient lying supine, the examiner positions the limb to be examined in flexion, abduction, and external rotation so that the foot rests on the opposite thigh just above the knee; the examiner then slowly and passively presses the side to be examined toward the table while stabilizing the opposite anterior superior iliac spine.
Burn's Test	Have the patient kneel on a chair and touch the floor with their fingertips. They should be able to reach within 15 cm of the floor without difficulty.

WEB REFERENCES

- Bernstein RM, Cozen H. 'Evaluation of Back Pain in Children and Adolescents', American Family Physician. 2007 Dec 1; 76(11); 1669–1676, retrieved from http://www.aafp.org/afp/2007/1201/p1669.html
- Fritz JM and Clifford SN. 'Low Back Pain in Adolescents: A Comparison of Clinical Outcomes in Sports Participants and Nonparticipants', Journal of Athletic Training. 2010 Jan-Feb; 45(1); 61–66, retrieved from http:www.ncbi.nlm.nih.gov/pmc/articles/PMC2808757/
- Olsen TL, *et al.* 'The Epidemiology of Low Back Pain in an Adolescent Population', American Journal of Public Health. April 1992; 82(4); 606–608, retrieved from http://www.ncbi.nlm.nih.gov/pmc/articles/PMC1694113/pdf/amjph00541-0104.pdf
- Pub Med Health, Spondylolisthesis (last reviewed 7/11/2012) retrieved from http://www.ncbi.nlm.nih.gov/pubmedhealth/PMH0002240/
- Rodriguez DP and Poussaint TY. 'Imaging of Back Pain in Children', American Journal of Neuroradialogy, 2010; 31; 787–802, retrieved from http://www.ajnr.org/content/31/5/787.full

Additional Clinician and Patient Resources:

- American Academy of Orthopedic Surgeons, OrthoInfo, 'Back Pain in Children' (last reviewed February 2010), retrieved from: http://orthoinfo.aaos.org/topic.cfm?topic=a00036
- Scoliosis Research Society (SRS), Adolescent Back Pain, retrieved from http://www.srs.org/patient_and_family/spondylolisthesis/adolescent_lumbar_back_pain.html
- Stanford Hospital and Clinics, SPondylolysis/Spondylolisthesis, retrieved from http://standfordhospital.org/clinicsmedServices/COE/orthopaedics/spineCenter/patientEducation/spondylolysis.html

29

SPORTS MEDICINE: MUSCULOSKELETAL INJURIES

Nailah Coleman

TEST YOUR KNOWLEDGE

41. When evaluating a young athlete with ankle pain, which of the following should be done first?

    A. Have the patient point to the location of pain with one finger.
    B. Ask the patient to walk and observe his/her gait before palpating the injured ankle.
    C. Palpate the injured area.
    D. A and B.
    E. A and C.

Refer to end of chapter for answer on page 319.

A 15 year old male comes to the office limping. He is a basketball player and presents with acute left ankle pain since twisting his foot on a rebound yesterday. He has an important championship game in a couple of days that he "can't miss."

BACKGROUND

- Adolescents often present for injury-related office visits in the following situations:
  - Something hurts (acutely or chronically) and affects athletic participation.
  - Something looks or feels different from before (i.e. a deformity) and affects athletic participation.
  - Something does not work the way it used to work (i.e. weakness).
  - They were hit in the head and now feel or act differently (i.e. a concussion).
- This chapter will focus on the consult for ankle pain following an injury: the related concepts can all be extrapolated to other extremity injuries sustained by teens.

ASSESSMENT

HISTORY

History of Present Illness

- Determine the nature of the injury. The most common mechanism of ankle sprains is an inversion injury.
- Determine the exact location of pain. The teen should point with one finger to the point of maximal pain and areas to where the pain radiates. The two most commonly injured ligaments of the ankle are located on the lateral aspect of the ankle (anterior talofibular and calcaneofibular ligaments).
- Determine the pain characteristics. Is the pain sharp, aching, burning, throbbing, or pulling? Is it better, worse or unchanged since injury? It is always best to have the teen use his own words.
- Does the pain cause sensation changes? **Ankle sprains** are associated with normal sensation.

- Is the pain associated with other concerning symptoms (e.g. swelling, redness, bruising, popping or cracking)? Swelling can typically occur with an ankle sprain, but swelling that *does not improve over time* with supportive measures may be associated with more serious ankle injuries.
- Does the pain affect the patient's function? Can the teen bear weight after suffering a lower limb injury? Does the pain affect the patient's ability to participate in school or athletics, and does it interfere with sleep?
- Determine factors that alleviate (e.g. ice, rest, elevation, compression and/or medication) and aggravate (e.g. weight-bearing or direct pressure).
- Has the patient sought treatment for this injury such as physical therapy, complementary and/or alternative medicine, or been evaluated by a chiropractor or certified athletic trainer?

Past Medical History

- Are there any past or present medical conditions that might clarify the diagnosis or affect the treatment or treatment response? Has the patient been diagnosed with:
  - Other musculoskeletal disorders (i.e. fibromyalgia or osteoarthritis).
  - Rheumatologic disorders (i.e. juvenile rheumatoid arthritis, systemic lupus erythematosis (SLE) or psoriasis).
  - Endocrinopathies (i.e. diabetes mellitus, thyroid disorder or obesity).
  - Neurologic or psychiatric disorders (i.e. complex regional pain syndrome, anxiety or depression).
  - Cardiac, pulmonary or gastrointestinal disease.
  - Has the patient had any past surgeries?

Family History

- Does any family member have a similar problem (e.g. frequent ankle sprains), other bone or joint disorders, arthritis, SLE, sarcoidosis or other pertinent conditions that might relate to the patient's condition and/or treatment?

Review of Systems

- Assess for systemic causes of joint pain and swelling, including infection, inflammation and metabolic concerns.
- Determine if there are:

- Constitutional symptoms such as fevers, chills, weight changes or fatigue.
- Neurologic symptoms such as headaches, changes in vision or balance disturbance.
- Cardiovascular symptoms such as chest pain.
- Respiratory symptoms such as shortness of breath or chest tightness.
- Gastrointestinal symptoms such as vomiting, diarrhea, weight loss or abdominal pain.
- Dermatologic changes including skin, hair or nails.

PHYSICAL

First: Observe without touching.

- Observe the patient's general behavior before, during and after the exam. Does the teen appear comfortable? Are the patient's movements easy or strained?
- Expose the injured area and compare it to the opposite extremity. Note asymmetry.
- Look at the overlying skin for erythema, swelling, bruising, deformity and asymmetry. Swelling is common with ankle sprains.
- Observe gait and ability to perform weight-bearing maneuvers (i.e. heel and toe walking).
- Evaluate the patient's range of motion, noting any variation from the opposite extremity. Determine whether limited motion is due to pain, restriction or both.

Second: Perform the exam.

- Palpation should occur at the end of the exam to avoid irritating a painful area that if manipulated early, could limit the remainder of the exam.
- Feel for edema.
- If a deformity is noted, determine its size, mobility and if there is tenderness to palpation.
- Determine the exact location of tenderness.
- Evaluate joint functions including strength and stability.
- Strength testing can be difficult to assess on a teen in acute pain.
- Evaluate sensation and neurovascular status distal to the area of injury.

- Perform joint-specific special tests based on history and exam findings. There are specific tests to consider when evaluating an injured ankle (Table 1).

STUDIES

Further diagnostic testing might be necessary to establish the diagnosis.

- The Ottawa ankle and foot rules were created to guide the clinician's decision to obtain an x-ray (Table 2).
- When deciding if a radiologic study of a joint is warranted, consider the presenting symptoms (i.e. trauma, deformity, inability to use, unexplained pain) and understand that the joint involved, as well as nature of injury, should dictate which studies should be ordered (Table 3).

X-ray of Injured Joint or Limb

- When obtaining an x-ray to evaluate an injury, always obtain at least two views, usually AP/PA and lateral.
- When evaluating the ankle, a third view should be obtained in the inverted position, also known as the Mortise view. The AP/PA view is limited by the distal overlap of the tibia and fibula, thereby obscuring part of the joint line. The Mortise view allows for complete observation of the tibia-fibular-talar interface.
- When reading an x-ray, note the view, joint space symmetry and appearance, any deformity (i.e. fracture) and its exact location.

MRI with or without Contrast

- Useful to evaluate soft tissues and bone trauma.
- Imaging can be affected by implanted devices, posing a potential safety concern.

CT with or without Contrast

- To evaluate more detailed bony anatomy and imaging of hardware.
- Typically contrast is used when there is a concern for infection or tumor, which can underlie a pathologic fracture.

- Clinicians should consult with a radiologist or a specialist before ordering any advanced study to ensure that the appropriate views and contrast versus no contrast are ordered.

Arthrography

- To evaluate the joint capsule and articular surface integrity.
- Can be used in combination with other modalities (i.e. MRI and CT).

Bone Scan (Scintigraphy)

- To evaluate blood flow and metabolic activity.
- Can identify infection, neoplasm or occult fracture.
- Can be used in combination with other modalities (i.e. CT).

Ultrasound

- To evaluate soft tissue.
- Can be used for interventional procedures.

TREATMENT

- Encourage supportive care, the **PRICE** regimen, until the swelling decreases:
  - Protect the ankle from further injury.
  - Rest the ankle.
  - Ice the ankle to reduce swelling.
  - Compress the ankle with an ace bandage to immobilize and reduce swelling.
  - Elevate the ankle to reduce swelling.
- Additional measures:
  - Crutches can be used until the patient is able to bear weight with a normal gait.
  - NSAID's have been associated with improved pain control, decreased swelling and more rapid return to activity in patients with ankle sprains.
  - A lace-up ankle brace can provide additional support to the ankle while ambulating. It should initially be worn continuously with usage decreased

as the teen regains full strength, at which point it should be worn only during athletic activity.

- When weight bearing is difficult, consider a walking fracture boot that has a rocker bottom allowing added ankle stability during ambulation.
- Within 48 to 72 hours of an injury, and insofar as pain will allow, range of motion exercises that progress to strength training and balance exercises should be initiated.
- Return to sports should progress gradually once the patient is able to bear weight with a normal gait. Teens should progress from light jogging to sports-specific drills to practice sessions to scrimmaging and finally to full game play.

What is unique about musculoskeletal injuries in adolescents?

- Adolescents often harbor misconceptions such as "walk through pain" or "no pain, no gain."
- Counsel patients that playing on an injured joint could potentially lead to more serious injury. Additionally, the disincentive of poor performance caused by pain may deter athletes from playing on an injured joint.
- Adherence to recommendations, such as icing, resting and limb elevation may be inconsistent.
- Many teens will put pressure on the clinician to return them to the game before adequate rehabilitation has taken place.
- Firm and kind guidance is often required for the injured athlete. Referral to a sports medicine specialist and/or physical therapist is often invaluable for the prevention of disabling re-injury.

TEST YOUR KNOWLEDGE ANSWER

41. D. When evaluating an athlete with ankle pain, it is useful to observe the gait and ask the patient to point with one finger to the area of pain. Palpation should be done at the end of the exam to avoid irritating a painful area and making subsequent examination difficult.

Table 1. Special Testing: Ankle.

Drawer Testing	• Stabilize the tibia, cup the heel and pull anteriorly in an attempt to anteriorly sublux the talus (compare to unaffected side). • Tests stability of the anterior talofibular ligament.
Talar Tilt Testing	• Stabilize the tibia, grasp the midfoot, and invert and evert the ankle (compare to unaffected side). • Tests stability of the calcaneofibular ligament (CFL).

Table 2. Getting X-rays: Ottowa Ankle and Foot Rules.

Ankle	• Pain in malleolar zone (medial or lateral) *Plus at least one of the following*: • Inability to bear weight immediately, at the ER or in the physician's office • Tenderness at the posterior medial or lateral maleolus and distal tibia/fibula
Foot	• Pain in the midfoot zone (medial or lateral) *Plus at least one of the following*: • Inability to bear weight immediately, at the emergency department or physician's office • Tenderness at the base of the fifth metatarsal or at the navicular bone

Table 3. Standard Radiographic Views (Obtain Images of the Entire Bone in 2 or More Planes.)

Region	Views	Special Considerations
Hand	PA and Lateral	
Wrist	PA and Lateral	Scaphoid view for scaphoid fracture
Elbow/Forearm	AP and Lateral	+/− Comparison of opposite arm
Shoulder	AP, True AP and Axillary	+/− Scapular Y view (if axillary not available)
Cervical Spine	AP and Lateral	+/− Swimmer's view
Thoracic Spine	AP and Lateral	+/− Swimmer's view
Lumbar Spine	AP and Lateral	+/− Spot L5 lateral for closer view
Pelvis	AP	
Hips	AP and True Lateral (Frog Leg)	
Knee	AP and Lateral	• Merchant (sunrise) views for patellar pathology • Oblique views for alternate angles • Tunnel views for osteochodritis dessicans
Ankle	AP, Lateral and Mortise (Ankle Inversion)	
Foot	Weight Bearing AP and Lateral, Supine Oblique (Foot Inversion)	+/− Eversion oblique for alternate angles

WEB REFERENCES

- American Academy of Pediatrics (pediatrics.aappublications.org)
  - Brenner JS, and the Council on Sports Medicine and Fitness. 'Overuse Injuries, Overtraining, and Burnout in Child and Adolescent Athletes', Pediatrics. 2007; 119(6); 1242–1245, retrieved from http://pediatrics.aappublications.Org/content/119/6/1242.full?sid=9d652a53-2fcl-4226-b563-6belc22a4137

- Cheng TL, *et al.* 'Sports Injuries: An Important Cause of Morbidity in Urban Youth', Pediatrics. 2000; 105(3); e32, retrieved from http://pediatrics.aappublications.org/content/105/3/e32.full?sid=9d652a53-2fcl-4226-b563-6belc22a4137
- Martin, TJ. 'Technical Report: Knee Brace Use in the Young Athlete', Pediatrics. 2001 Sugust; 108(2); 503–507, retrieved from http://pediatrics.aappublications.org/content/108/2/503.full

- Cassas KJ and Cassettari-Wayhs A. 'Childhood and Adolescent Sports-Related Overuse Injuries'. American Family Physician. 2006 March; 73(6); 1014–1022, retrieved from http://www.eteamz.com/bangoreastll/files/Yourhsportsinjury.pdf
- Fong DTP, *et al.* 'Understanding acute ankle ligamentous sprain injury in sports', Sports Medicine, Arthoscopy, Rehabilitation, Therapy and Technology. 2009. 1(14), retrieved from http://www.smarttjournal.com/content/1/1/14
- Kennedy JG, *et al.* 'Sports injuries of the foot and ankle in the adolescent athlete', International SportMed Journal. 2006; 7(2); 85–97, retrieved from http://www.jamestownsoccerclub.com/docs/foot%20and%20ankle%20injuries%20in%20adolescent%20athletes.pdf

Additional Clinician and Patient Resources:

- American College of Sports Medicine (http://www.acsm.org/)
  - Ibrahim V, Meylet Z and Panagos A. 'Ankle Sprains and the Athlete's patient handout, retrieved from http://www.acsm.org/docs/current-comments/anklesprainstemp.pdf
- American Medical Society of Sports Medicine (http://www.amssm.org/)
- Relay Health, Ankle Sprin: Teen Version (last modified 2/8/2011), retrieved from http://www.cpnonline.org/CRS/CRS/pa_anksprai_sma.htm
- Sundberg S. 'Returning to Sports After an Ankle Injury', A Pediatric Perspective. 2003; 12(5), retrieved from http://www.gillettechildrens.org/fileUpload/Vol12No5.pdf
- Teens Health from Nemours. Ankle Sprains, retrieved from http://kidshealth.org/teen/safety/firstaid/ankle_sprains.html
- Wheeless' Orthopaedics Online Textbook, Ankle Sprain (last updated December 19, 2012), retrieved from http://www.wheelessonline.com/ortho/ankle_sprain

30

ACNE

Karen Rosewater and
Harshita J. Saxena

TEST YOUR KNOWLEDGE

42. All the following statements are true *EXCEPT*:
    A. Topical tretinoins are considered first line therapy against comedonal lesions.
    B. Benzoyl peroxide has both keratolytic and bactericidal properties making it an ideal agent to treat inflammatory acne.
    C. When evaluating teens for routine physical exam, if they do not raise acne as a concern, it usually means that they are not bothered by their acne.
    D. *Propionibacterium acnes* is one of the causes of acne in teens.
    E. Acne lesions can occur in many different areas of the body including the face, torso and extremities.

Refer to end of chapter for answer on page 330.

"My daughter doesn't want to go to school because of her skin problem ... kids make fun of her."

BACKGROUND

- Acute skin eruptions, such as hives and allergic reactions, will often be brought to clinicians' attention. By contrast, acne vulgaris may not be verbalized as a concern, even though the diagnosis of acne, followed by appropriate treatment may profoundly affect a teen's life.
- Acne is caused by
  - hormonal influences of adrenal and gonadal androgens which increase sebum production.
  - abnormal keratinization of sebaceous and follicular epithelium causing clogged pores.
  - growth of bacteria, namely *Propionibacterium acnes.*
  - inflammatory responses caused by the breakdown of triglycerides into free fatty acids by bacterial lipase enzymes.
- While acne is common in adolescence, it may be exacerbated by an underlying medical condition (i.e. an endocrine disorder associated with hyperandrogen state), use of anabolic steroids, some medications or cosmetics.

ASSESSMENT

HISTORY

History of Present Illness

- How old was the teen when they first noticed the lesions? Age of onset and relationship to Tanner stage are important to assess, as earlier onset may indicate the potential for a more severe disease course.
- How severe is the problem and what effect is it having on the teen's life?

Past Medical History

- Has there been any history of manipulations to the skin (i.e. popping, picking, rubbing or squeezing)? These manipulations may lead to secondary infections and scarring.
- What skin treatments has the teen used in the past and what were the results?

Menstrual History

- Has the teen noticed worsening of lesions at or around the time of menses?

Family History

- Genetics likely play a role in the severity of disease so it is important to ascertain other family members with a known history of acne.

Medications

- Medications such as lithium, some seizure medications (i.e. dilantin), steroids and anti-tuberculosis treatment with isoniazid may cause an increase in acne.
- Birth control pills often improve acne although some progesterone dominant pills may worsen acne.
- Certain cosmetics (that are not "non-comedogenic") and hair products (i.e. oils and pomades) may cause or exacerbate acne.
- Be alert for the possibility of anabolic steroid use that may cause or worsen acne.

Review of Systems

- Hirsutism, irregular menses and acne are all evidence of increased androgen production.
- Acne may be a clue to **polycystic ovarian syndrome** (PCOS), a condition which typically is associated with elevated androgens.

PHYSICAL

Acne is characterized by a variety of lesions: closed/open comedones, papules, pustules, nodules and cysts. A careful exam and accurate description of the lesions, will help guide therapy.

Skin

- Assess the location of acne lesions. Acne most commonly occurs on the face but can also appear on the chest, back, buttocks or even extremities.

Characteristic lesions

Non-inflammatory microcomedones:
- Closed comedones, or "whiteheads," are accumulations of keratin, lipids and bacteria trapped within hair follicles right below the skin surface.
- Open comedones, or "blackheads," are lesions that open to the surface of the skin over a follicular sac that is plugged with stratum corneum cells. The oxidation of melanin in these cells leads to the characteristic black appearance.

Inflammatory lesions:
- Papules are well circumscribed lesions that result from a break in the follicular wall with subsequent localized inflammatory response. These lesions can be inflammed, red and tender to touch.
- Pustules, or "pimples," occur when inflammatory cells lead to the collection of pus.

Severe lesions:
- Nodules are larger lesions that are often hard and painful to touch. These lesions can lead to significant scarring including skin pitting or raised knots.
- Cysts appear similar to nodules but are filled with pus and can also lead to significant scarring. For this reason, teens with cystic acne should receive immediate and definitive treatment.

Severity of lesions
- Mild: small number of papules and/or pustules with no nodules.
- Moderate: many papules and/or pustules but few nodules.
- Severe: widespread papules and/or pustules with significant nodular component.
- Acne should be differentiated from other acne-like lesions (Table 1).

STUDIES

- Acne vulgaris is a clinical diagnosis and laboratory tests are only indicated if the patient has additional symptoms that warrant concern.
- Consider if the teen has signs of hyperandrogenism (acne, hirsutism or irregular menses):

Testosterone (Free and Total), Dehydroepiandrosterone Sulfate (DHEAS), Luteinizing Hormone (LH) and Follicle Stimulating Hormone (FSH)

TREATMENT

- The primary goals of acne therapy include:
  - Reducing the number of comedones using keratolytic agents.
  - Treating inflammation with antibiotics and products that have anti-inflammatory properties.
- The therapeutic approach may include topical, systemic or a combination of topical and systemic medications depending on the severity and duration of acne lesions.
- Treatment vehicle is also an important consideration when prescribing topical agents and should take into account patient's skin type (Table 2).
- Most topical regimens offer varied formulations (i.e., cream, gel, lotion and solutions) to provide optimal coverage regardless of skin type.
- Combination therapy is often prescribed as most teens have comedonal and inflammatory acne.

Keratolytics

Topical retinoids:

- Considered first line therapy for comedonal acne.
- Effective prescription retinoids include tretinoin, adapalene and tazarotene.
- Increase the turnover of follicular epithelial cells, normalize keratinization and thereby extrude comedones.
- Side effects include redness, peeling, irritation and increased sun sensitivity.
- To decrease side effects, patients may be advised to apply to the skin once every other day when they initiate treatment, and to increase frequency of application to once daily as patient's are able to tolerate.

- Tretinoin (retinoic acid), is available as a microgel or in combination with a polymer cream which are the least irritating formulations.
- Adapalene is made from naphothoic acid, a less irritating retinoid type compound which has anti-inflammatory properties.
- Tazarotene is a synthetic acetylenic retinoid with more rapid penetration of skin and also has anti-inflammatory properties.

Salicylic acid products:

- Available over the counter, they work by sloughing dead skin skin cells and penetrating the follicle to clear comedonal plugs.
- Does not have any activity against *P. acnes.*

Sulfur based products:

- Available over the counter. Prescribed less frequently to treat acne but known to be effective against inflammatory lesions as a result of keratolytic action.
- Can cause skin discoloration.

Keratolytic and Bactericidal Compounds

Benzoyl peroxide:

- Very effective agent against *P. Acnes* with better efficacy than topical antibiotics.
- Can cause skin irritation, more common at higher doses. Improves with use.
- An oxidizing agent, this has the potential to bleach clothing and linens.

Azelaic acid:

- Exact mechanism of action is unknown but also known to have both keratolytic and bactericidal properties.
- Less irritating to the skin than benzoyl peroxide.
- Can cause hypopigmentation Use with caution in teens with darker complexions.

Antibiotics

Have both antibacterial properties that reduce *P. acnes* and anti-inflammatory properties that reduce the amount of free fatty acids.

- Topical antibiotics: Erythromycin and Clindamycin

  - Available alone or in combination with other products (i.e. Benzoyl peroxide, tretinoin, adapalene, etc.). Rarely used alone due to bacterial resistance.

- Oral antibiotics
  - Erythromycin and clindamcyin are not typically prescribed orally due to gastrointestinal (GI) upset.
  - Moreover, oral erythromycin is associated with bacterial resistance while long-term clindamycin use is associated with pseudomembranous colitis.
  - Tetracycline is also associated with GI upset, and has rare serious side effects such as neutropenia and anemia.
  - Expired tetracycline can induce renal tubular acidosis.
  - Doxycycline is associated with esophageal irritation, reflux and photosensitivity.
  - Minocycline is associated with GI upset, dizziness and tinnitus (at higher doses). A unique side effect is a lupus like reaction.
  - All these antibiotics may cause pseudotumor cerebri in teens as well as tooth discoloration if used in younger children.
  - Contraindicated in pregnancy.

Isotretinoin (Accutane)

- Isotretinoin is used to treat recalcitrant nodular acne that has not responded to oral antibiotics and is often prescribed by a dermatologist but can also be prescribed by any clinician who has registered and activated with the iPLEDGE program to prevent fetal exposure to isotretinoin.
- Requires close monitoring for associated side effects including elevated liver enzymes.
- Usually started at a low dose, increased incrementally as tolerated and treatment course usually lasts 16–20 weeks.

DISPOSITION

- Most teens with mild to moderate acne (comedonal and inflammatory lesions) can be treated by their primary care physician.

- Teens with severe acne, characterized by cystic and/or nodular lesions with scarring potential may be referred to a dermatologist for further evaluation and management.
  - Isotretinoin should be used cautiously in women of reproductive age because of its teratogenic potential.
  - Additionally, this medication has been associated with serious side effects and doctors prescribing this medication often check baseline and periodic laboratory studies to monitor lipid profile and liver function.
  - Curative in up to 50% of patients who are prescribed this medication, when used over 4–5 months.

What's unique about acne in adolescents?

- Acne can have a devastating affect on a teen's sense of self and self-image.
- Teens with acne may be embarrassed or shy to raise it as a concern during routine visits.
- Some teens and parents may believe that acne is a normal aspect of adolescence that will pass with time and not seek the needed treatment.
- Teens should be counseled that acne treatments take time to work and never work "overnight."
- Teens should be aware that some topical regimens (i.e. topical tretinoins) may lead to worsening of acne soon after initiation, with optimal affects not witnessed for up to 8–12 weeks after initiating therapy.
- Advise teens to NOT manipulate lesions as this can lead to scarring and hyperpigmentation.

TEST YOUR KNOWLEDGE ANSWER

42. C. Although teens may not complain about their acne or raise it as a concern, most teens are profoundly affected by their acne and may be embarrassed or shy to address the issue directly during routine and other visits. Treatment options should be discussed and offered to teens with acne, regardless of severity of lesions. All other statements are true.

Table 1. Acne-Like Skin Conditions.

Rosacea	Chronic skin condition involving inflammation of the face. Typically includes flushing or redness and skin eruptions that are acne-like. May also have telangiectasias, or spider-like blood vessels.
Flat warts	Papular lesions that are usually non-tender and are not associated with inflammation.
Perioral dermatitis	Marked by erythematous papules and/or pustules that occur periorally and worsened by topical steroids.
Folliculitis	Manifested by small follicular based pustules with erythema but associated with other bacteria (i.e. *Staphylococcus aureus*).
Hidradenitis supperativa	Typically occur in the axilla, groin and buttocks, and are usually large tender nodules.
Adenoma sebaceum	Angiofibromas that appear as erythematous fleshy papules of the face. A manifestation of tuberous sclerosis. Lesions mimic acne. These patients have other characteristic features including ashleaf spots, seizures and connective tissue lesions. Severe cognitive impairment may occur.

Table 2. Topical Medication Vehicle.

Vehicle	Skin Type
Cream	Sensitive or dry skin. Good choice for teens who require a nonirritating formulation that won't dry out the skin.
Gel	Oily skin. Can have a drying effect. Make-up applied to the skin after gel application may not adhere as well.
Lotion	Any skin-type. Contain propylene glycol which can burn and have a drying effect.
Solution	Oily skin. Primarily used with topical antibiotics.

WEB REFERENCES

- Dunn LK, O'Neill JL, Feldman SR. 'Acne in Adolescents: Quality of life, self-esteem, mood, and psychological disorders', Dermatology Online Journal. January 2011. 17(1), retrieved from http://dermatology.cdlib.org/1701/l_review/l_10-00256/feldman.html
- Pappas, A. 'The relationship of diet and acne', Dermatoendocrinology. 2009; l(5); 262–267, retrieved from http://www.ncbi.nlm.nih.gov/pmc/articles/PMC2836431/

- Russell JJ. 'Topical Therapy for Acne', American Academy of Family Physicians. 2000 Jan; 61(2); 357–365, retrieved from http://www.aafp.org/afp/20000115/357.html
- Tom WL and Barrio VR. 'New Insights into adolescent acne', Current Opinion in Pediatrics. 2008; 20; 436–440, retrieved from http://peds.Stanford.edu/Rotations/adolescent_medicine/documents/NewInsightsIntoAdolescentAcne.pdf
- Webster GF. 'Acne Vulgaris', BMJ. 2002 August 31; 325(7362); 475–479, retrieved from http://www.ncbi.nlm.nih.gov/pmc/articles/PMC1123998/
- Woodard, I. 'Adolescent Acne: A Stepwise Approach to Management', Topics in Advanced Practice Nursing eJournal. 2002; 2(2), retrieved from http://www.medscape.com/viewarticle/430534_5

Additional Clinician and Patient Resources:

- Acne.com, Treatment Options, retrieved from http://www.acne.com/treatment/treatment-options/salicylic-acid/
- Acne.org, What is acne?, retrieved from http://www.acne.org/types-of-acne.html
- American Academy of Dermatology, AcneNet (last updated 5/9/2011), retrieved from http://www.skincarephysicians.com/acnenet/
- American Osteopathic College of Dermatology, Accutane, http://www.aocd.org/skin/dermatologicdiseases/accutane.html
- Fulton, J., 'Acne Vulgaris', Medscape Reference (updated Jun 28, 2012), retrieved from http://emedicine.medscape.com/article/1069804-overview
- Pub Med Health, Rosacea: http://www.ncbi.nlm.nih.gov/pubmedhealth/ PMH0001882/
- Teens Health from Nemours, Why Do I Get Acne, retrieved from http://kidshealth.org/teen/yourbody/skinstuff/acne.html

31

VAGUE SOMATIC COMPLAINTS

Tomas J. Silber

TEST YOUR KNOWLEDGE

43. A 15 year old female has had frequent medical visits for vague somatic complaints including abdominal pain, leg cramps and dizziness. She has accumulated 25 days of school absenteeism. She usually feels worse on Sunday evenings and Monday mornings.
    Which one of the following is the next *BEST* step you can take to help her?
    A. In view of the school absenteeism, parents should be advised to home school the patient to attenuate her intense anxiety about "falling behind."
    B. Firmly explain that these are psychosomatic symptoms and immediately refer the patient to a psychiatrist, for the longer these symptoms last, the more entrenched they will become.
    C. Incorporate into the initial discussion of possible causes, a word about "stress reaction" that can be exacerbated by anxiety.
    D. A and B.
    E. All the above.

Refer to end of chapter for answer on page 342.

"I am very worried about my daughter. She has had bad stomach pains on and off for a long time and now she complains of frequent headaches and is missing so much school."

BACKGROUND

- Vague somatic complaints and functional symptoms are common in adolescents: 10% of teens report frequent headaches, chest pain, nausea and fatigue.
- Somatization has been recognized as a tendency to experience and communicate physical distress and describe symptoms that cannot be explained by pathological findings.
- The central feature of somatoform disorders is that they present with symptoms suggestive of an underlying medical condition, yet such a condition either is not found or does not fully account for the level of impairment.
- Somatization disorders:
  - Exhibit a gender disparity in the prevalence of somatic symptoms during adolescence (11% of girls and 4% of boys) that persists into adulthood.
  - Occur more often in adolescents of lower socioeconomic backgrounds.
  - Are seen in genetically predisposed teens with concordance seen in identical twins.
  - Occur more often in adolescents who exhibit anxiety.
  - Cluster above what would be expected by chance in families where there is attention deficit disorder and alcoholism.
- Stress is an important contributing factor: the possibility of bullying and physical or sexual abuse needs to be considered.
- Somatization is a learned behavior. The "psychosomatic pathway" begins with somatic complaints, more easily noticed or accepted in the household than are expressions of strong feelings such as fear, jealousy and anger.

- This pathway is reinforced when an emotionally distressed child repeatedly gets more attention for physical symptoms that often accompany the disturbed emotional state (i.e. "Are you hurting, darling?").
- Through frequent reinforcing, a spectrum of somatization disorders develops that can range from the mild "somatic complaint variation" (transient complaints that do not interfere with normal functioning) to more severe "somatoform disorders" (associated with significant social and academic problems).

- Environmental factors are significant and may include "illness models" in the family.

ASSESSMENT

- Children and adolescents with vague somatic complaints present two challenges:
  - The risk of "missing" another medical diagnosis.
  - The risk of alienating the patient and family when explaining the nature of the condition.
- The diagnosis of somatoform illness should be based on a set of positive psychosocial findings and not on the process of exclusion.
- Establishing the diagnosis evolves over time along three *simultaneous* tracks:
  - Ruling out an organic disease as the cause of the symptoms.
  - Identifying psychosocial dysfunction.
  - Recognizing and alleviating stressors.
- Doctors baffled by the onslaught of symptoms may feel frustrated by the never-ending recurrent complaints, or become annoyed by the time consumed in caring for patients who are "not really sick." Take a deep breath and begin taking the history!

HISTORY

History of Present Illness

- A detailed biopsychosocial assessment (HEEADSSS) can be therapeutic and is often followed by improvement and sometimes even resolution of symptoms.

- Findings that suggest somatization disorder include: a history of multiple somatic complaints, numerous physician visits and/or specialty consultations, a family member with chronic/recurrent symptoms, and dysfunction in the primary areas of life (i.e. family, peers and school).
- Determine if symptoms described are feigned, suggesting **malingering** or **factitious disorder**, or are better explained by mental illness such as **depression** or **anxiety**.
- Explore the source of stress as this is often a triggering factor.
  - Stress may be bound to parental anxiety.
  - The most common form of stress consists of pressure on the teen to perform.
- More serious problems, such as physical or sexual abuse or being bullied may present with vague somatic complaints, sometimes progressing to **school phobia.**
- When the symptoms are severe, look for "la belle indifference," an attitude of disinterest by the patient despite the serious nature of their complaint: it suggests a **conversion reaction.**
- Assess if a parent has concerns about the child's behavior or emotional well-being.
  - This question often elicits a positive response, suggesting that at least one of the parents is making the connection between symptoms and emotional distress.
- A detailed school history will uncover the number of missed school days.

Past Medical History

Somatization follows a developmental sequence.

- During childhood and early adolescence abdominal pain predominates.
- During middle to late adolescence, headaches increase in frequency.
- As age increases, insomnia and fatigue tend to emerge.

Family History

Is there a family history of psychiatric disorder?

- Psychiatric disorders such as depression and anxiety often initially present with physical complaints such as poor concentration, fatigue, weight loss, headaches, stomach aches, and/or chest pain.

- There is frequently a model for the symptoms, such as a grandparent with cardiac symptoms. Sometimes, the patient may serve as his or her own model, as happens with pseudoseizures in patients with epilepsy.
- The presence of a family member with somatization disorder is not uncommon.

PHYSICAL

- A complete physical exam should be performed with a focus on organ systems associated with the patient's physical complaints.
- The physical exam often reveals discrepancies: e.g. severe pain on abdominal palpation, but not with applied stethoscope pressure during abdominal auscultation.

Pelvic Exam

- Pelvic pain requires a pelvic examination: adhesions and endometriosis are often late diagnoses following years of "functional pelvic pain."

Musculoskeletal Exam

- Conversion symptoms are usually self-limited, often resolving within 3 months of onset, but may persist longer and be associated with sequelae, such as contractures following an episode of hysterical paralysis.

Neurologic Exam

- A comprehensive neurologic exam should be performed to offer reassurance and because up to 1/3rd of patients diagnosed with conversion reaction show evidence of a neurological disorder over time.
- In conversion disorders, one or more symptom/deficit affect a sensory or voluntary motor function (i.e. blindness or paresis), suggesting a medical or neurologic condition; yet findings on exam are inconsistent with known neuroanatomic or pathophysiologic conditions.

STUDIES

- When evaluating somatic complaints, clinicians should avoid the temptation to perform unnecessary, often repetitive testing, in attempts to demonstrate to the family that complaints are of psychosomatic origin.
- A cost-effective method to determine the extent of laboratory and radiology studies is to base the decision on the presence of red flags: complaints or findings that suggest an organic pathology (i.e. syncope on exercise, asymmetric location of pain, anemia or weight loss).
- When history suggests somatization, basic laboratory screening suffices, including a complete blood count, erythrocyte sedimentation rate or C-reactive protein, urine dipstick, basic metabolic panel and occasionally stool for occult blood.
- Other tests should be ordered on a case by case basis.
  - For example, persistent epigastralgia may indicate *H. pylori* gastritis requiring tests for *H. pylori* antigen in the stool.

TREATMENT

Central to any successful treatment strategy is the untiring effort to motivate patients and parents towards a partnership with their clinician to deal with the complaints and symptoms.

- Treatment begins at the time of the initial patient evaluation.
  - Explicitly discuss stressors detected and list functional disorder as one diagnostic possibility. This helps ensure easier "disclosure" of the diagnosis in the future.
- A detailed history and careful physical exam IS treatment. This conveys a sense of specialness to the teen and their family, and may later serve as a buffer to the narcissistic injury stemming from having to recognize that "something is wrong" in the teen's life.
- Eventually, the clinician needs to "bite the bullet" to make and disclose the diagnosis, usually best done during a well planned "last patient of the day" follow up visit:
  - Precede disclosure with a clear assurance that one has taken the complaint very seriously.
  - During disclosure, remind the family of earlier visits, referring to your comments that symptoms may be related to stress, temperamental

sensitivity, anxiety, or whatever term may be tolerated by the family to facilitate acceptance of a behavioral intervention or request for mental health consultation.

- The diagnosis of somatization should never lead a patient or parent to believe that this will be raised as a barrier to preempt future complaints.
- Most families, even when disagreeing with their physicians, can accept treatment recommendations if they are assured proper attention, open-mindedness and regularly scheduled follow-up appointments.
- Use cognitive and behavioral interventions, positive and negative reinforcements, and recommend self-monitoring techniques such as hypnosis, relaxation and biofeedback.
- Judicious use of psychopharmacologic therapy in somatoform disorders may be appropriate when there is comorbid depression or anxiety, and/or the severity of symptoms has led to significant and prolonged impairment.

DISPOSITION

- Clinicians should recognize their response to family resistance or reluctance to lay aside the "search for disease," and not inadvertently convey, by word or body language, their frustrations about the difficult and time-consuming task faced when treating teens with somatic complaints.
- A primary reason that many adolescents and their parents become angry and reject the diagnosis of somatization is because they feel disrespected and/or not believed:
  - "You think it is all in my head, but I know I hurt and that there is something wrong."
  - The displeasure may sometimes relate to the term "psychosomatic," which for some implies being crazy or "psycho."
- Understand that correct identification of somatization, though necessary, may not be sufficient to help families, as they are often reluctant to accept the explanation.
- Successful communication about the condition and the need for treatment is a crucial but elusive goal. Patients are more willing to listen to their clinicians only if they feel that *they* have been listened to first.

- Before disclosure, it is useful to ask the teen and parents about their fears.
  - This can elicit surprising answers, such as a fear that the teen has cancer or heart disease.
  - Conversely, the reply may reveal a harbored parental suspicion or understanding of the problem, such as "it may be a case of stress" or "nerves."
- A clear, supportive, matter-of-fact discussion needs to include assurances to the family that the physician will remain available.
- It is important to convey that the "functional versus organic" paradigm is old-fashioned and does not reflect current thinking: that there is a complex interplay of multiple factors including genetic and biochemical components predisposing to and underlying the patient's symptoms.
- The physician must convey an appreciation that the patient's pain is real: pain has a neural nociceptive component and an affective component, both processed by the central nervous system and influenced by personal experience, genetics and the environment.
- Patients and parents can be reminded of how themes in our everyday language acknowledge the connection between emotions and bodily processes: we have a "gut reaction," describe "butterflies in my stomach," "feel choked up," or that a situation "makes me want to vomit."
- Call attention to visible changes and their relation to strong emotions: embarrassment can manifest as blushing, fear as cold sweat, and anger as stiffening muscles and clenching teeth, thus facilitating explanations such as "blushing of the gut" and "spastic colon."
- Another way to help understand somatization is as a sensitivity, a phenomenon of "amplification" of otherwise normal body sensations, similar to the role of an amplifier in the transmission of music.
- Families often worry that the diagnosis of somatization will be followed by physician abandonment. This concern can be dispelled by frequent follow-up visits, which have the potential to "preempt" the emergence of new symptoms, prevent emergency department visits and ease the overall management of symptoms.
- Emphasize that all forthcoming symptoms will be examined with the attention they deserve because somatizing under stress is very common but does not "provide immunity" against appendicitis, flu, pneumonia and other conditions.

- With appropriate intervention, the prognosis for most somatization disorders in adolescents is very good; however, untreated adolescents risk continuous somatization as adults.

What is unique about somatization in adolescents?

- Rapid body transformations, social challenges and new transitions add complexity to the lives of teens and prove fertile ground for the development of vague somatic complaints.
- Adolescents are anxious about their symptoms and often resent the diagnosis of a functional disorder: they feel insulted by what they perceive is the clinician saying that their symptoms are "all in their head."
- Simultaneously, they worry that this diagnosis will be followed by rejection or abandonment by their physician. Many will urge their parents to "doctor shop."
- Somatic complaints may lead to school absenteeism, which in turn can develop into a full blown school avoidance syndrome. This is often not recognized by parents because "my child loves school and wants to go" (which may be true).
    - Family counseling and good communication between the clinician and the school can "turn things around" in most cases of school phobia.
    - Parents should be instructed to take the teen to school, but not necessarily to class: it is important that the *adolescent stay in the building.*
    - Class attendance is not mandatory but going to school is: if necessary the adolescent can rest in the school infirmary, library or any other quiet area.
    - This agreement can be facilitated when one parent is often able to help the other. Single parents may enlist a friend or relative to assume this role.
    - Parents need to be prepared for difficult days, specifically Sundays and the last day of vacation before returning to school.
    - Consistency in fulfilling the contract will result in return to school, even though a period of "testing" with increased symptoms may initially take place.
- Adolescents will eventually grudgingly accept that there will be no returning home unless febrile. Attendance in class then follows spontaneously.

TEST YOUR KNOWLEDGE ANSWER

43. C. Home schooling ought to be avoided because it reinforces the secondary benefit obtained from symptoms. The treatment of physical manifestations of school avoidance consists of precisely the opposite: assuring an effective plan for going to school in spite of the symptoms. This can be done in a staged way: in time or place (e.g. less hours at school, initially staying in the library and then moving to class). A direct or blunt recommendation for mental health consultation before the family is ready to accept it is problematic. They may perceive this as dismissive of their concerns, or even as rejection and abandonment. Following a thorough initial assessment, and at the time of requesting basic tests, it is helpful to comment that the presenting symptoms could be related to stress. This could then be taken up again at a later visit, introducing further concepts, such as "pain amplification syndrome" to ease family acceptance of the diagnosis and seek appropriate counseling.

WEB REFERENCES

- Fremont WP. 'School Refusal in Children and Adolescents', American Family Physician. Oct 2003;68(8);1555-1561, retrieved from http://www.aafp.org/afp/2003/1015/pl555.html
- Poikolainen K, Janerva R, Lonnqvist J. 'Life Events and Other Risk Factors for Somatic Symptoms in Adolescence', Pediatrics. 1995 July; 96(l); 59–63, retrieved from http://pediatrics.aappublications.org/content/96/1/59.short
- Viner R and Christie D. 'Fatigue and somatic symptoms', BMJ. 2005 April; 330(7498); 1012–1015, retrieved from http://www.ncbi.nlm.nih.gov/pmc/articles/PMC557154/

Additional Clinician and Patient Resources:

- Agency for Healthcare Research and Quality, Somatic symptoms: mental health approach and differential diagnosis, retrieved from http://www.guideline.gov/content.aspx?id=l5096
- Vorvick LJ, Rogge T, Zieve D. 'Somatization Disorder', Medline Plus. Updated 9/9/2012, retrieved from http://www.nlm.nih.gov/medlineplus/ency/article/000955.htm
- UCLA School Mental Health Program, Physical and Somatic Complaints, retrieved from http://smhp.psych.ucla.edu/qf/somatic.htm

32

SLEEP DISORDERS

Jose J. Casas-Rivero

TEST YOUR KNOWLEDGE

44. Which one of the following statements is true?
    A. Adolescents need less sleep than adults, which is why they stay up late.
    B. At puberty onset, teens are sleepier in the morning and have difficulty waking up.
    C. Adolescents should do more stimulating activities in the late evening, when they are most active.
    D. All the above.
    E. None of the above.
45. Which one of the following statements is true?
    A. Mood instability, irritablility and poor school performance can be due to sleep problems.
    B. Driving accidents are more frequent in sleep deprived adolescents.
    C. Mood disorders, suicidal ideation and substance abuse (legal and illegal) have to be ruled out in an adolescent with sleep problems.
    D. All the above.
    E. None of the above.

Refer to end of chapter for answers on page 349.

"My 17-year old son will not get out of bed in the morning! It is impossible to wake him and he is always late to school. He stays up on the computer late at night complaining that he can't fall asleep anyway and says that everybody else is connected then."

BACKGROUND

- The sleep-wake cycle undergoes significant reorganization during the transition to adolescence.
  - At puberty onset, there is a sleep-wake "phase delay" of about 2 hours that is associated with later bed and rise times.
  - Teens tend to sleep for shorter periods, and have associated increased daytime sleepiness.
  - There is a decrease in slow-wave sleep time (decreased by 40% pre-puberty to late puberty), an increase in the amount of stage 2 sleep and a decrease in latency to the first episode of rapid eye movement (REM) sleep.
  - There is a steep decrease in delta REM sleep, also associated with increased sleepiness.
  - Maturation leads to a greater tolerance for sleep deprivation or extended wakefulness.
- Adolescents need about 9 hours of sleep per night and most only get 7–7.5 hours, resulting in considerable sleep debt over time. Attempts to catch up with sleep occur over the weekend with a temporal shift of wake and sleep times (social jet-lag).
- There are a wide range of conditions that cause sleep problems in teens (Table 1) but the most common cause is sleep deprivation.

ASSESSMENT

HISTORY

History of Present Illness

- The BEARS acronym can be a helpful tool to obtain a sleep history (Table 2).

- Ascertain the quantity and quality of sleep. With delayed sleep phase, teens get normal quantity and quality of sleep but timing is the problem (sleep onset after 2 a.m.) and conflicts with school schedules.
- Assess for extra-curricular activities or work that the teen is engaged in after school and/or during weekends. There may not be enough time in a 24 hour day to fit in all activities and at least 9 hours of sleep per night.
- Determine the number of electronic devices (i.e. cell phone, computers or game systems) in the teen's room as well as the time and duration of their use.
- Determine caffeine intake, especially in the afternoons and evenings. **Caffeine intake** can lead to delayed sleep.
- Excessive daytime sleepiness, with episodes of profound sleepiness, suggests **narcolepsy** (25% also have a family history).
- Does the patient sleep walk or have nightmares?
- "Crawling" and motor restlessness in the lower extremities that increase in the evenings suggest **restless leg syndrome.**
- Fatigue that interferes with normal activities and marked sleep-phase delay following a flu-like episode suggests **chronic fatigue syndrome.**
- Snoring can be a sign of **obstructive sleep apnea (OSA).**

Review of Systems

- Fatigue, day time somnolence, irritability, aggressive behavior, impulsivity, hyperactivity, short attention span and poor academic performance can result from disrupted or fragmented sleep. Investigate snoring and sleep-apnea, ADHD, and sleep related movement disorders (restless leg syndrome or periodic limb movement disorder).
- **Anxiety** and **depression** can co-exist, precede or follow a sleep problem.
- Complaints of feeling sick or fatigued may indicate **chronic or serious illness.**
- Hair loss, fatigue, heat intolerance, palpitations or insomnia suggest **hyperthyroidism.**
- Weight loss and malnutrition, as seen with anorexia nervosa, can result in insomnia secondary to delayed clearance of cortisol and/or hunger.
- Nocturnal eating, such as a binge eating disorder, may interfere with sleep.

Social History

- Decline in school performance, things disappearing from home, change of friends and increased time spent away from home suggest **stimulant abuse.**
- Investigate friends' bedtimes. Friends with later bed times increase the risk of sleep deprivation and substance abuse in a teen.
- Inquire about anxiety, depression and suicidal ideations.
- Is there a history of any driving accident? This could be the result of increased sleepiness on the road, but it is also important to assess for signs and symptoms of ADHD.

PHYSICAL

- There are no findings on physical exam that are pathognomonic for sleep problems.

Anthropometric Measurements

- Assess height and weight and calculate BMI. A high BMI is associated with **OSA.**
- Plot changes over time on a growth curve with the aid of old records.

Vital Signs

- Search for low body temperature, bradycardia, hypotension and orthostasis.
- Tachycardia and hypertension are red flags that suggest **stimulant use** (i.e. cocaine or amphetamines) or **hyperthyroidism.**

General Appearance

- Obesity, nasal obstruction, nasal speech and high arched palate raise the concern for **OSA.**
- There may be enlarged tonsils on physical exam.
- Although rare, it may be possible to catch the patient having an episode of cataplexy, falling down asleep and becoming completely hypotonic.

STUDIES

Complete Blood Count

- Elevated hemoglobin and hematocrit may indicate **chronic poor oxygenation.**
- The presence of marked anemia is suspicious for an **organic cause.**

Sedimentation Rate and C Reactive Protein

- Elevation suggests inflammation and the clinician should evaluate for systemic disease.

SPECIAL TESTS

Polysomnogram (PSG)

- Will diagnose **OSA.**
- Documents abnormal muscle movements in **periodic limb movement disorder.**
- An overnight PSG with a sleep latency test is needed to diagnose **narcolepsy.** It shows a shortened sleep onset latency and REM sleep immediately following sleep onset.

Ferritin

- Low levels have been associated with **restless leg syndrome.**

Thyroid Studies

- Low TSH and high T3/T4 indicate **hyperthyroidism.**

Urine Drug Test

- A positive test for any drug should prompt search for more risk-taking behaviors.

CSF

- Low cerebrospinal fluid hypocretin-1 levels is diagnostic for **narcolepsy.**

DISPOSITION

- Support and educate parents and teens about adolescent sleep needs (Table 2) and guide parents on how to help their teens improve sleep hygiene.
  - Teach adolescents to comply with parental set bedtimes. Earlier bedtimes protect against depression and suicidal ideation.
  - Limit amount of caffeine intake, especially later in the day.
  - Keep electronic devices out of the bedroom.
  - Advise teens that the bed is a place to sleep, not to work or use the computer.
- A few patients may need to be referred for sleep study testing and results may require referral to specialists to help treat the sleep abnormality.
- An otolaryngology consultation may be indicated if patients are suspected to have OSA secondary to enlarged tonsils or adenoids.
- Referral to a sleep disorder specialist may be required, especially if there is a behavioral component to the sleep disorder.

What is unique about sleep problems in adolescents?

- Today's teens lead busy lives and are often involved in multiple extracurricular activities. While they need over 9 hours of sleep per night, most teens are only getting between 7–7.5 hours of sleep per night or less, thereby incurring a "sleep debt."
- Teens undergo dramatic changes to their sleep cycle in early adolescence with constant changes through the adolescent years. Maturation and the emergence of new interests during these years also compete with sleep time.
- Some abnormal behaviors and academic problems can be explained by sleep deprivation and can be corrected by addressing the sleep problem. Sleep deprivation may mimic ADHD.
- Widespread sleep problems among teens are raising issues concerning current school policies. Changing school start time from 8 to 8:30 am

has been found to improve class attendance, is associated with decreased sleepiness and improved mood.

- Exposure to bright light in the morning and shifting more difficult classes to after 10 a.m. also improve wakefulness during the day.

TEST YOUR KNOWLEDGE ANSWERS

44. B. At puberty onset, there is a sleep-wake "phase delay" of 2 hours. Adolescents have a decreased propensity to fall asleep in the evening and an increase in midday sleepiness. The extreme manifestation of this maturation in sleep is the Delayed Sleep Phase Syndrome (DSP). Adolescent sleep needs are about 9 hours/night and most only obtain 7–7.5 hours/night. Encourage teens to "calm down" with relaxing activities before going to bed. Regular bed-time, bright light in the morning and a change of school start from 8.00 to 8.30 a.m. can all improve adolescent quality of life.
45. D. Anxiety, depression and suicidal ideations can coexist with, precede or follow a sleep problem. Adolescents with psychological problems tend to have later bed times and poorer compliance with parental set bed times. The same is true for stimulant use (caffeine) or drug abuse. If friends also have late bed times, the risk of sleep deprivation and substance abuse is higher. Sleep-related crashes are most common in young people, who tend to stay up late, sleep too little, and drive at night. In a North Carolina state study, 55% of fall-asleep crashes involved people 25 years old or younger. Seventy-eight percent were males and the peak age of occurrence was 20.

Table 1. Sleep Disorders*.

Insomnia: Problems Falling or Staying Asleep	Psychophysiological Insomnia (Conditioned Insomnia) Adjustment Sleep Disorder (Transient Insomnia) Inadequate Sleep Hygiene Idiopathic Insomnia Insomnia Due to Other Known Conditions Insomnia Due to Substance Abuse Insomnia Due to Adverse Drug Effect Insomnia Due to Psychiatric/Behavioural or Medical Condition
Sleep-Related Breathing Disorder	Obstructive Sleep Apnea Sleep Related Breathing Disorder Due to Cardiorespiratory Disease
Hypersomnia NOT due to a Sleep-Related Breathing Disorder	Narcolepsy with Cataplexy Narcolepsy without Cataplexy Recurrent Hypersomnia (Kleine-Levyn syndrome) Idiopathic Hypersomnia with Long Sleep Time Idiopathic Hypersomnia without Long Sleep Time Behaviourally Induced Insufficient Sleep Syndrome Other Hypersomnia Due to Substance Abuse Other Hypersomnia Due to Adverse Drug Effect Hypersomnia Due to Psychiatric/Behavioural or Medical Condition
Primary Circadian Rhythm Sleep Disorder	Delayed Sleep Phase Type (Delayed Sleep Phase Syndrome) Advanced Sleep Phase Type (Advanced Sleep Phase Syndrome) Irregular Sleep-Wake Type Non-entrained Type Other Primary Circadian Rhythm Sleep Disorder Due to Other Known Conditions
Behaviorally-Induced Circadian Rhythm Sleep Disorder	Jet-lag Type Shift-work Type Circadian Rhythm Disorders Due to Substance Abuse Circadian Rhythm Disorders Due to Adverse Drug Effect
Parasomnias	Confusional Arousals Sleepwalking REM Sleep Behavior Disorder, including Parasomnia Overlap Disorder Recurrent Isolated Sleep Paralysis

(*Continued*)

Table 1. (*Continued*)

	Nightmare Disorder Parasomnia Due to Substance Abuse Parasomnia Due to Psychiatric Disorders
Sleep Related Movement Disorders	Restless Legs Syndrome Periodic Limb Movement Disorder Sleep-related Leg Cramps Sleep-related Bruxism Sleep-related Rhythmic Movement Disorder
Isolated Symptoms and Normal Variants	Long Sleepers Short Sleepers Snoring Sleeptalking Sleep Starts, Hypnagogic Jerks

*Reproduced and modified from *Kohrman M. Principles and Practice of Pediatric Sleep Medicine, with permission from Elsevier (2005).*

Table 2. "BEARS": A Sample Sleep History.

B	Bedtime problems: Do you have any problems falling asleep at bedtime?
E	Excessive daytime sleepiness: Do you feel sleepy during the day? In school? While driving?
A	Awakenings during the night: Do you wake up often during the night?
R	Regularity and duration of sleep: What time do you usually go to be on school nights? Weekends? How much sleep do you usually get?
S	Sleep disordered breathing: Parent: Does your teen snore more loudly or nightly? Teen: Has anyone ever told you that you snore loudly at night?

Reproduced with permission from the American Academy of Pediatrics: Millman RP and the Working Group on Sleepiness in Adolescents/Young Adults, Excessive sleepiness in adolescent and young adults: causes, consequences, and treatment strategies, *Pediatrics* **115**: 1774–1786 (2005).

WEB REFERENCES

- Meltzer LJ, *et al.* 'Prevalence of Diagnosed Sleep Disorders in Pediatric Primary Care Practices', Pediatrics. 2010; 125; el410, retrieved from http://pediatrics.aappublications.org/content/125/6/el410.full.pdf+html?sid=lfe9f980-d26c-4005-8a3c-9el497fl5a2c
- Millman RP. Working Group on Sleepiness in Adolescents/Young Adults, and the Committee on Adolescence. 'Excessive Sleepiness in Adolescents and Young Adults: Causes, Consequences, and Treatment Strategies', Pediatrics. 2005; 115(6); 1774–1786, retrieved from http://pediatrics.aappublications.Org/content/115/6/1774.full?sid=lfe9f980-d26c-4005-8a3c-9el497fl5a2c
- Mindell, JA, *et al.* 'Pharmacologic Management of Insomnia in Children and Adolescents: Consensus Statement', Pediatrics. 2006 June; 117(6); el223–1232, retrieved from http://pediatrics.aappublications.org/content/117/6/el223.full?sid=lfe9f980-d26c-4005-8a3c-9el497fl5a2c
- National Center on Sleep Disorders Research, National Sleep Disorders Research Plan, retrieved from http://www.nhlbi.nih.gov/health/prof/sleep/res_plan/contents.html
- Okawa, M, *et al.* 'Orcadian rhythm sleep disorders in adolescents: Clinical trials of combines treatments based on chronobiology', Psychiatry and Clinical Neurosciences. 1998 September; 52(5); 483–490, retrieved from http://onlinelibrary.wiley.com/doi/10.1046/j.1440-1819.1998.00449.x/full

Additional Clinician and Patient Resources:

- American Academy of Sleep Medicine: www.aasmnet.org
  - A listing of accredited sleep disorders centers can be obtained from this site
- American Sleep Medicine Foundation: www.discoversleep.org
- Associated Professional Sleep Societies, LLC (APSS): www.apss.org
- Journal of Clinical Sleep Medicine (JCSM): www.aasmnet.org/JCSM
  - Official publication of the American Academy of Sleep Medicine (AASM)
- National Sleep Foundation: www.sleepeducation.com
- SLEEP: www.journalsleep.org
  - ©SLEEP is the official publication of the Associated Professional Sleep Societies
- SleepCenters.org: www.sleepcenters.org
  - The online directory of sleep centers and labs has a map that enables visitors to search for help by state.
- Teens Health from Nemours, Common Sleep Problems, retrieved from http://kidshealth.org/teen/your_body/take_care/sleep.html

33

TICS AND TOURETTE SYNDROME

Jonathan Fanburg

TEST YOUR KNOWLEDGE

46. A fearful parent comes to you with her 12 year old child for evaluation of tics. After diagnosing a classic history and presentation of tics, the *MOST* accurate advice would be the following statement:
    A. "We need to obtain an MRI to rule out a neurologic cause for this problem."
    B. "Medications always work in patients with tic disorders."
    C. "It is likely that your child will outgrow tics with time."
    D. "Tell your child to not make the movement and she should be able to comply. After a while, tics will disappear."
    E. "Strep infection may have caused your child's Tourettes syndrome."
47. The diagnosis of Tourettes is more likely to exist with all the following *EXCEPT*:
    A. Coexisting ADHD.
    B. Symptoms that have occurred for over a year and started in early childhood.
    C. Suppression of tics that occurs briefly with effort.
    D. Patients express not remembering having had a tic.
    E. History of both verbal tics and motor tics.

Refer to end of chapter for answers on page 357.

A 12 year old male presents to the office with an intermittent facial twitch that has gradually become more noticeable in class and at home over the last 3 months.

BACKGROUND

- **Tics** are characterized as sudden, rapid, involuntary, movements of a single muscle group (simple tics) or multiple motor groups (complex tics).
- Tics can be **motor** or **vocal**. Motor tics typically involve the face, neck, shoulders, trunk, and/or hands, and can change location over time.

ASSESSMENT

HISTORY

History of Present Illness

Assess current symptoms: are the patients movements/vocalizations voluntary or involuntary?

- **Seizures** are involuntary repetitive movements of muscle groups, accompanied by the complete inability to suppress the movement and amnesia about the event.
- Tics are involuntary, but a key diagnostic feature that distinguishes tics and **Tourettes syndrome** (**TS**) from other movement disorders is the patient's ability to transiently suppress the behavior.
  - Does the patient have vocal tics, motor tics or a combination of both?
  - There are unique types of vocal/motor tics listed below:
    - Coprolalia (obscene words)
    - Echolalia (repetition of words)
    - Palilalia (repetition of phrase with increasing rapidity)
    - Copropraxia (obscene gestures)
    - Echopraxia (mimicking of gestures)
- Determine the age of onset of current symptoms.
  - TS commonly presents between 2–15 years, and almost all manifest symptoms by 11 years with an average age of 6 years.

- **Tics** resolve by age 18 years in 50% of teens, but may also persist into adulthood (with gradually diminishing symptoms). Rarely, some violent tics may become disabling.
- Determine the duration of symptoms.
    - To diagnose **TS**, patients must have BOTH motor AND vocal tics occurring for more than one year on a regular basis, although not necessarily at the same time.
- Assess when tics typically occur.
    - **Dyskinetic movements and dystonias** occur during both wakefulness and sleep while tics and **TS** do not occur during sleep.

Past Medical History

- Patients with **TS** are likely to have a comorbid behavioral disorder.
    - Eighty-eight percent of teens with TS have a coexisting diagnosis of ADHD, OCD, learning disability (LD), compulsive disorder (CD), sleep difficulties, and/or ODD.
    - If there is no comorbid condition, a diagnosis of TS should be questioned.
- Determine if the patient has had a recent strep infection.
    - **PANDAS** (Pediatric Autoimmune Neuropsychiatric Disorders Associated with Streptococcal Infections) results in acute onset tic like movements associated with elevated Group A strep antibodies and strep infections. It is a distinct from TS and does not cause TS.

Medications

- Some medications (i.e. **carbamazepine, phenytoin, phenobarbital, antipsychotics**) can cause tic-like movements that are less rapid and are accompanied by other slowed behaviors such as slurred speech.

PHYSICAL EXAM

Physical exam findings are initially more important than history to categorize the type of movement disorder.

General Appearance

- Observe patient for vocal and/or motor tics.

STUDIES

- There is little role for studies in the diagnosis of Tics/TS.

Electroencephalogram (EEG)

- May provide assistance if there is a concern for a seizure disorder.

TREATMENT

- Treatment strategies exist, yet most work only partially and none are dependable. Research is evolving in this field and data is conflicting.
- Medications are reserved for patients whose symptoms interfere with social function.
- Options include: risperidone, clonidine, guanfacine and traditional neuroleptics (side effects outweigh benefit for most people).
- Botulism has been used primarily for the treatment of facial tics.
- In patients with co-morbid conditions, consider the following treatment options:
  - For ADHD and Tics: Clonidine (0.1 mg/day) or Guanfacine (1 mg/day)
  - For OCD and Tics: Fluoxetine (20 mg/day)
- Behavioral interventions can also help to reduce symptoms:
  - Advise teens to reduce caffeine intake.
  - Patients should get proper sleep at night and avoid over-fatigue.
  - Minimize stress by helping teens find alternative coping mechanisms such as exercise.

What is unique about Tics and TS in adolescents?

- Most teens will outgrow tics with time and patients and families can be reassured.
- The best treatment may be educating people about tic behaviors to promote tolerance and understanding of these behaviors.
- This is especially important in the school setting, where teachers may misinterpret symptoms as misbehavior or mocking, and punish the teen.

TEST YOUR KNOWLEDGE ANSWERS

46. C. Most teens outgrow their tics over time, typically by age 18 years. MRIs are not indicated unless there are other findings on history or neurological exam that suggest a brain tumor. Medications may only partially reduce the frequency and intensity of tics. Tics can be intermittently briefly suppressed, yet recurrent reminders do not work and developing a level of tolerance in the patient's community may be more effective. Strep antibodies can cause tic like behaviors, but is not the cause of Tourette syndrome.
47. D. Amnesia about tics should make one think about seizure activity. All other choices are typically seen with people who have Tourette syndrome.

WEB REFERENCES

- Centers for Disease Control and Prevention. 'Prevalence of Diagnosed Tourette Syndrome in Persons Aged 6–17 Years — United States, 2007.' MMWR 2009; 58(21); 581–608, retrieved from http://www.cdc.gov/mmwr/PDF/wk/mm5821.pdf
- Harris, E and Wu SW. 'Children with tic disorders: How to match treatment with symptoms', Current Psychiatry. March 2010;9(3);29-36, retrieved from http://www.currentpsychiatry.com/pdf/0903/0903CP_Aiticle2.pdf
- Kenney C, Kuo SH, Jimenez-Shahed J. 'Tourette's Syndrome', American Family Physician. 2008 Mar; 77(5); 651–658, retrieved from http://www.ncbi.nlm.nih.gov/pubmed/18350763
- Ludolph AG, *et al.* 'Tourette Syndrome and Other Tic Disorders in Childhood, Adolescence and Adulthood', Deutsches Arzteblatt International. 2012 November; 109(48); 821–828, retrieved from http://www.ncbi.nlm.nih.gov/pmc/articles/PMC3523260/
- Metzger H, Wanderer S & Roessner V. Tic Disorders. In Rey JM (ed), IACAAPAP e-Textbook of Child and Adolescent Mental Health. Geneva: International Association for Child and Adolescent Psychiatry and Allied Professions 2012, retrieved from http://iacapap.org/wp-content/uploads/H.2-TIC-DISORDERS-072012.pdf
- Robertson MM. 'Tourette syndrome, associated conditions and the complexities of treatment', Brain. 2000; 123; 425–462, retrieved from http://brain.oxfordjournals.org/content/123/3/425.full.pdf+html

Additional Clinician and Patient Resources:

- American Academy of Child and Adolescent Psychiatry (2010), Tourette's Syndrome, http://www.aacap.org/cs/root/resources_for_families/glossary_of_symptoms_and_illnesses/tourettessyndrome
- Freedman JL and Duckworth K. 'Tourette's Syndrome', National Alliance on Mental Illness (September 2012), retrieved from http://www.nami.org/Template.cfm?Section=By_Illness&Template=/ContentManagement/ContentDisplay.cfm&ContentID=23053
- National Institute of Neurological Disorders and Stroke (2012), NINDS Tourette Syndrome Information Page, retrieved from www.ninds.nih.gov/disorders/tourette
- National Tourette Syndrome Association: www.tsa-usa.org
- Robertson WC. 'Tourette Syndrome and Other Tic Disorders', Medscape Reference. Updated Jun 15, 2011, retrieved from http://emedicine.medscape.com/article/1182258-overview#aw2aab6b2b4

34

ATTENTION DEFICIT HYPERACTIVITY DISORDER (ADHD)

Barbara K. Snyder

TEST YOUR KNOWLEDGE

48. Which of the following statements about diagnosing ADHD in adolescents is *NOT* true?

    A. Information about the adolescent's educational history and behavior should be obtained from the adolescent, parents and teachers.
    B. A brain MRI and EEG are most accurate to diagnose ADHD because of their specificity.
    C. ADHD is more common in boys.
    D. The core symptom of hyperactivity often decreases by the time the child reaches adolescence.
    E. The most common psychiatric comorbidity in young people with ADHD is oppositional defiant disorder.

49. Which of the following statements is/are true about the treatment of ADHD?

    A. Behavioral interventions alone may provide adequate treatment.
    B. Stimulants are considered first line pharmacotherapy for ADHD.
    C. Stratera (atomoxetine) is a first-line medication for teens with a known substance abuse.
    D. Prescribing medication for ADHD requires an individualized, stepwise approach.
    E. Common side effects of stimulants include decreased appetite and insomnia.
    F. All the above are true.

Refer to end of chapter for answers on page 366.

"My 16 year old daughter is not doing nearly as well in school as her teachers say she could. She is disorganized, forgets to write down assignments and loses things all the time! She has been like this since she was a little girl and we think she is just not trying hard enough."

BACKGROUND

- Attention deficit hyperactivity disorder (ADHD) is a common neurobehavioral disorder that is characterized by core symptoms of inattention and/or impulsivity and/or hyperactivity.
- These behavioral symptoms are developmentally inappropriate for the teen's age.
- About 11% of 12–17 year olds in the United States meet criteria for the diagnosis of ADHD.
- Formal diagnostic criteria require that symptoms be present by age 7 and cause significant impairment most days in at least two settings (e.g., home and school).
  - There are three subtypes based on predominant behaviors:
    - Inattentive type (predominantly seen in females)
    - Hyperactive/impulsive type
    - Combined type (most common)
- Though symptoms of ADHD begin in childhood, they usually persist into adolescence and adulthood; some symptoms, notably hyperactivity, improve with age and maturity.
- Although the cause is unknown, genetics may play a large role. Underlying mechanisms likely include an imbalance in the norepinephrine and dopamine systems.
- Numerous risk factors have been identified (Table 1) and a wide variety of conditions may mimic ADHD (Table 2).

ASSESSMENT

HISTORY

- Diagnosis requires a comprehensive clinical evaluation, including detailed history from the adolescent, parents and teachers (Table 3).

History of Present Illness

- Have school personnel, parents or the adolescent noticed poor school performance or underachievement, problems staying focused and attentive, mood lability, problems with peer relationships or impulsiveness?
- Difficulty with a specific subject or activity, but not others, suggests a **learning disability.**
- The diagnosis of **oppositional defiant disorder** (ODD) should be considered in a teen who is argumentative, defiant, deliberately breaks rules or has frequent anger outbursts.
- **Conduct disorder** should be considered if the teen's disruptive behavior is severe and if the teen harms or threatens other people, animals or property.
- Persistent sadness, loss of interest in activities or preferring to be alone suggest **depression.**
- Unusually strong fears, difficulty with separation or a history of panic attacks suggests an **anxiety disorder.**
- Conditions other than ADHD may explain academic or behavioral difficulties (Table 2).
  - Consider **decreased intellectual ability** or **inappropriate class placement** if the teen has academic difficulties with minimal or no behavioral impairment.
  - Difficulty concentrating, mood lability, irritability, depression or restlessness could be **side effects of medications.**
  - Undiagnosed **vision or hearing problems** could explain inattention and poor academic performance.
  - Consider **obstructive sleep apnea** as the cause of inattention and hyperactivity in an obese adolescent who snores.
  - Teens with **autism spectrum disorders** have social and communication difficulties that first become evident in early childhood.
- Sleep deprivation can mimic ADHD.

Past Medical History

- Does the adolescent have a history of any psychiatric, medical or learning disorders? About 2/3rd of teens with ADHD have at least one coexisting disorder (Table 4).
- These disorders can precede the diagnosis of ADHD, co-occur with the ADHD, or be mistaken for ADHD.
- About 1/2 of teens with **bipolar disorder**, characterized by periods of depression and periods of elated mood or volatile behavior, will also have ADHD.
- A history of sudden, repetitive, involuntary movements or vocalizations suggests **Tourette syndrome (TS).**
  - The majority of patients with TS have ADHD, but a much smaller proportion of patients with ADHD will have tics.

Social History

- Has the teen had any changes to peer group or increase in high risk activities?
- **Substance abuse disorder** should be considered in a teen with frequent somatic complaints, delinquent behavior, marked moodiness, agitation, increased time spent with peers who use drugs or alcohol or deteriorating school performance.
- Occasionally, a teen who never had a childhood history of ADD may claim "difficulty in focusing" seeking a prescription for a stimulant for abuse purposes.

PHYSICAL EXAM

- An adolescent with ADHD will have a normal exam unless there is an underlying neurodevelopmental condition, such as a genetic syndrome or TS.
- Some teens will have soft neurological signs such as "spooning," a concavity seen when extending fingers.

STUDIES

- There is no laboratory, imaging or neuropsychiatric test that can diagnose ADHD.

- Neuroimaging studies and EEG neither diagnose ADHD nor differentiate patients with and without ADHD.
- These tests are not indicated unless there are concomitant abnormal neurological findings.

ADHD Specific Questionnaires and Rating Scales

- Assess and quantify ADHD symptoms.
- Some are designed to be completed by parents and others by teachers.
- Though not diagnostic, these are often useful tools in the evaluation of ADHD.
- Rating scales can help describe the teen's functioning and degree of impairment in key areas of life (e.g. school and home).
- Sequential rating scales can help monitor progress after treatment has begun.

Psycho-educational Testing

- Useful to evaluate intellectual ability or rule out possible learning disabilities.

TREATMENT

- The most effective treatment is a combination of medication and behavioral interventions.
- Parents may resist medication for fears it will become a "crutch" or lead to drug dependence.
- Ongoing follow-up of the response to treatment is essential and should lead to changes if the desired outcomes are not seen.

Pharmacotherapy (Table 5)

- Stimulants (amphetamine, dextroamphetamine and methylphenidate) are first line therapy.

- Dosing strategies:
  - Long-acting formulations have advantages over short-acting ones.
  - Medication effects last well into the late afternoon and early evening (for completion of homework, focus on evening activities, etc.).

- Teens are able to avoid the stigma or disruption of going to the nurse for medication during the school day.
- From the starting dose, increase stepwise every 3 to 7 days to achieve the maximal benefit without significant side effects.
- There is significant individual variation in response to these medications.
- Teens with poor or sub-optimal response on an appropriate dose should be switched to another formulation.
- There is no reason to take "drug holidays," or days off medication. Many teens benefit from continued medication on weekends, vacation days or other days off school because it improves attention and decreases impulsivity; thereby, potentially decreasing social or family conflicts.

- Adverse effects:
  - Most are mild and resolve with time.
  - In spite of the potential for stimulants to suppress appetite, there is no significant effect on growth in adolescents.
  - In 2008, the American Heart Association recommended a routine EKG before starting medications for ADHD.
  - There is no evidence that those taking ADHD medications are at increased risk of sudden cardiac death or that an EKG will identify those at risk.
  - The American Academy of Pediatrics and the American Association of Child and Adolescent Psychiatry concluded that an EKG is not needed before starting medication, and that all teens should be routinely screened for cardiac abnormalities through history and physical exam.
- There remains the risk of medication misuse or abuse:
  - Stimulant abuse or dependence among adolescents or young adults taking prescribed ADHD medication is very low.
  - Misuse of stimulants (especially short-acting formulations) is increasing, especially among older teens and college students. Reasons for use include a desire to improve academic performance or to get high.
  - Some patients may sell or give away their medication, or it might be stolen.

- Instead of a stimulant, atomoxetine (Strattera) might be first line treatment for a patient with a history of substance abuse.

Behavioral Interventions (Table 6)

- May consider first line treatment when ADHD symptoms are mild and/or the family does not want to use medication.
- Behavioral strategies include those directed to the adolescent, family and school.
- As with pharmacotherapy, treatment needs to be individualized and there should be close follow up with the primary care physician to assess treatment success or failure.

Complimentary and Alternative Medicine Approaches

- There are limited data and research on the effectiveness of these approaches for ADHD management, but most are safe and may be helpful as adjuncts to other treatment options.
- Examples include: acupuncture, homeopathy, yoga, meditation, cognitive behavioral therapy, biofeedback and massage.
- There is no evidence that nutritional supplements or elimination diets (e.g., sugar or dye free) help treat ADHD.

What is unique about ADHD in adolescents?

- Teens may deny a problem with attention and resist all suggested treatments. They need to be engaged in the process and believe that the recommended treatment will be of help to them.
- Teens with ADHD are at increased risk to engage in impulsive high-risk behaviors including: smoking, using alcohol or other drugs, having unsafe sex, repeating a grade, dropping out of school, having a poor driving record or losing a license or having difficulties at work.
- Teens whose ADHD is adequately treated do *NOT* have higher rates of substance abuse or mood disorders than the general population.

- ADHD impulsivity increases the risk for suicide, especially with comorbid mood disorders.
- Adolescent females may have less hyperactivity with only inattentive features, often resulting in a late diagnosis. These teens have remarkable academic improvement on medication.

TEST YOUR KNOWLEDGE ANSWERS

48. B. There are no diagnostic tests that discriminate reliably between teens with and without ADHD. While there seem to be some differences in brain morphology in those with ADHD (especially in brain areas involved with executive function), neuroimaging studies are neither sensitive nor specific enough to diagnose ADHD. ADHD can only be diagnosed after a comprehensive clinical evaluation with information obtained from the adolescent, parents and teachers.
49. F. In cases where the adolescent has mild ADHD symptoms or the family is very resistant to medication, well-designed behavioral interventions may be sufficient. In the vast majority of cases, stimulants should be tried first. However, if there is a history of substance abuse, Strattera might be the best first-line treatment because there is no known abuse potential with Strattera. Because there is great individual variation in response to a particular medication and dose, trials of different medications at different doses may be needed before an optimal outcome is achieved. Common side effects of stimulants include headaches, abdominal pain, decreased appetite and difficulty falling asleep.

Table 1. Risk Factors for ADHD.

Genetic	• There is often a family history of ADHD. • More prevalent in males than females (2:1). • Genes involved in catecholamine regulation have been associated with ADHD.
Other risk factors	• Prematurity. • Low birth weight. • Prenatal exposure to nicotine or alcohol. • Traumatic brain injury. • Parenting style and family functioning do not *cause* ADHD but can influence the severity of the symptoms and the outcomes. • A parent with ADHD may have more difficulty facilitating the child's organization.

Table 2. Differential Diagnosis of ADHD in Adolescents.

Psychiatric Disorders Listed in Table 4
Sleep Disorder/Sleep Deprivation
Learning Disability
Inappropriate Class or School Placement
Medication Side Effects
Impaired Vision or Hearing
Autism Spectrum Disorders

Table 3. ADHD Symptoms and Behaviors.

Symptoms	Common Behaviors
Inattentiveness	• Forgetful, often losing things • Disorganized • Difficulty with or procrastinating about tasks that require sustained attention (e.g. long reading assignments) • Poor time management skills • Poor attention to details, especially following directions • Easily distracted
Impulsivity	• Easily bored • Impatient • Easily frustrated • Loses temper easily • Difficulty making and/or keeping friends • Engages in high risk activities
Hyperactivity	• Difficulty being quiet or sitting still when the setting requires it • Restless, fidgety • Prefers very busy or intense activities (e.g. video games)

Table 4. Co-morbid Conditions.

	Disorder	Estimated Prevalence in Teens with ADHD (%)
Psychiatric	ODD	35–50
	Conduct Disorder	25–30
	Depression	20
	Anxiety	25–50
	Bipolar Disorder	15
	Substance Abuse	15
Neurodevelopmental	Learning Disability	30
	Tourettes Syndrome	5–10

Table 5. FDA-approved Medications for ADHD.

Medication	Starting Dose* (mg)	Duration of Action (Hours)	Common Side Effects
<u>STIMULANTS</u>			
Amphetamine and Dextroamphetamine	5 (QD or BID)	4–6	
• Adderall	10 (QD/BID)	10–12	
• Adderall XR	10	4–6	
• Dexedrine spansules	10 (QD/BID)	6–10	Headaches Insomnia
• Vyvanse			Abdominal pain
Methylphenidate	30	10–12	Decreased appetite
			Jitteriness
• Concerta	18–27	8–12	Jitteriness
• Focalin	2.5 (BID)	3–5	Anxiety
• Focalin XR	10	8–12	Irritability
• Metadate ER	20	6–8	Agitation
• Metadate CD	20	8–9	
• Methylin	5 (BID)	3–5	
• Methylin ER	10	6–8	
• Ritalin	10 (BID)	3–5	
• Ritalin SR	20	6–8	
• Ritalin LA	20	8–9	
<u>SNRI**</u>			
Strattera (Atomoxetine)	18–25	24	Sedation Dry mouth Dizziness Nausea Constipation Decreased appetite ***<u>Black box warning:</u>*** *Increased risk of suicidal ideation*
<u>ALPHA-2 AGONIST</u>			
Intuniv (Guanfacine)	1–2	6–12	Hypotension Bradycardia Dizziness Sedation Decreased appetite Constipation *Approved for up to age 17 yrs*

*All doses are once per day unless otherwise specified.
**Selective Norepinephrine Reuptake Inhibitors.

Table 6. Behavioral Interventions for ADHD.

Directed to the...	Interventions
Adolescent	• Learn better study, time management and organizational skills. • Establish a time and place to do homework. • Use a calendar or assignment book to track assignments, due dates, etc. • Get adequate and regular sleep since fatigue can exacerbate ADHD symptoms. • Limit screen time (TV, video games, computer, etc.) because these can interfere with academics and increase social isolation.
School setting	• Individualize approaches to facilitate learning (e.g. smaller classes and extra teacher in the classroom) • Allow students to keep an extra set of books at home. • Make a contract with expected behaviors and provide regular feedback to the student and parents. • If ADHD causes significant impairment or if there are associated problems (e.g. learning disability), the student should be evaluated by a child study team, and an individualized education plan (IEP) should be devised. • If ADHD greatly affects learning, but no other disability is present, a "504 Accommodation Plan" can be written to ensure the student gets some accommodations to ensure future success.
Family	• Work closely and regularly with school personnel to monitor the student's progress. • Learn to replace frequent arguments and criticism about the teen's behaviors and grades with more positive communication and problem-solving discussions.

WEB REFERENCES

- Setlik J, Bond GR and Ho M. 'Adolescent Prescription ADHD Medication Abuse Is Rising Along with Prescriptions for These Medications', Pediatrics. September 2009; 124(3): 875–880, retrieved from http://pediatrics.aappublications.Org/content/124/3/875.full?sid=236dcb20-433a-4001-8324-6b4b88e71227

- Subcommittee on Attention-Deficit/Hyperactivity Disorder, Steering Committee on Quality Improvement and Management. 'ADHD: Clinical Practice Guideline for the Diagnosis, Evalutaion, and Treatment of Attention-Deficit/Hyperactivity Disorder in Children and Adolescents', Pediatrics. Novemeber 2011; 128(5): 1007–1022, retrieved from http://

pediatrics.aappublications.org/content/128/5/1007.full?sid=236dcb20-433a-4001-8324-6b4b88e71227

- Visser SN, Lesesne CA. 'Mental Health in the United States: Prevalence of Diagnosis and Medication Treatment for Attention-Deficit/Hyperactivity Disorder-United States, 2003', MMWR. Spetember 2005;54(34);842-847, last reviewed 8/31/2005, retrieved from http://www.cdc.gov/mmwr/preview/mmwrhtml/mm5434a2.htm

Additional Clinician and Patient Resources:

- Attention Deficit Disorder Association; information for adults with ADHD: www.add.org
- Centers for Disease Control and Prevention: www.cdc.gov/ncbddd/adhd/
- Children and Adolescents with ADHD: www.chadd.org
- National Resource Center on ADHD: www.help4adhd.org

35

ANXIETY DISORDERS

Michele D. Wilson

TEST YOUR KNOWLEDGE

50. Which of the following statements about anxiety disorders is true?
    A. They are more common among males than females.
    B. They subside in late adolescence and have no long term effects on function.
    C. Obsessive compulsive disorder is no longer considered to be an anxiety disorder.
    D. Post traumatic stress is an anxiety disorder.
    E. Beta agonists and antihistamines have proven helpful to alleviate anxiety.
51. Effective treatment modalities for anxiety disorders in adolescence include:
    A. Education of the patient and family about the condition.
    B. Cognitive behavioral therapy.
    C. Selective serotonin reuptake inhibitors.
    D. All the above.
    E. None of the above.

Refer to end of chapter for answers on page 378.

A 15 year old female patient complains of chronic abdominal pain. She has had an extensive workup with no significant findings. On questioning, she reports that she has missed 50 days of school this academic year. She says she feels anxious at school and in social situations.

BACKGROUND

- Anxiety disorders are one of the most common psychiatric disorders affecting adolescents; yet, they are often under-diagnosed and inadequately treated.
- Anxiety disorders are characterized by fear in specific environments, anticipatory fear and autonomic arousal.
- Anxiety disorders are more common in females than males (2:1 to 3:1 ratio) and have an earlier age of onset for females, although the average age of onset is 11 years.
- The prevalence of anxiety disorders ranges from approximately 6 to 20% of teens.
- Many teens may experience mild, transient worries without significant impairment; this is *not* consistent with a diagnosis of an anxiety disorder. It is important to distinguish normal fears and worries from those that impair functioning.
- Teens living with anxiety disorders have symptoms that are excessive and severe, and adversely impact their functioning at school, home, in social circumstances and/or with peers.
- Symptoms of anxiety disorders are longstanding and cause significant distress to the teen.

RISK FACTORS

- There is a genetic or familial tendency to anxiety disorders so that teens with family history of either anxiety or mood disorder are more likely to develop an anxiety disorder.
- An anxious or inhibited temperament increases the risk for anxiety disorder.
- Environmental factors including parental modeling of anxious or fearful behaviors, significant stress or violence in the home are also risk factors.

ASSESSMENT

HISTORY

- To make an accurate diagnosis, it is important to know all seven anxiety disorders (Table 1).

History of Present Illness

- Ask if the teen has any specific fear and determine if that fear is excessive or pathologic.
- Assess if there have been any changes to their performance in school or relationships with peers and family as these may become impaired due to the anxiety.

Medications

- Review all prescribed medication use. Medications that may cause symptoms of anxiety include: beta agonists, sympathomimetic agents, steroids, selective serotonin reuptake inhibitors, antipsychotic medications, diet pills and antihistamines.

Social History

- Assess for substance use, abuse and dependence. Use or withdrawal from cocaine, amphetamines, caffeine, alcohol or marijuana may cause anxiety.

Family History

- Obtain a family history inquiring about mood, anxiety or other psychiatric disorders.
- May reveal genetic loading or disclose a situational reaction to abuse or violence that can mimic an anxiety disorder but will resolve with adequate intervention.

Review of Systems

- Adolescents with anxiety disorders may present with somatic complaints; inquire about hyperventilation, palpitations, abdominal pain, headaches, muscle pains, fatigue, sleep disturbance, difficulty breathing or dizziness.

PHYSICAL

Vital Signs

- Anxious patients may be mildly tachycardic or tachypneic.
- Patients anxious in doctors' offices may experience "white coat hypertension."

General

- May present with dizziness, faintness, sweaty palms or hyperventilation.

STUDIES

- Screening questionnaires can be very useful. The Screen for Child Anxiety Related Disorder (SCARED) questionnaire can be given to adolescents with suspected anxiety disorders. It is relatively short and can guide the clinician.
- There are no laboratory findings specific for anxiety disorders; however, they can be helpful in cases where a diagnosis is suspected that can mimic an anxiety disorder such as hypoglycemia, hyperthyoidism, pheochromocytoma or arrhythmias.

SPECIAL TESTS

Throat Culture, ASO Titers and Antineuronal Antibodies

- In acute onset OCD with a clinical history of sore throat, these labs may help identify Pediatric Autoimmune Neuropsychiatric Disorder Associated with Streptococcal infections (PANDAS).

DISPOSITION

- The primary care provider can initiate early treatment.
- Teens with more serious symptoms or functional impairment require a mental health referral.
- Prompt treatment can improve functioning at school and socially.

Multimodal treatment is often indicated.

- Education of the teen and parents or guardians is important and may be adequate for those with mild anxiety disorder of recent onset.
  - Education should include information regarding the disease, symptoms, course and treatment options.
- Cognitive behavioral therapy has been shown to be effective.
  - Facing the fear is a key aspect of healing.
  - The teen must learn new ways of reacting to situations that cause anxiety by managing their somatic symptoms and facing their fear through exposure techniques.
- Medications may be initiated.
  - If indicated, selective serotonin re-uptake inhibitors (SSRIs) are first line medications.
  - Beta blockers may be used for short-term anxiety such as performance anxiety.
  - Benzodiazepines are rarely used due to their addictive potential, but may be used for a short course to treat severe anxiety.
  - Buspirone is a less common medication prescribed for anxiety.

What is unique about anxiety disorders in adolescents?

- Some anxiety disorders will resolve, but teens with more serious disease are more likely to have persistent symptoms.
- Untreated anxiety can negatively impact normal psychosocial development.
- Those with anxiety disorders risk exacerbating symptoms with life changes or stress.
- Studies have shown that adolescents with anxiety disorders are at increased risk for depression, drug abuse and educational underachievement as young adults.
- Adolescents with untreated panic attacks are at increased risk for suicide.
- Anxiety disorders may be comorbid with other psychiatric disorders including depression, substance abuse and attention deficit hyperactivity disorders.

TEST YOUR KNOWLEDGE ANSWERS

50. D. Anxiety disorders occur more commonly in females than males and can have significant long-term effects on functioning. Obsessive compulsive disorder and post-traumatic stress are part of the spectrum of anxiety disorders. Beta agonists, sympathomimetic agents, steroids, selective serotonin reuptake inhibitors, antipsychotic medications, diet pills and antihistamines may all cause anxiety.
51. D. Treatment of anxiety disorders is multimodal and may include education of the patient and family, cognitive behavioral therapy and use of medications.

Table 1. Anxiety Disorders.

All Anxiety Disorders are Characterized by Fear in Specific Environments, Anticipatory Fear and Autonomic Arousal.	
Separation Disorder	• Excessive and developmentally inappropriate fear about separation from the home or from parents. • School avoidance is common due to somatic complaints such as abdominal pain or headaches.
Specific Phobia	• Persistent fear of a specific situation that is excessive, irrational and not developmentally appropriate. • Common fears include heights, small animals or storms.
Social Phobia (Social Anxiety Disorder)	• Excessive fear of one or more social situations such as public speaking, parties or standing up in class. • May appear shy and at times refuse to speak in class due to fear of embarrassment. • May be associated with school avoidance. • At increased risk for substance abuse and for academic & social underachievement.

(*Continued*)

Table 1. (*Continued*)

All Anxiety Disorders are Characterized by Fear in Specific Environments, Anticipatory Fear and Autonomic Arousal.	
Generalized Anxiety Disorder (GAD)	• Characterized by uncontrollable, excessive and chronic worry associated with emotional distress and functional impairment. • Patients worry about multiple aspects of their life, most commonly school performance, health, safety, family or social issues. • Patients may be irritable or restless and may have somatic complaints such as headaches, abdominal pain or fatigue. • Distress may be internal and therefore not evident to family, friends or teachers. • May result in academic and social underachievement.
Panic Disorder	• Typically has its onset in middle adolescence to mid 20's. • Characterized by recurrent panic attacks with sudden unexpected onset of intense fear and sense of dread and symptoms of autonomic hyperarousal including racing heart, shaking, trouble breathing, dizziness and nausea. • Episodes are so uncomfortable that teens experience anticipatory anxiety and may avoid situations that have led to panic attacks, resulting in agoraphobia.
Obsessive Compulsive Disorder (OCD)	• Consists of recurrent and intrusive repetitive thoughts, impulses or images called obsessions and repetitive physical or mental rituals or movements called compulsions. • Obsessions and compulsions cause marked distress and functional impairment at school and home, taking up significant parts of the day. • Acute onset can occur in the setting of PANDAS.
Post-Traumatic Stress Disorder (PTSD)	• Occurs after a severe traumatic event (i.e. threat of death or serious injury of self or others). • Subsequently, there are recurrent and intrusive flashbacks to the traumatic event. • This leads to avoidance of associated places, events or people and hyperarousal associated with functional impairment.

WEB REFERENCES

- Connolly SD, Bernstein GA, *et al.* 'Practice Parameter for the Assessment and Treatment of Children and Adolescents With Anxiety Disorders', American Academy of Child and Adolescent Psychiatry. February 2007; 46(2), 267–283, retrieved from http://www.aacap.org/galleries/PracticeParameters/JAACAP Anxiety 2007.pdf
- Geller DA, March J, *et al.* 'Practice Parameters for the Assessment and Treatment of Children and Adolescents with Obsessive Compulsive Disorder,' American Academy of Child & Adolescent Psychiatry, retrieved from http://www.aacap.org/galleries/PracticeParameters/OCDRevisedAug2011.pdf
- Seligman LD, Ollendick TH. 'Cognitive Behavioral Therapy for Anxiety Disorders in Youth', Child Adolescent Psychiatr Clin N Am. 2011 April; 20(2): 217–238, retrieved from http://www.ncbi.nlm.nih.gov/pmc/articles/PMC3091167/

Additional Clinician and Patient Resources:

- American Academy of Child and Adolescent Psychiatry, Anxiety Disorders Resource Center, retrieved from http://www.aacap.org/cs/AnxietyDisorders.ResourceCenter
- Anxiety Disorders of America Association: www.adaa.org
  - Practice Guidelines, Screening & Teach Tools, Videos, retrieved from http://www.adaa.org/resources-professionals/practice-guidelines
- National Institute of Mental Health, Anxiety Disorders: http://www.nimh.nih.gov/health/topics/anxiety-disorders/index.shtml
  - Anxiety Disorders in Children and Adolescents (Factsheet), retrieved from http://www.nimh.nih.gov/health/publications/anxiety-disorders-in-children-and-adolescents/index.shtml

36

DEPRESSION

Michele D. Wilson

TEST YOUR KNOWLEDGE

52. Which of the following statements is *NOT* true?
    A. Teen females are more likely than males to experience major depression.
    B. The risk of depression is lower in patients with ADHD.
    C. Teens with bipolar disorder often initially present with depression.
    D. Adolescent depression in males can manifest as irritability, fighting and acting out.
    E. All the above are true.

Refer to end of chapter for answer on page 388.

A previously straight "A" student, active in many extracurricular activities, is brought to clinic by her concerned mother. She reports that her daughter recently quit the track team and her grades have been slipping: "She just doesn't seem interested in anything anymore!"

BACKGROUND

- Depression often has its onset during adolescence and is a leading cause of disability for teens.
- Depression is characterized by sadness, irritability and loss of interest or pleasure in most things that persists for more than two weeks.
- The estimated prevalence of major depressive disorder among adolescents aged 13 to 18 years is 5.6% with a lifetime prevalence as high as 20%.
- Adolescent females are twice as likely as males to suffer from depression.
- Depression is often under-recognized. Only 40.3% of teens with a major depressive episode in the previous year received any treatment for this disorder.
- It is especially important to screen for bipolar disorder in any depressed teen since patients with bipolar disorder often initially present with a major depressive episode.
  - 20–40% of adolescents diagnosed with depression will eventually develop bipolar disorder.

RISK FACTORS

- Depression in a parent.
- Previous episode of depression.
- Co-morbid mental health conditions including anxiety disorder.
- Chronic medical conditions such as hypothyroidism, diabetes mellitus or cancer.
- Experience of a significant negative life event including abuse.
- Alcohol and substance abuse.
- Medications.

ASSESSMENT

HISTORY

- A diagnosis of depression is made by the clinical history (Table 1).
- Teens should be screened routinely for depression at well visits including questions about suicide risk such as past or current ideation or attempts.

History of Present Illness

- Determine the extent and duration of symptoms.
- Depressed teens often have pessimistic or sad outlooks with a focus on death or dying.
- Does the teen report feeling worthless, hopeless or helpless?
- Has there been any increase in agitation or restlessness?
- Inquire about active or passive suicidal ideations. Is there a plan?
- If suicidal thoughts are present, what has stopped the adolescent from acting on them?
- Assess for the presence of co-morbid mental illnesses that may be present in up to 40% of teens diagnosed with depression. These include:
    - Anxiety disorders
    - Substance abuse disorders
    - Eating disorders
    - Attention deficit hyperactivity disorder (ADHD)
- Any depressed teen should also be screened for bipolar disorder. Characteristic symptoms include: decreased sleep, racing thoughts or hyperactivity, pressured speech, impulsive behavior or irritability, hypersexuality, grandiose thinking and/or psychotic symptoms.
- Assess for behaviors that suggest "acting out." Clinicians should be concerned if teens are getting into trouble at home, school or in the community with legal authorities.

Past Medical History

- Teens diagnosed with chronic medical conditions adversely affecting quality of life are more likely to suffer from symptoms of depression and should be screened routinely.

- Some depressive symptoms may also occur in the context of other illnesses:
  - Weight loss or weight gain, temperature intolerance, skin and hair changes suggest **thyroid disease**.
  - Fatigue and low energy in a menstruating female should raise concern for **iron deficiency anemia**.
  - Long standing fatigue following a viral syndrome suggests **infectious mononucleosis**.
- Has the teen been diagnosed or treated with difficult to manage ADHD in the past? This is suspicious for bipolar disorder.
- Has there been any suicidal attempt?
- Any prior psychiatric hospitalizations?

Family History

- Ask about the history of psychiatric disorders in family members.
- The risk of depression or bipolar disorder is increased in those with a family history of these illnesses.
- Ask about family members who have attempted or successfully completed suicide.

Medications

- Some medications can cause depressive symptoms as a part of their side effect profile (i.e. propanolol).
- It is also important to determine current medications used by the teen as many drugs used to treat depression can have potential dangerous interactions with other medications (e.g. prolonging the QT interval) that could affect treatment efficacy or lead to patient harm.

Social History

A detailed HEEADSSS assessment may alert the clinician to red flags that would otherwise be missed, such as insomnia or frequent fights.

- Ask about the home environment, school successes and challenges, the teen's support network and high risk behaviors that could represent "acting out."

- Parents should be alert to signs of potential substance abuse as teens may choose to use drugs or alcohol to self-medicate for depression.
- Alternatively, substance abuse may lead to or mimic depression.
- Teens with depression are at risk for higher health care costs, early pregnancies and suicide.

Review of Symptoms

- Teens with depression may have a range of psychosomatic complaints including: headaches, abdominal pain, musculoskeletal pain, increased nausea and fatigue.

PHYSICAL

- Teens being assessed for depression should have complete physical exams to exclude other medical causes of depressive symptoms.

Vital Signs

- Bradycardia and/or hypotension in the context of lost weight and depressive symptoms suggests an underlying **eating disorder**.
- Tachycardia may suggest **stimulant** or other **substance abuse**.
- Fever suggests infectious etiology (i.e. mononucleosis).

HEENT

- Assess for cervical adenopathy: multiple enlarged notes in the context of fatigue suggests **infectious mononucleosis**.
- Palpate thyroid gland for size and nodularity: **hypothyroidism** can cause severe depression.

Skin

- Pallor suggests anemia.
- Observe for signs of self-injury such as cutting scars on arms or other parts of the body.

STUDIES

Complete Blood Count (CBC)

- Consider if anemia is suspected.

Thyroid Studies

- TSH and T4 if history and physical exam findings are consistent with hypothyroidism.

Drug Testing

- Consider in cases of suspected substance abuse.

Screening Instruments

- Clinicians are in the unique role of identifying depression in teens since these patients often seek care from their primary care provider rather than mental health providers.
- The primary care provider can screen for and identify depression aided by screening tools that are easily administered to teens in a clinical setting:
    - Patient Health Questionnaire for Adolescents (PHQ-A)
    - Beck Depression Inventory-Primary Care Version (BDI-PC)

DISPOSITION

- Clinicians can monitor, counsel and provide medications to patients.
- Referrals when necessary, should be made to mental health professionals, preferably a child and adolescent psychiatrist with expertise in the field.
- Treatment should be based on severity of symptoms.

Mild Depression

- It is often reasonable to provide education and monitor before initiating medications.
- Follow up visits, usually weekly, should occur to assess risk for suicide.
- Families should ensure teen safety by removing weapons and any medications that could be used for self-harm, from the teen's environment.

- Teens who do not respond to treatment within four to six week of initiation, merit more intensive evaluation and referral to a mental health professional.

Moderate to Severe Depression

- In cases of moderate to severe depression, coexisting substance abuse or psychosis, teens should be referred to a mental health professional for further evaluation and treatment.
- For adolescents with moderate or severe depression, intensive treatment is important.
- Psychotherapy, specifically cognitive behavioral therapy and interpersonal therapy, have been shown to be beneficial treatments.
- Research has demonstrated the effectiveness of selective serotonin reuptake inhibitors (SSRIs), specifically fluoxetine, for depression in adolescents.
  - At this time, fluoxetine is the only SSRI approved by the Food and Drug Administration (FDA) to treat depression in teens.
  - The FDA-issued black box warning regarding SSRIs and suicide risk in adolescents led to increased safety concerns and decreased prescribing of medication for teens with depression.
  - Subsequent analysis has suggested that the overall benefits of SSRIs for teens with depression outweigh their risks.
  - The FDA recommends weekly evaluation for the first month when teens begin SSRIs.
  - When medications reach optimal effectiveness, treatment should be continued for a minimum of six to nine months.
  - Use of antidepressants not approved for teens is reasonable, especially if a parent has responded to such a medication.
  - The combination of medication and cognitive behavioral therapy has been shown to be most effective in The Treatment of Adolescent Depression Study (TADS).

Bipolar Disorder

- Teens with suspected bipolar disorder should be referred to a mental health professional for further evaluation and treatment.

- Individuals with bipolar disorder may have worsening symptoms of agitation and decreased sleep. Mania may be triggered by antidepressants prescribed for what initially appears to be a major depressive disorder.

What is unique about depression in adolescents?

- The diagnosis of depression in adolescents is often challenging since even normal teens may experience moodiness or sadness that is short-lived and does not affect overall function.
- Substance abuse in depressed adolescents increases the risk for suicide.
- Adolescents are often reluctant to accept a mental health referral because "I am not crazy"; hence, some educational counseling regarding depression can facilitate a referral.
- A call to the mental health consultant and a follow up call to the patient and family are essential steps toward a successful treatment of more severe cases of depression.
- Teens often improve quickly and hospitalization during the crisis may be life saving.

TEST YOUR KNOWLEDGE ANSWER

52. E. Patients with ADHD have a higher rate of smoking, substance abuse and depression then the general population. Females are more likely than males to experience major depression. The majority of patients with bipolar disorder that begins in adolescence may initially appear to have major depression. Depression in male adolescents may manifest as irritability, fighting and acting out.

Table 1. Common Symptoms of Depression.

Decreased school performance
Withdrawal from social interactions
Sleep disturbance (insomnia or hypersomnia)
Appetite disturbance (usually decreased appetite)
Anger and/or irritability
Nonspecific pain or somatic complaints
Trouble concentrating and/or making decisions
Anhedonia, or no longer enjoying things that were a source of happiness in the past
Suicidal thoughts

WEB REFERENCES

- Cheung AH, *et al.* 'Guidelines for Adolescent Depression in Primary Care (GLAD-PC):II. Treatment and Ongoing Management', Pediatrics. Nov 2001; 120(5): el313–el326, retrieved from http://pediatrics.aappublications.Org/content/120/5/el313.full
- Food and Drug Administration (revised 1/26/05), Medication Guide About Using Antidepressants in Children and Teenagers, retrieved from http://www.fda.gov/downloads/drugs/drugsafety/%20%E2%80%A8informationbydrugclass/UCMl61646.pdf
- National Survey on Drug Use and Health, The NSDUH Report (May 16, 2008) 'Depression among Adolescents', retrieved from http://oas.samhsa.gov/2k5/youthDepression/youthDepression.htm
- Ryan, ND. 'Treatment of depression in children and adolescents', Lancet. 2005; 366: 933–940, retrieved from http://www.mhfa.com.au/cms/wp-content/uploads/201l/03/2_depression_tab.pdf
- Stein REK, Zitner BA, Jensen PS. 'Interventions for Adolescent Depression in Primary Care', Pediatrics. August 2006; 118(2): 669–682, retrieved from http://pediatrics.aappublications.org/content/118/2/669.abstract?ijkey=0f6d6f56bbdl4049603f9f4b7a8a49250al7dfel&keytype2=tf_ipsecsha
- US Preventive Services Task Force. 'Screening and Treatment for Major Depressive Disorder in Children and Adolescents: US Preventive Services Task Force Recommendation Statement', Pediatrics. April 1, 2009; 123(4): 1223–1228, retrieved from http://pediatrics.aappublications.org/content/123/4/1223.full

Additional Clinician and Patient Resources:

- Mental Health America, Depression in Teens, retrieved from http://www.nmha.org/index.cfm?objectid=C7DF950F-1372-4D20-C8B5BD8DFDD94CFl

- Moreland CS, Bonin L. 'Patient information: Depression treatment options for adolescents (Beyond the Basics)', UpToDate (last updated Jan 31, 2013), retrieved from http://www.uptodate.com/contents/depression-treatment-options-for-adolescents-beyond-the-basics
- National Institute of Mental Health, Antidepressant Medication for Children and Adolescents: Information for Parents and Caregivers, retrieved from http://www.nimh.nih.gov/health/topics/child-and-adolescent-mental-health/antidepressant-medications-for-children-and-adolescents-information-for-parents-and-caregivers.shtml
- The Reach Institute, Guidelines for Adolescent Depression-Primary Care, retrieved from: http://www.glad-pc.org/

SECTION III

REPRODUCTIVE HEALTH CARE

37

BREAST PATHOLOGY: MASSES AND NIPPLE DISCHARGE

Amy L. Weiss

TEST YOUR KNOWLEDGE

53. A 16 year old girl presents with her mother. Both are extremely concerned about a breast mass she recently found. She discovered it about 3 weeks ago in the upper, outer quadrant of her left breast. Her LMP was last week. She is very healthy, but a maternal aunt was recently diagnosed with breast cancer. On exam, no masses are palpable in either breast. What will you tell the patient and her mom?

    A. Even though you cannot feel a mass today, she should be referred for ultrasound evaluation.
    B. Her lump was probably fibrocystic disease, and the enlarged tissue resolved during her period last week.
    C. Due to her family history, she should be referred to a breast surgeon.
    D. The lump was probably a fibroadenoma, which is the most common breast mass in adolescents.
    E. Recurrent breast lumps herald cystosarcoma phyloides.

54. Which one of the following statements is true?

    A. A pregnancy test should be obtained on a young woman with nipple discharge.
    B. Many medicines, especially psychiatric drugs, can be a cause of galactorrhea.

Refer to end of chapter for answer on page 403.

C. Thyroid functions and prolactin should be checked when a teen presents with nipple discharge.
D. It is common to detect nipple discharge following erotic stimulation.
E. All the above are true.

Fibrocystic Disease and Fibroadenomas

"I found a lump in my breast. I'm really worried that I have breast cancer."

BACKGROUND

- Fibrocystic disease, or fibrocystic changes, is a benign condition consisting of lumpy, nodular breast tissue that can be painful.
- The etiology of fibrocystic disease is unknown but thought to be due to an imbalance of estrogen and progesterone.
- Fibroadenomas are common, benign, solid, and typically painless breast masses.
- Fibroadenomas may be hormonally driven. They are common during reproductive years, can increase during pregnancy or with estrogen use, and often shrink post menopause.

ASSESSMENT

HISTORY

History of Present Illness

- Assess duration of symptoms. How long has the mass or lumpy tissue been present?
- Has the teen noticed any change in the size of the mass, becoming smaller or larger, since first noticed? Any variation in the size of lumpy tissue related to the menstrual cycle?
- Is the lump painful? If so, does the pain change throughout the menstrual cycle?
- Has the teen ever been pregnant or does she suspect a current pregnancy? Breast tenderness with a history of amenorrhea suggest **pregnancy.**
- Fever with breast tenderness, redness or warmth in a teen who has recently been pregnant or is currently breast feeding suggests **mastitis.**
- Bloody nipple discharge or overlying skin dimpling are more consistent with **malignancy.**

Menstrual History

- At what point in the menstrual cycle is the teen? When was the last menstrual period and are periods regular and once monthly? **Fibrocystic disease** varies through the menstrual cycle and is thought to be hormone related.

Past Medical History

- Ask about previous breast disease.
- Determine if there is a history of prior malignancy or radiation to the chest?

Family History

- Is there a family history of breast disease or breast cancer? Teens and their mothers are often anxious about cancer when there is a strong family history.

Medications

- Ask about all current medications including herbal supplements.

PHYSICAL

Vital Signs

- Fever in the context of breast warmth and/or tenderness suggests **mastitis.**

Breasts

- Inspect for Tanner staging and symmetry.
- Determine the location of the mass.
    - Is it central or peripheral?
    - In what quadrant is it located?
    - **Fibrocystic changes** and **fibroadenomas** are most typically found in the upper, outer quadrants of the breast.
- Determine mass consistency: nodular, cystic or solid? **Fibroadenomas** are solid and rubbery.
- Measure the size of the breast mass.

- Is the mass mobile or fixed? Mobility suggests **fibroadenoma.**
- Assess for tenderness or pain.
- Assess for nipple discharge as well as skin changes such as redness, thickening of the skin, and/or warmth which are consistent with inflammation, infection, or rarely malignancy.

Lymph Nodes

- Axillary, supraclavicular, and/or infraclavicular lymphadenopathy may be concerning for a malignant lesion and warrant further work up.

STUDIES

- Fibrocystic changes and fibroadenomas can be diagnosed clinically. No testing is needed if you are certain of the diagnosis.

SPECIAL TESTS

Ultrasound

- If uncertain of the diagnosis, this is the best modality to image adolescent breast tissue to confirm a diagnosis of fibrocystic disease or fibroadenoma. A fibroadenoma will be a solid, avascular and well-circumscribed mass on ultrasound.

MRI

- The next best imaging modality in cases where ultrasound results are inconclusive.

Needle Aspiration

- Can help to confirm the diagnosis of fibroadenomas or cysts.

Mammogram

- Is not recommended in adolescents due to the large amount of dense glandular tissue that make visualization difficult.

DISPOSITION

Fibrocystic Disease

- Reassure and educate teens about the benign nature of fibrocystic changes as well as the potential for variation of symptoms through the menstrual cycle.
- Recommend use of a supportive bra and NSAIDs to treat associated pain. Combination oral contraceptives can help in some cases.
- Caffeine and MSG food additive can worsen fibrocystic symptoms and should be avoided.

Fibroadenomas

- Can be managed with reassurance and close follow-up.
  - If less than 5 cm, they can be observed with serial exams.
  - If larger than 5 cm or rapidly growing, surgical removal can be considered.
  - The disadvantages of surgery include scarring, dimpling and damage to the breast's duct system.
- Rapidly growing breast masses and "giant fibroadenomas" may be due to a rare tumor, "cystosarcoma phyloides" that can be malignant.
- Breast cancer is almost unheard of in teens; however, primary tumors in other locations can metastasize to the breast and this should not be missed as patients tend to be quite sick.

What is unique about breast masses in adolescents?

- Fibrocystic changes are extremely common, occurring in over half of women of reproductive age.
- Fibroadenomas represent the majority (67–94%) of breast masses in adolescents.
- Two-thirds of fibroadenomas stay the same size or regress and can thus be managed conservatively.
- No reports exist of malignancy associated with a preexisting fibroadenoma.

Nipple Discharge/Galactorrhea

"I have something coming from my nipples, and it's staining my bra."

BACKGROUND

- Nipple discharge is a common complaint of women of reproductive age and can be categorized as lactation, physiologic discharge, galactorrhea or pathologic discharge.
- Most frequently, nipple discharge in adolescents is non-pathologic.
- Prolactinomas, though rare, always need to be considered in the differential of galactorrhea.
- There are a number of reasons teens could present with nipple discharge.
  - Hormones: pregnancy, post-abortion and birth control pills
  - Afferent nerve stimulation: erotic stimulation, irritation from tight clothing or "runner's nipple"
  - Medication or drug side effects (Table 1)
  - Ductal papilloma or prolactinoma

ASSESSMENT

HISTORY

History of Present Illness

- Ascertain if the discharge is unilateral or bilateral? Nipple discharge is often bilateral and multi-ductal.
- Does it occur spontaneously or only with manipulation?
- What is the appearance of the discharge? Is it clear, purulent, bloody or milky? Bloody discharge is more likely associated with **malignancy** while a purulent discharge is due to an underlying infection or **mastitis.**

Menstrual History

- Missed periods always warrant evaluation for pregnancy.
- A detailed menstrual history can pick up missed or irregular periods that may be associated with galactorrhea and suggest a **prolactinoma.**

- Has the teen recently given birth or had a termination of pregnancy? **Lactation** can occur in any of these situations.

Sexual History

- Is the adolescent sexually active? Is there is a history of stimulation of the breasts by a sexual partner?

Review of Systems

- Headaches, visual changes and secondary amenorrhea may suggest a **prolactinoma.** Other associated symptoms include loss of libido or painful intercourse secondary to increased vaginal dryness.

Past Medical History

- Has there been any repetitive trauma? Is the adolescent a long distance runner? **Jogger's nipple,** as a result of long distance running and chafing of the nipple, can cause serous or serosanguinous discharge.
- Are there any symptoms of hypothyroidism, such as weight gain, fatigue, cold intolerance, constipation or depression?

Medications

- Is the adolescent taking any medications, specifically psychiatric medications, such as antipsychotics or tricyclic antidepressants? These medicines, as well as Reglan, antihypertensives, and opiates, can all cause elevations in prolactin which can lead to galactorrhea (Table 1).

PHYSICAL

Breasts

- Inspect and palpate.
- Observe the symmetry and contour of the breasts and note any skin dimpling or retraction, erythema, discoloration, ulceration or crusting of the nipples.
- Attempt to elicit nipple discharge by massaging from the periphery of the breast toward the nipple/areolar complex. Gentle pressure should be applied to the base of the areola and not the nipple.

- Observe if discharge is coming from one or more ducts on the nipple, or from the areola. Flow from one duct is more concerning than that from multiple ducts.
- If discharge is identified, is it milky, purulent, serous, bloody or multi-colored?
- Eczema, skin diseases, or **apocrine chromohidrosis** (secretion of colored sweat from the apocrine glands on the areola) should be considered if discharge is from the areola.
- Breast masses and tender areas should be identified.

Lymph Nodes

- Axillary, infraclavicular or supraclavicular lymphadenopathy is concerning for malignancy.

Skin

- Examine for normal peri-areolar papules also known as **Montgomery tubercles**, or distension of the subareolar ducts which could be **mammary duct ectasia**. Both can occasionally lead to discharge.

STUDIES

Pregnancy Test

- Galactorrhea is common in pregnancy.

Prolactin

- Prolactinomas are associated with very elevated prolactin levels.
- Many medications can cause moderate prolactin elevations.
- Thyroid stimulating hormone (TSH) can cross-react with prolactin.

Thyroid Function Testing

- Evaluate for hypothyroidism.

Hemoccult or Guaiac Test

- Can be performed on bloody discharge for confirmation.

Culture of Fluid with Sensitivities

- If discharge is purulent, consider cellulitis or an abscess.

SPECIAL TESTS

- *Ultrasound.* Useful if a tumor is suspected.
- *Brain MRI*: In cases where prolactin levels are elevated and the patient has symptoms suspicious for a prolactinoma.
- *Cytology of the discharge:* Can be sent for testing by smearing discharge on a slide.
- *MRI Ductography*: Provides precise imaging of the breast tissue and ducts to localize a suspected mass or tumor.
- *Ductoscopy:* Allows for visualization of peripheral lesions.
- *Ductal Lavage:* To increase the amount of specimen obtained over simple expression.
- *Skin punch biopsy:* Helpful if a skin lesion on the nipple is thought to be the source of discharge versus true nipple discharge.

DISPOSITION

- Bilateral nipple discharge in teens is often due to a physiologic or endocrinologic process.
- If a medication is determined to be the cause of hyperprolactinemia, then the medication should be discontinued or changed.
- Once other lesions have been ruled out, nipple discharge can be managed by a terminal duct excision.
- Adolescents with prolactinomas should be referred to an endocrinologist.

What is unique about nipple discharge in adolescents?

- Nipple discharge in adolescence is typically associated with benign conditions.
- Attention needs to be paid to cases of erotic stimulation, contraceptive medication and pregnancy, even when the patient denies having had sexual intercourse.

- Psychotropic medications, increasingly used in teens with psychiatric conditions, are an increasing cause of galactorrhea.
- Galactorrhea with amenorrhea is suspicious for a prolactinoma.

TEST YOUR KNOWLEDGE ANSWER

53. B. The mass was likely due to fibrocystic changes which are hormonally responsive. It is not uncommon for fibrocystic changes to resolve by the time the teen presents, especially if she has had a menstrual period. These changes can recur, and should be treated symptomatically with NSAIDs and supportive bras for pain relief. Fibroadenomas are common masses in adolescents but do not resolve so rapidly.
54. E. All statements are true regarding nipple discharge in adolescents.

Table 1. Medications and Drugs that can cause Galactorrhea.

Typical Antipsychotics	Phenothiazine Drugs (Chlorpromazine, Clomipramine, Thioridazine)
	Haloperidol
	Pimozide
Atypical Antipsychotics	Risperidone
	Molindone
	Olanzapine
Anxiolytics	Benzodiazepines (Alprazolam)
	Buspirone
Neurologic Drugs	Sumatriptan
	Valproic Acid
	Dihydroergotamine
Antidepressant Drugs	Tricyclic Antidepressants (Amitriptyline, Clomipramine, Desipramine)
	Monoamine Oxidase Inhibitors
	Serotonin-Selective Reuptake Inhibitors (Fluoxetine, Paroxetine, Sertraline)
Opiates	Codeine
	Morphine
Drugs of Abuse	Amphetamines
	Cannabis
Gastrointestinal Drugs	Metoclopramide
	Cimetidine
Antihypertensive Drugs	Methyldopa
	Reserpine
	Verapamil
Hormones	Danazol
	Estrogen
	Medroxyprogesterone
	Oral Contraceptives
Herbal & Food Preparations	Anise
	Blessed Thistle
	Fennel
	Fenugreek Seed
	Marshmallow
	Nettle
	Red Clover
	Red Raspberry

WEB REFERENCES

- Alexander KCL, Pacaud D. 'Diagnosis and Management of Galactorrhea', American Family Physician. 2004 Aug 1; 70(3): 543–550, retrieved from http://www.aafp.org/afp/2004/0801/p543.html
- American College of Obstetrics and Gynecologists, Tool Kit for Teen Care (2nd Edition): Primary and Preventive Health Care for Female Adolescents (2010), retrieved from http://www.acog.org/~/media/Departments/Adolescent%20Health%20Care/Teen%20Care%20Tool%20Kit/ACOGPreventCare.pdf?dmc=1&ts=20130409T1344059349
- Arca, MJ. 'Pediatric Breast Disorders: Breast Disorders in Adolescent Girls', Medscape Reference (updated April 23, 2012), retrieved from http://emedicine.medscape.com/article/935410-overview#aw2aab6b6
- Arca MJ, Caniano DA. 'Breast Disorders in the Adolescent Patient' (updated February 22, 2005), retrieved from http://www.redorbit.com/news/health/129843/breast_disorders_in_the_adolescent_patient/
- FamilyPracticeNotebook.com, Galactorrhea: http://www.fpnotebook.com/gyn/sx/glctrh.htm

Additional Clinician and Patient Resources:

- The American College of Obstetricians and Gynecologists, FAQ: Benign Breast Problems and Conditions (November 2012), retrieved from http://www.acog.org/~/media/For%20Patients/faqo26.pdf?dmc=1&ts=20130409T1341203490
- Center for Young Women's Health, Children's Hospital Boston, Breast Lumps and Bumps (updated 7/8/2010), http://www.youngwomenshealth.org/breast_health_lumps.html
- MedicineNet.Com, Fibrocystic Breast Condition (reviewed 2/1/2012), http://www.medicinenet.com/fibrocystic_breast_condition/article.htm
- Medline Plus, Breast Diseases, retrieved from http://www.nlm.nih.gov/medlineplus/breastdiseases.html
- Pub Med Health, Fibroadenoma (last reviewed Nov 17, 2012), http://www.ncbi.nlm.nih.gov/pubmedhealth/PMH0004482

38

DYSMENORRHEA, PMS AND PMDD

Nneka A. Holder

TEST YOUR KNOWLEDGE

55. Which of the following statements is true?
    - A. Ovarian cysts are the cause of primary dysmenorrhea.
    - B. A pelvic ultrasound test is routinely recommended as part of the evaluation for new onset dysmenorrhea.
    - C. Sexually transmitted infections can be associated with dysmenorrhea.
    - D. All the above.
    - E. None of the above.
56. Which of the following statements is true?
    - A. As many as 80% of teens suffer from Premenstrual Syndrome (PMS).
    - B. Total hysterectomy can be a treatment for severe Premenstrual Dysphoric Disorder (PMDD).
    - C. Dietary supplements have been shown to help the symptoms of PMS/PMDD.
    - D. Selective serotonin re-uptake inhibitors are often used to successfully treat PMDD.
    - E. None of the above.

Refer to end of chapter for answers on page 414.

Dysmenorrhea

"My 14 year-old daughter misses school every time she has a period. Her cramps are just awful. Is there anything we can do to help her?"

BACKGROUND

- Up to 50% of menstruating females are affected by dysmenorrhea.
- Treatment is aimed at reducing symptoms and improving quality of life. Fortunately, there are successful treatment modalities for this very common condition.
- Patients are classified as having either primary or secondary dysmenorrhea.

Primary Dysmenorrhea:

- Cyclic pelvic pain with no underlying pathology.
- Usually associated with ovulatory cycles.
- Pain is thought to be caused by elevated uterine prostaglandins, leading to uterine dysmotility with secondary ischemia.
- Some patients also experience symptoms of bloating and nausea.

Secondary Dysmenorrhea:

- Cyclic pelvic pain with an underlying pathology such as infection, obstruction (i.e. genito urinary tract abnormalities), ovarian cysts, fibroids (rare in adolescence) and endometriosis.

ASSESSMENT

HISTORY

Menstrual History

- Determine the extent of symptoms. Does the teen have severe menstrual cramping that affects daily function (i.e. missed school or work), mood changes, bloating or nausea?

- Consider **endometriosis** when a patient presents with pelvic pain that occurs during or right before menses, lessens after menstruation and doesn't improve with standard therapy.
  - These patients often have dysmenorrhea that gets worse with each successive menstrual cycle.
- Assess timing of menarche. Most cycles are initially anovulatory; therefore, if pain is noted during menarche, especially if it is unilateral, **genital tract obstruction** should be ruled out.

Past Medical History

- A history of past surgeries or **pelvic inflammatory disease** (**PID**) may suggest **adhesions.**

Family History

- Ask about the menstrual history of female relatives. Dysmenorrhea, especially if due to **endometriosis**, has a genetic component.

Dietary History

- Dehydration and a high fat diet are thought to worsen symptoms.
- Caffeinated products can also worsen dysmenorrhea.

Review of Systems

- Consider secondary causes of dysmenorrhea if patients present with vaginal discharge which suggests a **sexually transmitted infection** (**STI**).

Social History

- Get a detailed sexual history. Fever and pelvic pain at menses suggests PID.
- Dyspareunia and cyclic pelvic pain suggests secondary dysmenorrhea.
- Nicotine can exacerbate symptoms of dysmenorrhea.

PHYSICAL

Vital Signs

- Fever suggests an infectious process.

Abdomen

- Exclude **masses** on abdominal exam.
- Pain in lower quadrants or rebound tenderness suggests **PID.**

Pelvic with Bimanual

- Consider if there is concern for an **STI** or **PID.**

STUDIES

CBC and Sedimentation Rate (ESR)

- If there is a high index of suspicion for an infectious etiology.
- If the white count and ESR are elevated, consider a pelvic ultrasound to rule out a **tubo-ovarian abscess** (**TOA**).

Urine Pregnancy Test

- Important to exclude the pain and bleeding associated with an ectopic pregnancy.

STI Screening

- Screen for gonorrhea and chlamydia in sexually active teens.

Pelvic Ultrasound or MRI

- Consider if an abdominal or pelvic mass is palpated, if the patient is hospitalized, a TOA is suspected or if the history suggests endometriosis.

SPECIAL TESTS

Laparoscopy

- May be indicated in cases of severe worsening dysmenorrhea, as it may be the only way to diagnose endometriosis or adhesions in a young adolescent.

TREATMENT

- For primary dysmenorrhea, non-steroidal anti-inflammatory drugs (NSAIDs) are considered first line therapy.
  - They act by interfering with prostaglandin production.
  - Advise teens to take NSAIDs at the first sign of symptoms, that may precede menses by 1–2 days.
- Supportive care measures such as applied topical heat can help alleviate symptoms.
- Hormonal therapy may be required to suppress ovulation and treat severe recurrent symptoms:
  - Combined oral contraceptives pills (COCs).
  - Progestin-only methods (i.e. medroxy progesterone acetate).
  - Other hormonal methods (i.e. transdermal patch or intra-vaginal ring) are also effective.
  - Newer formulations of COCs (lower estrogen-dosing and continuous dosing).
  - If symptoms persists after two cycles on hormonal therapy, consider switching hormonal methods (in cases where compliance or side effects are a concern).
- Preventive care measures can also help lessen the severity of symptoms over time such as moderate daily exercise, caffeine avoidance and proper hydration.
- Consider laparoscopic evaluation if symptoms progress and continue beyond 3 cycles despite adequate treatment.

Premenstrual Syndrome (PMS) and Premenstrual Dysphoric Disorder (PMDD)

"I don't know what's happening to my daughter. She acts like a completely different person when it's that time of the month and its causing problems for my family."

BACKGROUND

PMS

- Symptoms generally occur during the second half of the menstrual cycle (luteal phase) and resolve a few days after menses.
- The American College of Gynecology (ACOG) established diagnostic criteria in their practice bulletin released in 2000 (Table 1).
- There are no studies that definitively prove that PMS is related to cortisol, thyroid, follicle stimulating hormone, luteinizing hormone, insulin or prolactin levels.
- Nutritional deficiencies have not (to date) demonstrated a relationship to PMS.
- Symptoms resolve within 4 days of menses and recur 12 days into the next cycle.
- Symptoms adversely affect work or school function,

PMDD

- PMDD is a psychiatric diagnosis and may need to be co-managed by a psychiatrist.
- PMDD is distinct from PMS in that it is associated with significant psychiatric dysfunction.
- Symptoms include marked depression, anxiety, mood swings, irritability, anhedonia, fatigue, sleep problems and poor concentration.
- The etiology of PMS/PMDD is unclear. Many experts believe that hormonal fluctuations (of sex steroids) and interactions with central neurotransmitters play a significant role.
- Like PMS, PMDD can exist with other psychiatric problems and it must be clear that the symptoms are not due to the exacerbation of another psychiatric or medical condition.

- Psychiatric and medical conditions can mimic symptoms of PMDD and include: depression, bipolar disorder, panic disorder, substance abuse, anemia, chronic fatigue syndrome, autoimmune disorders, endometriosis and diabetes.

ASSESSMENT

HISTORY

Menstrual History

- Obtain a detailed menstrual history including symptoms that occur prior to menses.
- A documented log or diary of symptoms that have occurred for at least two cycles can help establish the diagnosis.

Family History

- Document the menstrual history of female family members and determine if others have experienced similar symptoms.

Social History

- Studies suggest that post-traumatic events may be a risk factor.

Mental Health History

- Obtain a detailed psychiatric history since the patient's symptoms may be related to an exacerbation of a pre-existing psychiatric condition versus new onset PMDD.

TREATMENT

- Published data regarding prevalence and treatment of PMS/PMDD in adolescents is lacking; however, several treatment strategies have been found to be beneficial in adults:
  - Selective Serotonin Re-uptake Inhibitors (SSRIs) can help alleviate the symptoms of PMS/PMDD and are considered first-line therapy.

- Hormonal contraception has been used to suppress ovulation. As with dysmenorrhea, most studies have examined the effect of COCs to induce regular menstrual cycles; however, other formulations and continuous dosing regimens may be used.
- Cognitive behavioral therapy and biofeedback have been shown to improve symptoms.
- Adhering to a healthy lifestyle by avoiding caffeine, increasing free water intake and exercising daily may help to lessen the severity of symptoms.
- Nutritional supplements have been studied but not enough to make recommendations.

- Anxiolytics, antidepressants and gonadotropin releasing hormone (GnRH) analogs can be used but should be done in consultation with psychiatry or gynecology, respectively.

What is unique about dysmenorrhea, PMS and PMDD in adolescents?

- Adolescents often underreport dysmenorrhea and may not seek care even if severely afflicted. Questions about menstrual symptoms need to be part of the history for all routine well visits.
- PMDD, a disabling condition, is often overlooked in teens because it is misinpterpreted as an "adolescent" attitude.

TEST YOUR KNOWLEDGE ANSWERS

55. C. Sexually transmitted infections (particularly, PID from *Neisseria gonorrhea)* can be associated with dysmenorrhea. It is not uncommon for a patient to present with dysmenorrhea caused by an infection due to *N. gonorrhea* since this bacteria has a high affinity to hemoglobin. In the United States, the prevalence for *Chlamydia trachomatis* is much higher than *N. gonorrhea*; hence it is prudent to get a sexual history and consider appropriate STI screening in a patient complaining of dysmenorrhea. Ovarian cysts are a cause of secondary, not primary dysmenorrhea. A pelvic ultrasound is warranted if PID, TOA or a uterine malformation is suspected.

56. D. Selective serotonin re-uptake inhibitors have been shown to be helpful in alleviating the symptoms associated with PMDD. Patients who are sexually active or who have many physical complaints may also benefit from hormonal contraception to suppress ovulation. Other antidepressant and anxiolytics can be used in consultation with psychiatry. GnRH analogs can be used in consultation with a gynecologist. The exact prevalence of PMS/PMDD in adolescents is unknown. Studies in adult women indicate the prevalence of 20–40% for PMS and only 3–8% for PMDD. Surgical management is not recommended for the treatment of PMS/PMDD during adolescence. Nutritional supplements have not demonstrated much efficacy treating symptoms related to PMS/PMDD.

Table 1. American Congress of Obstetricians and Gynecologists (ACOG) Diagnostic Criteria for PMS.[1]

Affective Symptoms	Depression Angry Outbursts Irritability Anxiety Confusion Social Withdrawal
Somatic Symptoms	Breast Tenderness Abdominal Bloating Headaches Extremity Swelling

[1] Diagnosis of PMS can be made if one of the above symptoms occurs in the 3 previous cycles during the 5 days preceding menses.

WEB REFERENCES

- Association of Reproductive Health Professionals, Managing Premenstrual Symptoms (June 2008), retrieved from http://www.arhp.org/publications-and-resources/quick-reference-guide-for-clinicians/pms
- Biggs WS, Demuth RH. 'Premenstrual Syndrome and Premenstrual Dysphoric Disorder', American Family Physician. 2011 Oct 15; 84(8): 918–924, retrieved from http://www.aafp.org/afp/2011/1015/p918.html
- Delara M, *et al.* 'Health realted quality of life among adolescent with remenstrual disorders: a cross-sectional study', Health and Quality of Life Outcomes. 2012; 10(l), retrieved from http://www.hqlo.com/content/10/1/1

Additional Clinician and Patient Resources:

- American College of Obstetricians and Gynecologists, Tool Kit for Teen Care (2nd Edition): Premenstrual Syndrome and Premenstrual Dysphoric Disorder Fact Sheet (2009), retrieved from http://www.acog.org/~/media/Departments/Adolescent%20Health%20Care/Teen%20Care%20Tool%20Kit/PMS.pdf?dmc=l&ts=20130409T1406165580
- Center for Young Women's Health, Boston Children's Hospital, Premenstrual Syndrome (PMS), retrieved from http://www.youngwomenshealth.org/menstrual7.html
- Endometriosis.org: www.endometriosis.org
- TeensHealth from Nemours, Coping with Common Period Problems, retrieved from http://kidshealth.org/teen/sexual_health/girls/menstrual_problems.html
- Womenshealth.gov, Menstruation, menopause and mental health (last updated March 29, 2010), retrieved from http://www.womenshealth.gov/mental-health/menstruation-menopause/

39

AMENORRHEA

Maria Trent

TEST YOUR KNOWLEDGE

57. Which of the following statements is *NOT* true?
    A. Early adolescents often experience irregular menses while their cycles are still anovulatory.
    B. Menses must be absent for more than six months before initiating an evaluation for secondary amenorrhea.
    C. Adolescents with polycystic ovarian syndrome may experience both dysfunctional uterine bleeding and amenorrhea.
    D. The primary treatment goal for management of amenorrhea is the treatment of underlying pathology that may be contributing to the amenorrhea.
58. Treatment of hirsutism may include which of the following:
    A. Oral contraceptive pills
    B. Eflornithine cream
    C. Spironolactone
    D. A and C
    E. All the above

Refer to end of chapter for answers on page 427.

"My periods disappear for months at a time, and when I do have one it is heavy. I have also gained weight and noticed more body hair. What's going on with me?"

BACKGROUND

- Primary amenorrhea, or delay in menstrual onset, as well as secondary amenorrhea, or cessation of menses, have many potential causes (Table 1).
- Moreover, several organ systems must effectively work together to maintain normal menstrual function in young teens. Disruptions in these organ systems may lead to amenorrhea (Table 2).

ASSESSMENT

HISTORY

Pubertal Growth and Development

- Menses is a relatively late pubertal event so assessment of pubertal development and overall growth will help to determine if menstrual patterns are within the normal range, part of overall pubertal delay or a deviation in menstrual function.

Sexual History

- **Pregnancy** is the most common cause of secondary amenorrhea in adolescent girls.
- A comprehensive menstrual disorder evaluation should include questions about sexual debut, last sexual intercourse, contraceptive use and pregnancy history.
- A negative history does not preclude pregnancy, since adolescents may fear disclosure and subsequent consequences.

Current and Past Medical History

- Chronic medical problems can stress the hypothalamic pituitary axis, particularly those that impair nutritional status such as malabsorption secondary to **inflammatory bowel disease.**

- Medications used to treat medical illness and/or potentially toxic treatments (e.g. irradiation or chemotherapy) can impair ovarian function.

Psychosocial/Mental Health History

- Significant psychosocial stressors (i.e. **grief**) and mental illness (i.e. **major depression**) can impair menstrual function due to a depressive effect on the hypothalamic pituitary axis (hypothalamic amenorrhea).
- Side effects of **medications** used to treat mental illnesses can impair menstrual regularity by creating hormonal abnormalities (e.g. elevated prolactin levels due to the use of atypical antipsychotics).

Dietary and Exercise History

- Nutritional status affects menstrual regularity. Malnutrition can lead to amenorrhea.
- Ascertain the presence of significant weight loss or gain, disordered eating patterns, body image distortion and intensity of athleticism (**female athlete triad**).
- Screening tools such as the Eating Disorders Attitude Test (EAT-26) may be helpful in determining the risk for an eating disorder.
- Loss of appetite and poor oral intake can be secondary to chronic illness and/or mental illness (i.e. **depression**).
- Loss of appetite may be due to medications used to treat **attention deficit hyperactivity syndrome** (i.e. stimulants).
- Smoking, co-occuring with eating disorders, can predispose the adolescent to osteoporosis.

Family History

- Assess for reproductive health disorders with a focus on menstrual, endocrine and genetic disorders as well as issues with infertility.
- Menstrual timing and pubertal status among first degree relatives can be useful in gauging abnormalities in the temporal progression of puberty including menses.
- A family history of osteroporosis is a risk factor for **osteopenia**.

Review of Systems

- Rule out **pituitary adenomas** or other **brain tumors** if the teen presents with a history of menstrual disorder and headaches.
- Consider **Kallman Syndrome** if the teen has anosmia.
- Galactorrhea may be due to psychiatric **medications, pregnancy** or **pituitary adenoma**.
- If the patient complains of excessive hair growth and acne, consider **polycystic ovarian syndrome** (PCOS) or other **androgen excess disorders**.

PHYSICAL

Anthropometric Measurements

- Plot height, weight and body mass index (BMI) to determine nutritional status and assess for nutritional deficiencies, eating disorders and overweight/obesity.
- If there is short stature that is incongruent with parental height, consider **Turner's syndrome**, even in the absence of other stigmata.

Vital Signs

- Bradycardia, orthostatic changes in the context of nutritional insufficiency, low body weight, lanugo, and evidence of disordered eating and body image may suggest a **restrictive eating disorder**.
- The HAMWI formula is a useful measure for determining proximity to ideal body weight and calculation of mid-parental height allows for final height prediction (Figure 1).

Neck

- Palpate the thyroid gland to assess for thyromegaly/goiter.
  - If present, the teen should be evaluated for the presence of tachycardia, hypertension, tremors, and exophthalmos as the presence of these symptoms suggests **hyperthyroidism** (i.e. **Grave's disease**).
  - Hoarseness, constipation, weight gain and depression are consistent with **hypothyroidism**.
- Webbed neck can be seen in patient's with **Turner's Syndrome**.

Chest

- Scant or absent breast development suggests **hypogonadism.**
- Widely spaced nipples can be seen in **Turner's Syndrome.**
- Patients with **Turner's Syndrome** may have underlying cardiac pathology such as coarctation of the aorta which can be picked up by a harsh sounding murmur.

Abdomen

- An enlarged womb may be the first sign of pregnancy.
- Examine the abdomen for evidence of a mass or structural abnormality such as **hematocolpos** which could be associated with an **imperforate hymen**.

Genital

- Determine Tanner stage
  - Menses normally occurs during Tanner Stage IV so teens who have not yet reached this degree of maturity may not be expected to have had menarche.
  - Significant delay in pubertal progression may represent a constitutional delay and/or be due to a pathological cause.
- External genital assessment is indicated for all patients to determine estrogen status, presence of congenital abnormalities that can be noted externally (e.g. **imperforate hymen**) and the presence of abnormal lesions that suggest other pathology such as a **sexually transmitted infection (STI)**.
- Pelvic examination may be indicated to exclude **congenital abnormality**.

Musculoskeletal

- Cubitus valgus (deformity: elbows are turned in) can occur in **Turner's syndrome.**

Skin

- Acne, male pattern alopecia and hirsutism suggest that the patient may have a disorder of androgen excess such as **PCOS** or **late onset congenital adrenal hyperplasia.**

- Ferriman Gallwey scoring is a valuable strategy to evaluate body hair at baseline and follow-up (http://www.gfmer.ch/Cours/Hirsutism_ferriman_gallwey_score.htm).
  - A score greater than 8 is considered abnormal.
  - Hirsute teens may remove body hair, so it is important to determine the location and degree of excess body hair before removal for accurate scoring.
- Acne scoring systems can also be used to assess the severity of acne.
- Acanthosis nigricans is a sign of **insulin resistance** usually observed in obese patients. While insulin resistance alone may result in menstrual dysfunction, the majority of teens with disorders such as **PCOS** present with **obesity.**
- New onset skin pigmentation or axillary freckling suggests **adrenal insufficiency** or **Addison's disease.**

STUDIES

Urine hCG

- Confirm pregnancy status before initiating other laboratory tests in sexually active teens.
- Caution must be used when interpreting negative pregnancy tests for patients who have had sexual intercourse within 1 week of evaluation-they may need to return for re-testing.

Follicle Stimulating Hormone (FSH) and Luteinizing Hormone (LH)

- Increased levels are consistent with **primary ovarian failure** (at ovarian level).
- Low levels are consistent with **secondary ovarian failure** (pituitary or hypothalamic problem).
- An elevation (2:1 to 3:1) in the LH: FSH ratio in the context of amenorrhea and evidence of androgen excess suggests a diagnosis of **PCOS**. It is important not to interpret LH to FSH ratios in isolation. Normal ratios have been observed in women with PCOS and elevations can be seen in women with regular cycles who are ovulating.

Prolactin

- Elevations are consistent with **hyperprolactinemia** and requires further work up.

Thyroid Stimulating Hormone (TSH) level and T4

- Screen for hypo- or hyperthyroidism.

Free and Total Testosterone and Dihydroepiandronsterone Sulfate (DHEA-S)

- Expect elevations in cases of hyperandrogen syndrome.

Pelvic Ultrasound

- Indicated for patients for whom bimanual examination is not possible or for those who have abnormal findings on bimanual examination.

Bone Age

- Indicated for patients presenting with absence of menses associated with signs of pubertal delay and short stature.
- In these patients, bone maturity often guides treatment.

SPECIAL TESTS

Assessment of Estrogen Status

- Several strategies can be used to assess estrogen status in patients with amenorrhea:
- **Progesterone challenge**
  - Medroxyprogesterone 10 mg daily for 5–10 days. Withdrawal bleeding confirms the presence of an estrogen primed uterus. Lack of response usually indicates a **hypoestrogenic state**; however, lack of response can also be observed in patients with **PCOS** who have been amenorrheic for greater than 6 months and among young women with a previously unsuspected pregnancy.
- **Estradiol level**
  - Interpret in the context of pubertal status and other clinical findings.

Repeat FSH

- To confirm the diagnosis of ovarian failure.
- Teens with elevations in FSH should be karyotyped and screened for autoimmune endocrinopathies.

A First Morning 17-Hydroxyprogesterone Level

- Indicated for patients who have significantly elevated DHEA-S.
- This suggests an adrenal disorder as the primary cause of menstrual dysfunction such as **late-onset congenital adrenal hyperplasia (21 hydroxylase deficiency).**

Thyroid Panel

- Include autoantibodies to further evaluate patients with evidence of hyper- or hypothyroidism based on initial TSH screening.

MRI

- *Head MRI*
    - Indicated for adolescents who have specific clinical findings (i.e. persistent headaches and projectile vomiting without nausea) and laboratory evidence (hyperprolactinemia) that suggest a **pituitary adenoma.**
- *Abdominal and/or Pelvic MRI*
    - Indicated for teens who are found to have tumor range androgen levels, to exclude **adrenal or ovarian tumors.**
    - Consider when congenital abnormalities are present in order to fully define the nature of the reproductive **structural defect.**

Dual-Energy X-ray Absorptiometry (DEXA) Bone Density Testing

- Indicated in patients with hypoestrogenic amenorrhea, associated with **ovarian failure, eating disorders** and **female athlete triad.**
- Used to detect bone demineralization, a precursor to **osteopenia and osteoporosis.**

Karyotype

- Send if patients are suspected of having Turner's syndrome or if they have elevated gonadotropins (even if they had an occasional period, as they could have mosaicism).

Vaginal Maturation Index

- An assessment of estrogenization. A vaginal smear is obtained by swabbing the vaginal wall with a moistened swab and affixing the sample to a slide for pathology evaluation.

TREATMENT

- Etiology dictates clinical management of amenorrhea.
- If **pregnant**, adolescents should receive a full clinical evaluation and options counseling with appropriate referrals based on the outcome of their decision-making process.
- Underlying endocrine disorders such as **hyperprolactinemia, hyperthyroidism,** and/or **hypothyroidism** should be fully evaluated and treated appropriately by an endocrinologist.
- Patients with a structural reproductive tract abnormality should be referred to a pediatric/adolescent gynecologist for further evaluation and possible surgical management.
- If the above are ruled out, treatment is dictated by estrogen status.
  - **Euestrogenic patients:**
    - Use medroxyprogesterone 5–10 mg for 12–14 days every 1–3 months.
    - Sexually active teens should be given a combined contraceptive method to achieve menstrual regulation while also protecting against unintended pregnancy pending return of ovulatory function.
    - Patients with disorders of androgen excess (e.g. PCOS) benefit from treatment with combined contraceptives due to the resultant increase in sex hormone binding globulin and binding of circulating testosterone.
    - Combined contraceptives decrease LH secretion, ovarian androgen production, and conversion of testosterone to the more active form, dihydrotestosterone (via inhibition of 5-α reductase), leading to a reduction in circulating androgens.

- Combined contraceptives improve mild acne, but may be insufficient to improve moderate to severe acne which may require additional topical and oral agents.
- Additional treatments for hirsutism include use of temporary (e.g. waxing, threading, tweezing) and permanent (e.g. electrolysis, thermolysis, laser) mechanical hair removal methods. Oral anti-androgens such as spironolactone can reduce hair growth but its use is off-label.
- Topical agents designed to reduce hair growth such eflornithine cream may improve overall clinical appearance.

- **Hypoestrogenic patients:**
    - Underweight adolescents need to normalize weight for height.
    - Athletic adolescents need to reduce athletic training and disordered eating should be evaluated and addressed.
    - Nutritional counseling should include recommendations to increase calcium intake.
    - Estrogen replacement therapy (ERT) is indicated for adolescents with ovarian failure; however, ERT for adolescents with restrictive eating disorders remains controversial due to data that questions its efficacy to treat osteopenia.
    - It may be difficult to interpret return of menses due to hormonal intervention versus nutritional repletion. Successful nutritional repletion with concurrent weight increases that result in reproductive function is a primary goal of treatment in this subset of patients.

What is unique about amenorrhea in adolescents?

- Menstrual disorders in adolescents can be caused by many medical and behavioral problems.
- The pubertal process adds another layer of complexity to the evaluation of menstrual disorders in adolescents.
- The key to determining the necessity of and approach to treatment depends on adequate understanding of the normal menstrual cycle and effective use of symptomatic clues.
- Parental support and education during the menstrual disorder evaluation is often essential for discerning details about pubertal development, past

medical history, familial lifestyle factors (e.g. mom buys menstrual supplies such as tampons or pads), and pertinent family history.

- Adolescents with eating disorders often know that amenorrhea may prompt parental or medical alerts that they wish to avoid; hence, they may prepare menstrual calendars documenting periods that never happened. Low estradiol levels can clarify this issue.
- Conversely, many adolescents terrified by the possibility of being pregnant may be in denial about their amenorrhea of pregnancy or simply try to delay the "moment of truth." Symptoms of weight gain, chloasma, nausea and vomiting, back pain and/or breast tenderness or lactation can end with the detection of an undisclosed pregnancy.

TEST YOUR KNOWLEDGE ANSWERS

57. B. Early adolescents and girls with PCOS often experience dysfunctional uterine bleeding (DUB) associated with anovulatory cycles. The primary approach to amenorrhea is to identify the underlying pathology that may be the cause. While the definition of secondary amenorrhea suggests that any adolescent with absence of menses for more than six months should be evaluated; any sexually active adolescent who has missed one or more cycles should be evaluated for pregnancy. Adolescents who have missed 3 periods and show evidence of disordered eating, nutritional insufficiency, and/or body image disturbance should be evaluated for a restrictive eating disorder.
58. E. Many adolescents who have menstrual disorders associated with hirsutism engage in temporary methods of mechanical hair removal (i.e. waxing, tweezing, or use of chemical depilatory agents) before seeking additional treatment. Oral contraceptives are used as a key treatment strategy because of their effects on circulating androgens resulting from overproduction by the ovaries or adrenal glands. More specifically, oral contraceptive pills increase levels of sex hormone binding globulin which reduces bioavailable androgens. Oral contraceptive pills also decrease secretion of luteinizing hormone, androgen production by the ovaries, and conversion of testosterone to the more active form (dihydrotestosterone) by inhibition of 5-α reductase. Spironolactone is an anti-androgen used

best in conjunction with combined contraceptives to reduce hair diameter in hirsute patients. It's use is off-label and does have a black box warning (as there is a risk for hyperkalemia). Eflornithine 13.9% cream is a topical agent used as an adjunct to mechanical hair removal methods. Eflornithine is an irreversible inhibitor of ornithine decarboxylase; an enzyme that mediates cell division and growth in hair follicles.

Table 1. Primary versus Secondary Amenorrhea.

Primary Amenorrhea	Defined by absence of menses by age 16 regardless of pubertal development. Evaluation should also be considered for adolescents who: 1. show no evidence of pubertal development by age 14, 2. have not had menses despite reaching Tanner stage V for at least a year or have had breast development for more than 4 years, *OR* 3. show stigmata of another disease process.
Secondary Amenorrhea	Pregnancy must be excluded in any girl who is late for her menstrual cycle. Defined by absence of menses of more than six months since the last menstrual cycle. Occurs when only 3 months have elapsed since the last cycle and an eating disorder is suspected (i.e. anorexia nervosa).

Table 2. Causes of Amenorrhea by Organ System.

Organ Systems	**Pathophysiological Causes**	
Central Nervous System	Eating Disorders Female Athlete Triad Head Trauma Idiopathic Physiologic Delay Infiltrative Disease Irradiation Kallmann Syndrome Laurence-Moon Biedl Syndrome	Pharmacologic Agents Post-Partum Necrosis Prader Willi Syndrome Psychological Stressors Surgery (e.g. tumor removal) Systemic Illness Tumors

(*Continued*)

Table 2. (*Continued*)

Organ Systems	Pathophysiological Causes
Thyroid	Hyperthyroidism Hypothyroidism
Adrenal	Addison's Disease Adrenal Tumor Cushing Syndrome Late-Onset Congenital Adrenal Hyperplasia
Ovaries	Autoimmune Oophoritis Galactosemia Ovary Destruction or Removal Ovarian Tumor (masculinizing) Polycystic Ovarian Syndrome Radiation or Chemotherapy Exposure Surgery Turner's Syndrome (Gonadal Dysgenesis or Streak Gonad with Mosaicism)
Uterus	Congenital Anomalies (e.g. Mullerian Agenesis) Pregnancy Uterine Synechiae
Vagina, Cervix, and Hymen	Imperforate Hymen Transverse Vaginal Septum Vaginal Agenesis

For individuals over 5 feet tall:

Males: 106 + 6 pounds for every inch over 60 inches

Females: 100 + 5 pounds for every inch over 60 inches

Add 10% if person has large frame, subtract 10% if person has small frame. If frame size is unavailable, assume medium.

Figure 1 The HAMWI Formula for Ideal Body Weight (IBW) Calculations.

WEB REFERENCES

- ACOG: Committee Opinion. 'Menstruation in Girls and Adolescents-Using the Menstrual Cycle as a Vital Sign', No 349, November 2006, retrieved from http://www.acog.org/Resources%20And%20Publications/Committee%20Opinions/Committee%20on%20Adolescent%20Health%20Care/Menstruation%20in%20Girls%20and%20Adolescents%20-%20Using%20the%20Menstrual%20Cycle%20as%20a%20Vital%20Sign.aspx
- Committee on Sports Medicine and Fitness. 'Medical Concerns in the Female Athlete', Pediatrics. 2000; 106(3): 610–613, retrieved from http://pediatrics.aappublications.org/content/106/3/6l0.full
- Braverman PK, Breech L. 'Gynecologic Examination for Adolescents in the Pediatric Office Setting', Pediatrics. 2010 Aug 30; 126(3): 583–590, retrieved from http://pediatrics.aappublications.org/content/126/3/583.full?sid=d78de583-ab17-400a-937a-01607adaf4cf
- Geneva Foundation for Medical Education and Research: Ferriman-Gallwey scoring tool to determine extent of hirsutism: http://www.gfmer.ch/Cours/Hirsutism_ferriman_gallwey_score.htm
- Master-Hunter T, Heiman DL. 'Amenorrhea: Evaluation and Treatment', American Family Physicia. 2006 April 15; 7398): 1374–1382, retrieved from http://www.aafp.org/afp/2006/0415/pl374.html
- Nutrition and Food Web Archive: HAMWI calculator retrieved from http://www.nafwa.org/hamwi.php

Additional Clinician and Patient Resources:

- Bielak KM. 'Amenorrhea', Medscape Reference (updated June 5, 2012), retrieved from http://emedicine.medscape.com/article/252928-overview
- Center for Young Women's Health, Boston Children's Hospital: Amenorrhea (updated 12/1/2010), retrieved from http://www.youngwomenshealth.org/amenorrhea.html
- Medline Plus, Amenorrhea-primary (Updated 5/31/2012), retrieved from http://www.nlm.nih.gov/medlineplus/ency/article/001218.htm
- Turner Syndrome Society of the United States: http://www.turnersyndrome.org/

40

VAGINAL BLEEDING

Maria Trent

TEST YOUR KNOWLEDGE

59. A 14 year old girl is fatigued and feels faint. On examination, she is found to be pale and tachycardic. Her hematocrit is 24. She reports several weeks of heavy bleeding including the passage of clots. All the following are possible causes *EXCEPT*:

    A. Von Willebrand Disease
    B. Polycystic Ovarian Syndrome (PCOS)
    C. Dysfunctional Uterine Bleeding
    D. Endometriosis
    E. Complication of an abortion

Refer to end of chapter for answer on page 437.

A 13 year old female presents for her annual well visit and complains that her periods are really heavy and can last up to 2–3 weeks.

BACKGROUND

- Dysfunctional bleeding (DUB) is abnormal uterine bleeding without structural uterine pathology or systemic disease.
- DUB is common in the early years post menarche when girls are still anovulatory.
- DUB can also occur with disorders associated with anovulation such as polycystic ovarian syndrome (PCOS). As with younger patients, the normal negative feedback system of the hypothalamic-pituitary-ovarian axis is disrupted such that increasing levels of estrogen do not decrease FSH secretion.
- Cycles also become anovulatory when the positive feedback loop is disrupted and the endometrium becomes thick and unstable resulting in uncoordinated and unpredictable shedding of the endometrial lining.
- Abnormal vaginal bleeding can be caused by anovulation, systemic disorders, endocrine abnormalities (e.g. thyroid disease, PCOS), disorders of pregnancy, sexually transmitted infections, tumors, foreign body (e.g. retained tampon), coagulopathies (e.g. von Willebrand disease, thrombocytopenia), and drugs (e.g. warfarin, withdrawal bleeding due to mismanagement of oral contraceptives, contraceptive side effects).

ASSESSMENT

HISTORY

Menstrual History

- Determine age of menarche, length of cycles, length of menses and the best estimate of amount of blood lost with each cycle.
- Quantify blood lost by number of pads or tampons used during a typical day of menses, degree of absorbancy of pad/tampon used (e.g. light, regular, heavy or overnight), and rate of flow (e.g. soak through pad and undergarment in less than 1 hour versus longer).

- Ask about the presence of blood clots (usually associated with significant bleeding).

Past Medical History

- Assess for bleeding disorders, such as **von Willebrand's disease,** which could present with symptoms such as bleeding gums, epistaxis or easy bruising.

Family History

- Assess for other female family members with abnormal menstrual bleeding history. Bleeding disorders may run in families and other female family members may have required hormonal therapy in their adolescence for similar problems or required blood transfusions during delivery secondary to an underlying bleeding disorder.
- Inquire about relatives with infertility or only one child (can be associated with PCOS).

Review of Systems

- Patient may report fatigue or decreased stamina (related to anemia secondary to blood loss) along with complaints of heavy menstrual bleeding of lengthy duration.

PHYSICAL EXAM

Vital Signs

- Measure heart rate and orthostatic changes in blood pressure for hemodynamic stability.
- If the blood loss is ongoing, rapid and heavy, patient may be tachycardic with a low blood pressure and may require urgent evaluation for severe anemia.

General Appearance

- Pallor of gums or oral cavity may indicate long-term anemia secondary to blood loss.

- Evaluate for evidence of PCOS characterized by signs of androgen excess such as acne, hirsutism, male pattern alopecia or deepening of voice.

Pelvic

- May be deferred by parent or patient, especially if the patient is virginal.
- The benefit of a speculum exam is that the cervical os can be visualized and magnitude of bleeding can be assessed.

STUDIES

Any patient with DUB alternating with amenorrhea should undergo the same laboratory assessment as described for patients presenting with amenorrhea.

Complete Blood Count (CBC) with Differential and Platelet Count

- Degree of anemia will dictate treatment strategy and patient disposition. Mild anemia can be managed outpatient while more severe anemia may require hospitalization.
- Abnormal platelet count may indicate underlying platelet disorder.

Urine hcG

- Heavy bleeding may indicate a threatened pregnancy or spontaneous abortion.
- Screen for sexually transmitted infections: **Neisseria gonorrhoeae, Chlamydia trachomatis,** and **Trichomonas vaginalis** can all present with abnormal uterine bleeding resulting from endometritis.

Coagulation Studies

- Consider in cases of profuse hemorrhage, menorrhaghia at menarche, prior history of bleeding (epistaxis) and/or family history of a bleeding disorder (e.g. von Willebrand disease).

Thyroid Stimulating Hormone (TSH) Level

- Screen for hypo- or hyperthyroidism.

Pelvic Sonogram

- Indicated if a mass is present, there is suspected structural abnormality, or if pelvic examination is difficult to perform.
- Provides information on the thickness of the endometrial stripe, indicating how much endometrium is left to be shed.

Androgen Levels (DHEAS and Testosterone Levels, Free and Total)

- Is diagnostic in suspected cases of PCOS.

TREATMENT

- Identify and treat the underlying pathology that may be contributing to the bleeding.
- Treatment goals for DUB include:
  - Termination of prolonged menstrual bleed and/or prevention of future abnormal bleeding.
  - Prevention of the progression of clinical symptoms associated with endocrine disorders such as PCOS.
  - Prevention of long-term sequelae such as the endometrial hyperplasia from prolonged unopposed estrogen exposure leading to an increased risk for endometrial cancer.
- Treatment strategies are dictated by the degree of anemia:

Mild Anemia (Hemoglobin >12 mg/dl)

- Irregular bleeding for more than 2 months with normal hemoglobin can be managed with reassurance, supplemental iron, non-steroidal inflammatory drugs (NSAIDS), use of a menstrual calendar, and outpatient follow-up in 3–4 months.
- Adolescents who present with clinical findings of PCOS can also be started on hormonal management with combined contraceptives in the setting of mild anemia.

Moderate Anemia (Hemoglobin 10–12 mg/dl)

- Moderately prolonged bleeding or shortened cycle length can be effectively treated with combined contraceptives and iron supplementation with close outpatient follow-up in 4-6 weeks.

Severe Anemia (Hemoglobin <9 mg/dl)

- Prolonged, heavy bleeding that is rapid and ongoing may require hospitalization for circulatory support.
- Use of monophasic (30–35 meg) combined oral contraceptive pills four times per day for 3–7 days usually results in control of menstrual bleeding.
- Use of monophasic combined contraceptive pills versus other methods facilitates titration of contraceptive dosing once the endometrium has been stabilized and the bleeding has ceased.
- Anti-emetics may be indicated for management of nausea or vomiting that can accompany use of combined pills for treatment.
- Use of intravenous conjugated estrogens is reserved for hospitalized patients with severe ongoing bleeding.
- An adolescent medicine specialist and/or gynecologist should be consulted to assist with management of hospitalized patients, particularly when there are concerns about hemodynamic instability, complicating medical or gynecologic issues, and/or bleeding that has not responded to treatment as anticipated.

What is unique about vaginal bleeding in adolescents?

- While many adolescents are credible historians and can provide details about their menstrual history and patterns, this is highly dependent on their developmental status, experience and comfort interfacing with the healthcare system.
- Some inexperienced adolescents who have not discussed menses with anyone may believe that their profuse abnormal bleeding is what is to be expected and may be surprised to learn that they have an abnormal bleeding pattern that may have gone on for many months.
- Out of shyness or guilt (about sexual touching or intercourse) teens may not report their profuse vaginal bleeding. Tragically, it is not uncommon to first detect DUB in a patient who comes to the doctor with fatigue, tachycardia

and even a syncopal episode with a hemoglobin of 4 mg/dl and a hematocrit of 14%. A similar scenario can occur with the menorrhagia associated with an ectopic pregnancy.

- Dilation and curettage is rarely indicated as hormonal treatment induces a "medical curretage."

TEST YOUR KNOWLEDGE ANSWER

59. D. Dysfunctional uterine bleeding (DUB) occurs mostly in young adolescents with anovulatory cycles. Older adolescents with polycystic ovaries often alternate between months without menses and those with marked uterine bleeding. Spontaneous and induced abortions can result in uterine bleeding, especially if endometritis develops. An ectopic pregnancy can also present initially with vaginal bleeding. A significant proportion of patients with severe vaginal bleeding requiring hospitalization and transfusion have an underlying coagulation disorder, predominantly Von Willebrand's Disease. Endometriosis is a cause of severe dysmenorrhea but not of DUB.

WEB REFERENCES

- Benjamins LJ. 'Practice Guidelines: Evaluation and Management of Abnormal Vaginal Bleeding in Adolescents', Journal of Pediatric Health Care. 2009; 23(3): 189–193, retrieved from http://www.medscape.com/viewarticle/704152
- Committee Opinion. Von Willebrand Disease in Women. ACOG Committee Opinion No. 451. American College of Obstetrics and Gynecologists. Obstet Gynecol 2009; 114: 1439–1443, retrieved from http://www.acog.org/Resources_And_Publications/Committee_Opinions/Committee_on_Adolescent_Health_Care/Von_Willebrand_Disease_in_Women
- Ely JW, *et al.* 'Abnormal Uterine Bleeding: A Management Algorithm', Journal of The American Board of Family Medicine. 2006 Nov-Dec; 19(6): 590–602, retrieved from http://www.jabfm.org/content/19/6/590.full
- Gray SH, Emans S Jean. 'Abnormal Vaginal Bleeding in Adolescents', Pediatrics in Review. 2007; 28; 175–182, retrieved from http://peds.Stanford.edu/Rotations/adolescent_medicine/documents/MenstrualDisordersArticlel.pdf
- Hertweck P, Yoost J. 'Pediatric and Adolescnt Gynecology: Common Problems: Dysfunctional Uterine Bleeding: Menorrhagia in Adolescents', Medscape Education (2010), retrieved from http://www.medscape.org/viewarticle/720869_5

Additional Clinician and Patient Resources:

- Association of Reproductive Health Professionals, 'Abnormal Uterine Bleeding' (updated July 2008), retrieved from https://www.arhp.org/publications-and-resources/clinical-fact-sheets/abnormal-uterine-bleeding
- Zacur HA. 'Patient Information: Abnormal uterine bleeding (Beyond the Basics), last updated August 13, 2012, retrieved from http://www.uptodate.com/contents/abnormal-uterine-bleeding-beyond-the-basics

41

VAGINAL DISCHARGE

Karen E. Simpson

TEST YOUR KNOWLEDGE

60. Which of the following statements is true?
    - A. All pubertal teens with white vaginal discharge before menarche need a pelvic examination to rule out sexual abuse.
    - B. Urinary frequency and dysuria may be caused by pelvic inflammatory endometriosis of Langerhans.
    - C. New onset dyspareunia and vaginal spotting suggest a sexually transmitted infection (STI).
    - D. All the above are true.
    - E. None of the above is true.

Refer to end of chapter for answer on page 445.

A 16 year old girl complains of vaginal discharge and itching. Her discharge is whitish-yellow when dry, and the vaginal itching extends to the external genitalia.

BACKGROUND

- Vulvovaginitis or inflammation of the vagina and vulva, often results in a vaginal discharge.
- Common symptoms include vaginal discharge, irritation, discomfort, itching and/or odor.
- These symptoms may be caused by bacteria, viruses, fungi, parasites, irritants or allergic reaction (Table 1).

ASSESSMENT

HISTORY

History of Present Illness

- What are the characteristics of the vaginal discharge?
  - Color? A yellow-green discharge is more likely associated with a **sexually transmitted infection** (STI).
  - Consistency? Thick white discharge characterizes vaginal **candidiasis.**
  - Associated symptoms? Itching or vaginal irritation are non-specific complaints that may indicate any number of causes.
- What type of clothing or undergarment does the teen wear? Spandex, tight fitting jeans or shorts, or use of non-breathable synthetic fabrics can lead to poor aeration of the perineal area and predispose to **candidal vulvovaginitis** and **bacterial vaginosis (BV).**
- Determine types of hygiene products used: soaps, shampoos, scented panty liners and sanitary napkins may be sources of irritation to the vulva for those with sensitive mucosa. Infrequent changing of panty liners or sanitary pads may also cause irritation.
- Does the patient douche?
  - This alters the bacterial flora of the vagina, predisposing to **BV.**
  - Douching can also lead to infections of the upper genital tract with STI's ascending from the lower genital tract.

- Does the patient report dyspareunia, or pain with sexual intercourse? Dyspareunia may indicate **cervicitis, pelvic inflammatory disease (PID), pelvic peritonitis** or **vulvovaginal lesions.**

Past Medical History

- Does the patient report a history of an STI or high risk sexual behaviors that put her at increased risk for an STI?
- Is there an underlying condition such as diabetes or is the patient immunosuppressed? These conditions are associated with **vulvovaginal candidiasis.**

Menstrual History

- When was the last menstrual period? Increased vaginal discharge at the end of, or soon after menses may occur with **gonorrhea.**
- Does discharge vary with the menstrual cycle? Patients may have increased secretions mid cycle, also known as **physiologic leukorrhea.** Discharge from **gonorrhea** and/or **chlamydia** may increase at the end of menses.
- Is there a change in menstrual pattern? Heavier or longer bleeding or unusual spotting? This can occur with **chlamydia, gonorrhea** or **trichomoniasis.**
- If tampons are used, are they used properly? Tampons can be a forgotten **foreign body** in the vagina associated with putrid, foul smelling discharge.

Medications

- Has the patient been taking antibiotics or birth control pills? If so, for how long have they been on these medications? Both are associated with **candidal vulvovaginitis.**

Review of Systems

- Is there urinary frequency or dysuria? Commonly associated with UTIs, these symptoms may also be caused by urethral irritation from STIs.

PHYSICAL

Vital Signs

- Fever may indicate infectious etiology.

Genital Exam

- A fishy odor suggests **BV** while a foul smelling discharge may occur with a **foreign body.**
- Examine for lesions:
  - Excoriations suggest a dermatologic condition such as eczema or contact dermatitis, but may also indicate **parasitosis** (i.e. scabies, pinworm) or **candidal vulvovaginitis.**
  - Papular, often painful, vesicular crusted lesions occur with **herpes genitalis.**
- Discharge characteristics:
  - Mucopurulent discharge suggests an **STI**.
  - White, thick "cottage-cheese" discharge suggests **candidal vulvovaginitis.**
- A pelvic examination may be indicated when there is lower quadrant pain and discharge.
  - **Cervicitis** is marked by a purulent or mucopurulent endocervical discharge and/or a friable cervix which bleeds easily by gentle passage of a cotton swab through the os. Either, or both signs, might be present.
  - Cervical motion tenderness, adnexal pain or fullness and/or peritoneal signs indicates an upper genital tract infection such as **PID** or **tuboovarian abscess** (**TOA**).

STUDIES

- In clinical settings where there is access to a microscope and equipment, collecting a vaginal swab for pH testing and wet mount can be useful diagnostic tools.

pH Test of Vaginal Discharge

- pH < 4.5 is consistent with normal physiologic leukorrhea or candidal vulvovaginitis.
- pH > 4.5 is consistent with bacterial vaginosis and trichomoniasis.
- The presence of blood can alter vaginal pH making this test less accurate.

Vaginal Swab for Wet Mount

- Greater than 5 leukocytes per high power field (×1000) suggests gonorrhea and/or chlamydia infection. The absence of white cells is not uncommon with chlamydia.
- Greater than 20% clue cells (epithelial cells coated with bacteria) is consistent with BV.
- Pseudohyphae, branching spores or spores are consistent with candidal vulvovaginitis.
- Motile or immotile trichomonads may be visualized and confirm trichomoniasis.
- If the wet mount is negative for trichomonads but symptoms persist despite therapy, then a culture for trichomoniasis can be done.

Gonorrhea and Chlamydia Testing

- Nucleic acid amplification test (NAAT) of vaginal/cervical secretions or a urine sample can be used to diagnose *C. trachomatis* and *N. gonorrhoeae* in women with cervicitis.
- Endocervical discharge may also be sampled for gonorrhea/chlamydia culture or PCR testing but the practicality and accuracy of urine testing has made this practice less common.

ADDITIONAL TESTS

CBC, ESR and CRP

- May be indicated to support a diagnosis of PID.

Urine analysis

- The presence of leukocytes on a clean catch specimen may indicate UTI or vaginitis/cervicitis caused by chlamydia, gonorrhea or trichomoniasis.

Other Tests

- All sexually active teens should be screened for HIV and syphilis.
- Investigations for diabetes or immunocompromised state are usually not required but may be warranted if a patient presents with recurrent and or extensive candidal vulvovaginitis.

TREATMENT

- History, physical exam and study findings dictate treatment strategies (Table 2).
- Patients with physiologic leukorrhea can be reassured and advised on coping strategies including use of sanitary pads if the discharge is copious.
- If dermatologic conditions such as contact dermatitis are the cause of vaginal irritation, patients should be advised to remove the offending agent and avoid potentially irritating products such as perfumed soaps or other feminine hygiene products.
- Presumptive treatment for STIs is justified in areas of high prevalence for patients who engage in high risk behaviors.
- Empiric treatment can be initiated based on CDC STI guidelines, pending test results.
- Patients should receive clear instructions on how to take their medications and always use condoms to prevent the spread of STIs.
- Partner notification is an important aspect of STI counseling.
    - Patients need to inform partner(s) of the past 2–3 months so that they can seek testing and treatment.
    - Patients should abstain from sexual intercourse for at least 7 days after treatment and at least 7 days after their sexual partner(s) has been treated — whichever is longer.
    - Expedited partner therapy should be considered if necessary.
- Patients should be advised to follow up with their clinicians to ensure resolution of symptoms and appropriate treatment.
    - Patients with vulvovaginitis of any etiology should follow up if symptoms are not improved after 2 weeks of therapy.
    - Given high prevalence rates, teens diagnosed with chlamydia or gonorrhea should have repeat testing 3 months post therapy.

What is unique about vaginal discharge in adolescents?

- Teens with vaginal discharge may be embarrassed by their symptoms, worried that their sexual activity may be "found out," or fear the possibility of a pelvic examination; hence, they often delay consultations and are more prone to complications such as upper genital tract infections.

- Young adolescents may be confused and frightened by normal physiologic leukorrhea, often requiring education and reassurance.
- Vaginitis often leads to dysparuenia, which in turn may lead to sexual dysfunction and partner conflict. Adolescents need to be encouraged to discuss sexual matters with their partners.
- A consult for vulvovaginitis may often be the first opportunity to provide comprehensive reproductive health care services to a teen.
- Adolescents with vaginal discharge in areas with high prevalence of *C. trachomatis* and *N. gonorrhoeae* should be treated for both infections.

TEST YOUR KNOWLEDGE ANSWER

60. **D.** Pubertal teens presenting with premenarchal white vaginal discharge most likely have physiologic leukorrhea and do not require pelvic examinations. Urinary frequency and dysuria can be manifestations of a UTI, urethritis secondary to a STI, or both. The acute onset of vaginal discharge, painful intercourse and spotting are highly suspicious for a STI and require testing for chlamydia and gonorrhea. There is no such thing as pelvic inflammatory endometriosis of Langerhans.

Table 1. Causes of Vulvovaginitis.

Physiologic Leukorrhea	Starts 1–2 years before menarche. Usually white or transparent, odorless and may be thick. May increase mid cycle once ovulatory cycles begin.
Candidal Vulvovaginitis	May be associated with a thick, white/yellow cottage cheese-like discharge. Often presents with itching and no odor. May have erythema or excoriation of the vagina, vulvar edema, perineal irritation or fissures. More frequent in teens who are diabetic, immunosuppressed, use OCP or are on antibiotics.
Bacterial Vaginosis	A non-specific vaginitis caused by overgrowth of *Gardnerella vaginalis*. Not necessarily an STI, but more common in those who are sexually active. Common in females who have sex with females. Patients who douche may present with symptoms as douching alters normal vaginal flora.
Cervicitis	Inflammation of the cervix and teens may or may not be symptomatic. Common etiologic organisms are *Chlamydia trachomatis, Neiserria gonorrhea* and *Trichomonas vaginalis*. Cases may result from *M. genitalium* and *Gardnrella vaginalis*. May present with abnormal vaginal discharge, intermenstrual vaginal bleeding or bleeding after sexual intercourse.
Dermatologic Conditions	Eczema, psoriasis, seborrhea or irritants may result in vaginal itching and/or lesions. Vaginal discharge may be present from the irritation and weeping of the skin.
Genital Herpes	Commonly caused by herpes simplex type 2 (genital) but may be caused by type 1 (oral). Recurrence rate is greater with herpes simplex type 2. Presents with papular, vesicular or ulcerated lesions or a combination. Symptoms include burning and stinging of perineum, and there may also be vaginal discharge.

Table 2. Treatment of Vaginal Discharge.*

Diagnosis	Pharmacologic Therapies
Bacterial Vaginosis	First Line Therapies Metronidazole 500 mg BID × 7 days or Metrogel 0.75% intravaginally QHS × 5 days or Clindamycin Cream 2% intravaginally QHS × 7 days Alternative Therapies Tinidazole 2 gm QD × 7 days or Tinidazole 1 gm QD × 5 days or Clindamycin 300 mg BID × 7 days or Clindamycin ovules 100 mg intravaginally QHS × 3 days Pregnancy Metronidazole 500 mg BID × 7 days or Clindamycin 300 mg BID × 7 days
Candidal Vulvovaginitis	Prescription Intravaginal Agents Butoconazole 2% cream, 5 g intravaginally ONCE or Nystatin 100,000 units, one table intravgainally for 14 days OR Terconazole 0.4% cream, 5 g intravaginally for 7 days Terconazole 0.8% cream, 5 g intravaginally for 3 days OR Terconazole 80 mg vaginal suppository, one suppository for 3 days Oral Agent Fluconazole 150 mg one table, one tablet in a single dose by mouth ONCE.
Chlamydia	First Line Therapies Azithromycin 1 gm × 1 dose or Doxycycline 100 mg BID × 7 days Alternative Therapies Erythromycin base 500 mg qid × 7 days or Erythromycin EES 800 mg qid × 7 days or Levofloxacin 500 mg once per day × 7 days or Ofloxacin 300 mg bid × 7 days or Pregnancy Azithromycin 1 gm PO × 1 dose or Amoxicillin 500 mg PO TID × 7 days

(*Continued*)

Table 2. (*Continued*)

Diagnosis	Pharmacologic Therapies
	Alternative: Erythromycin base 500 mg QID × 7 days or Erythromycin base 250 mg QID × 14 days or Erythromycin EES 800 mg QID × 7 days or Erythromycin EES 400 mg QID × 14 days
Gonorrhea	Ceftriaxone 250 mg IM × 1 dose or Azithromycin 1 gram × 1 dose or Doxycycline 100 mg 2×/day × 7 days
Trichomoniasis	First Line Therapies Metronidazole 2 gm × 1 dose or Tinidazole 2 gm × 1 dose Alternative Therapy Metronidazole 500 mg 2×/day × 7 days
Genital Herpes (first episode)	Acyclovir 400 mg TID × 7–10 days or Acyclovir 200 mg PO 5×/day × 7–10 days or Famciclovir 250 mg PO 3×/day × 7–10 days or Valacyclovir 1 gm PO 2×/day × 7–10 days

*See CDC guidelines for suppressive therapies for genital herpes in immunocompetent and immunocompromised patients and OTC preparations for candidal vulvovaginitis.

WEB REFERENCES

- Barousse MM, *et al.* 'Vaginal yeast colonizsation, prevalence of vaginitis, and associated local immunity in adolescents', Sexually Transmitted Infections 2004; 80: 48–53, retrieved from http://sti.bmj.com/content/80/1/48.full.pdf+html
- Burnstein G, Jacobs A, Kissin D, Workowski K. 'Changes in the 2010 STD Treatment Guidelines What Adolescent Health Care Providers Should Know', ACOG, retrieved from http://www.acog.org/About_ACOG/ACOG_Departments/Adolescent_Health_Care/Changes_in_the_2010_STD_Treatment_Guidelines_What_Adolescent_Health_Care_Providers_Should_Know
- Centers for Disease Control and Prevention. 'Sexually Transmitted Diseases Treatment Guidelines, 2010. MMWR 2010; 59(No. RR-12): l–110, retrieved from http://www.cdc.gov/std/treatment/2010/STD-Treatment-2010-RR5912.pdf
- Committee on Adolescence. 'Sexually Transmitted Diseases', Pediatrics 1994; 94: 568–572, retrieved from http://pediatrics.aappublications.org/content/94/4/568.full.pdf+html?Sid=f6856de9-e81e-462f-9919-97c38b6bl743
- Hainer BL, Gibson MV. 'Vaginitis: Diagnosis and Treatment', American Family Physician. 2011 Apr l; 83(7): 807–815, retrieved from http://www.aafp.org/afp/2011/0401/p807.html
- Syed TS, Braverman PK. 'Vaginitis in adolescents', Adolescent Medicine Clinics. 2004; 15: 235–251, retrieved from http://pediatrics.uchicago.edu/chiefs/adolescent/documents/vaginitisadol.pdf

Additional Clinician and Patient Resources:

- American College of Obstetricians and Gynecologists, FAQ: Vaginitis (August 2011), retrieved from http://www.acog.Org/~/media/For%20Patients/faq028.pdf?dmc=l&ts=20130409T1521339476
- Center for Young Womens Health, Vaginal Infections (Vaginitis), last updated 11/20/2012, retrieved from http://www.youngwomenshealth.org/vaginitis.html
- KidsHealth from Nemours, What's Vaginal Discharge (last reviewed September 2011), retrieved from http://kidshealth.org/kid/grow/girlstuff/discharge.html
- WebMD, Women's Health: Vaginal Discharge: What's Abnormal? (reviewed August 2012), retrieved from http://women.webmd.com/guide/vaginal-discharge-whats-abnormal

42

PELVIC INFLAMMATORY DISEASE (PID)/ TUBOOVARIAN ABSCESS (TOA)

Avril Melissa Houston

TEST YOUR KNOWLEDGE

61. All the following organisms cause PID/TOA *EXCEPT*:

    A. *T. vaginalis*
    B. *Anaerobes*
    C. *Gardnerella vaginalis*
    D. Enteric Gram negative rods
    E. All the above
    F. None of the above

62. Which of the following presenting symptoms can be a manifestation of PID/TOA?

    A. Abnormal uterine bleeding
    B. Dyspareunia
    C. Right upper quadrant abdominal pain
    D. Mucopurulent vaginal discharge
    E. All the above

Refer to end of chapter for answers on page 458.

Your 16 year old female patient presents complaining: "I have had stomach pain all week long and it hurt a lot when I had sex yesterday."

BACKGROUND

- Sexually transmitted infections (STIs) occur at disproportionately higher rates among adolescents and racial or ethnic minorities.
- Left untreated, they can result in serious conditions: Pelvic Inflammatory Disease (PID) and Tuboovarian Abscesses (TOA).
- Many organisms can cause PID and/or TOA. Sexually transmitted organisms as well as normal vaginal flora have been associated with these disease processes (Table 1).

ASSESSMENT

HISTORY

History of Present Illness

- Ascertain the onset, location, frequency, and degree of abdominal pain.
- Recent onset of pain that increases with sexual intercourse or jarring movements suggests **PID.**
- Assess if there are any precipitating, alleviating or aggravating factors.
- Does the pain limit activities?
- Lower abdominal pain is often associated with PID/TOA in the sexually active teen.
- If a sexually active teen presents with right upper quadrant (RUQ) abdominal pain, consider **Fitz-Hugh-Curtis Syndrome**, or **perihepatitis** ("violin string adhesions"), a gonococcal or chlamydial infection of the liver capsule.
- Generalized severe abdominal pain that gradually becomes more localized to the lower right side could suggest **appendicitis.**

Sexual History

- Determine the teen's risk for STI acquisition (Table 2).
- Obtain a thorough sexual history including gender, number and type (i.e. oral, genital, rectal) of sexual contacts.
- Determine if the teen consistently uses barrier methods of protection.

Menstrual History

- Determine the timing and character of the last menstrual period: did it differ from previous months, come at an unexpected time or was it heavier than usual?
- Abnormal uterine bleeding is a common presentation of PID.
- Crampy abdominal and/or back pain that occurs monthly during the first couple of days of menses suggests **dysmenorrhea**, while new onset pain at the 3rd or 4th day of menses suggests early PID.
- Inquire if the adolescent douches post menses or at other times of the month. Infections of the vagina or cervix can track up to the endometrium and fallopian tubes with douching.
- Pain that occurs at the end of or immediately following menses suggests gonococcal endometritis.
- **Ectopic pregnancy or complications of an intrauterine pregnancy** must always be considered in adolescents with abdominal pain and/or irregular bleeding.

Review of Systems

- **Acute gastroenteritis** may present with pain preceded by vomiting while **intestinal obstruction** should be considered if a patient presents with bilious vomiting; however, vomiting can also be a presenting symptom of PID/TOA.
- RUQ abdominal pain accompanied by jaundice suggests **cholecystitis.**
- Pain with diarrhea and rectal bleeding suggest **inflammatory bowel disease.**
- Abdominal pain associated with painful and infrequent bowel movements may be a sign of **constipation.**

- Determine the presence of unusual vaginal discharge: malodorous, discolored discharge may be associated with **cervicitis/PID.**
- Ascertain if the patient has been febrile.
  - Fever, abdominal pain, and costovertebral angle tenderness are frequently found with upper urinary tract disease such as **pyelonephritis.**
  - Abdominal pain associated with urinary frequency, urgency or dysuria suggests **cystitis.**
  - It is not uncommon to have both an STI and UTI simultaneously.
- Ascertain onset, location, and pattern of dyspareunia: This may be a symptom of infection, ovarian cyst, trauma, skin lesions, or emotional or psychological factors (e.g. history of sexual abuse, anxiety or depression).

PHYSICAL

- PID is a clinical diagnosis based on (1) pelvic or abdominal pain with no other cause identified and (2) cervical motion tenderness, uterine tenderness OR adnexal tenderness.

Vital Signs

- Fever and or tachycardia suggest infectious etiology.

Abdomen

- Abdominal tenderness to palpation, greatest in the lower quadrants is usually present.
- Rebound tenderness and decreased bowel sounds may be present and are more ominous signs. Progression to **TOA**, **severe peritonitis** and death can occur in untreated patients.

Pelvic

- Evaluate:
  - Character of vaginal or cervical discharge.
  - Appearance of cervix.
  - Presence of pelvic mass or adnexal tenderness (suggests TOA).

- Cervical motion tenderness ("chandelier sign") is present in greater than 80% of patients with PID.
- Uterine tenderness.

Back

- Percuss back to evaluate for costovertebral angle tenderness suggesting **pyelonephritis.**

Skin

- Evaluate conjunctiva and skin for jaundice which suggest **gallbladder disease.**

STUDIES

Pregnancy Test

- Rule out ectopic pregnancy or other complications of intrauterine pregnancy.
- A positive pregnancy test in a patient with PID calls for a different treatment plan than for the non-pregnant teen, including hospitalization as well as different antibiotic selection.

Microscopic Examination of Vaginal Discharge

- The presence of leukocytes in vaginal fluid correlates with the diagnosis of PID.
- The presence of gram negative intracellular diplococci in a cervical sample suggests the possibility of PID.
- Leukocytes may not be present on wet mount in cases of chlamydia infection.

Complete Blood Count

- An elevated leukocyte count suggests an infection: PID, TOA, appendicitis and pyelonephritis should be considered and clinically correlated.

Erythrocyte Sedimentation Rate (ESR)/C-Reactive Protein (CRP)

- An elevated ESR or CRP suggests an inflammatory process and supports the diagnosis of PID. If markedly elevated, suggests of TOA.

Urinalysis

- The presence of leukocytes and/or nitrites on clean catch specimen is suggestive of a **urinary tract infection.**
- Microscopic examination of clean catch urine that reveals more than ten organisms per oil emersion field correlates well with positive culture results.
- The presence of bacterial casts can occur in cases of **pyelonephritis.**

SPECIAL TESTS

Pelvic or Transvaginal Ultrasound

- Evaluate for thickened fluid-filled fallopian tubes, free pelvic fluid or tuboovarian complex.

CT scan or Magnetic Resonance Imaging (MRI)

- Generally reserved for masses.

Endometrial Biopsy

- Rarely necessary, it provides histopathologic evidence of endometritis.

Laparoscopic Evaluation

- Usually a last resort measure.
- Abnormalities consistent with PID include edema, adhesions and a purulent exudate.

TREATMENT

- Mild to moderate PID can be treated with oral antibiotics on an outpatient basis, provided social circumstances allow for appropriate follow up.
- The Centers for Disease Control and Prevention recommended medical treatment regimens are summarized in Table 4.

- Patients should be counseled on completing the entire course of treatment.
- All sex partners of teens diagnosed with PID/TOA (within the preceding 60 days), should be examined and treated for *N. gonorrhea* and *C. trachomatis*.
- Expedited Partner Therapy (EPT) should be considered for the treatment of gonorrhea and chlamydia when other management strategies are impractical.
- If medical treatment of the TOA is unsuccessful or a very large abscess is identified, a gynecologic consult needs to be obtained to consider drainage procedures.

DISPOSITION

- Patients with mild to moderate PID should be reevaluated 48–72 hours following diagnosis and treatment. In cases where there is no clinical improvement, hospitalization is necessary for IV antibiotics, further testing or even surgical intervention.
- Criteria for hospitalization are summarized in Table 3.
- All adolescents with suspected TOA should receive inpatient management.

What is unique about PID/TOA in adolescents?

- Rates of *N. gonorrhea* and *C. trachomatis* infections are highest among teens and young adults.
- The risk of PID is greater among adolescents when compared to older women.
- Several factors place adolescents at higher risk of developing PID/TOA including:

Biologic risk factors:

- Cervical ectropion occurs when the normal squamo-columnar junction is extended outward from the its normal position at the cervical os. This occurs more often in young adolescent women and makes them more vulnerable to infection.
- Lack of local immunity.

Behavioral risk factors:

- Delays in seeking medical care.
- Fear of disclosure of sexual activity to parents or other caretakers.
- Exposures to multiple sex partners.
- Inconsistent condom use.
- Multiple obstacles to accessing health care.
- Gaps in communication (i.e. adolescents may refer to pelvic pain as "stomach pain").
- Patient education and partner notification are key components of adolescent treatment plans to prevent long term sequelae and re-infection.
- Complications of PID/TOA can have significant future consequences including increased risk for infertility, ectopic pregnancy and chronic pelvic pain (adhesions).
- Many cases of infertility due to tubal scarring do not have a history of PID, which indicates the possibility of indolent infection and necessitates STI screening of all sexually active teens.

TEST YOUR KNOWLEDGE ANSWERS

61. A. T. vaginalis does not cause PID/TOA *per se*. However, this traveling parasite can carry chlamydia and gonorrhea to the upper genital tract. Gardnerella and enteric gram negative rods have been occasionally implicated in PID. Anaerobic vaginal flora is a typical secondary invader of the upper genital tract organs and can lead to TOA.
62. E. Abnormal uterine bleeding occurs in approximately 1/3 of patients with PID. All sexually active teens should be asked about dyspareunia as it may be the initial presenting symptom of PID. Right upper quadrant abdominal pain may be a symptom of perihepatitis (Fitz-Hugh-Curtis Syndrome), which can occur when infection ascends from the genital tract into the peritoneal cavity. The presence of vaginal mucopurulent discharge is one of the criteria that can be used to support a diagnosis of PID.

Table 1. Organisms Associated with PID.

Sexually transmitted infections	*Neisseria gonorrhea*
	Chlamydia trachomatis
Normal vaginal flora	*Gardnerella vaginalis*
	Anaerobes
	Enteric gram negative rods
	Haemophilus influenza
	Streptococcus agalactiae
	Bacteroides fragilis
Other organisms	*Mycoplasma genitalium*
	Mycoplasma hominis
	Ureaplasma urealyticum

Table 2. Factors that Increase Risk for STI and PID.

Age less than 25 years
Young age at first sexual experience
Inconsistent use of barrier protection
New, multiple, or symptomatic sexual partners
Previous episode of PID
Vaginal douching
IUD insertion while actively infected

Table 3. Criteria for Hospitalization for PID Treatment.

Surgical emergencies cannot be excluded
Pregnancy
No response to outpatient oral antibiotic therapy OR
Patient unable to follow or tolerate outpatient oral therapy
Severe illness (nausea, vomiting or high fever)
Suspected TOA

Table 4. Recommended Treatment Regimen for PID.

	Outpatient Regimens	
Ceftriaxone 250 IM × 1 *PLUS*	Cefoxitin 2 g IM × 1 and Probenecid 1 g PO × 1 *PLUS*	Other third-generation cephalosporin (i.e. cefotaxime) *PLUS*
Doxycycline 100 mg PO BID × 14 days *WITH OR WITHOUT*	Doxycycline 100 mg PO BID × 14 days *WITH OR WITHOUT*	Doxycycline 100 mg PO BID × 14 days *WITH OR WITHOUT*
Metronidazole 500 mg PO BID × 14 days.	Metronidazole 500 mg PO BID × 14 days.	Metronidazole 500 mg PO BID × 14 days.
	Inpatient Regimen A:	
Cefotetan 2 g IV q 12 hours OR Cefoxitin 2 g IV Q 6 hours *PLUS* Doxycycline 100 mg PO or IV Q 12 hours.		
	Inpatient Regimen B:	
Clindamycin 900 mg IV q 8 hours *PLUS* Gentamicin loading does IV or IM (2 mg/kg of body weight), followed by maintenance dose (1.5 mg/kg) Q 8 hours.		

*IV therapy can be discontinued 24 hours after clinical improvement. Oral therapy with doxycycline should be continued to complete 14 days of therapy. When TOA is present, clindamycin is added to provide better anaerobic coverage.

WEB REFERENCES

- Burnstein G, Jacobs A, Kissin D, Workowski K. 'Changes in the 2010 STD Treatment Guidelines What Adolescent Health Care Providers Should Know', ACOG, retrieved from http://www.acog.org/About_ACOG/ACOG_Departments/Adolescent_Health_Care/Changes_in_the_2010_STD_Treatment_Guidelines_What_Adolescent_Health_Care_Providers_Should_Know
- Centers for Disease Control and Prevention. 'Sexually Transmitted Diseases Treatment Guidelines, 2010. MMWR 2010; 59 (No. RR-12): 1–110, retrieved from http://www.cdc.gov/std/treatment/2010/STD-Treatment-2010-RR5912.pdf
- Crossman SH. 'The Challenge of Pelvic Inflammatory Disease', American Family Physician. 2006 Mar l; 73(5): 859–864, retrieved from http://www.aafp.org/afp/2006/0301/p859.html

Additional Clinician and Patient Resources:

- Girlshealth.gov, Teen Survival Guide: Sexually transmitted diseases (STDs), last updated February 12, 2008, retrieved from www.girlshealth.gov/teenguide/reproductive/stds.cfm

- American Sexual Health Association, Inc., I Wanna know!: http://www.iwannaknow.org/teens/index.html
- National Institute of Allergy and Infectious Disease, Sexually Transmitted Diseases: www.niaid.nih.gov/factsheets/stdpid.htm
- TeensHealth from Nemours, Pelvic Inflammatory Disease (PID), retrieved from http://kidshealth.org/teen/infections/stds/std_pid.html

43

URETHRITIS IN MALES

Karen E. Simpson

TEST YOUR KNOWLEDGE

63. Which one of the following statements is true?

    A. The most common cause of urethritis in males is *E. coli* UTI.
    B. Most cases of urethritis in young males are secondary to vigorous masturbation.
    C. Urethritis that is secondary to a sexually transmitted infection always manifests with a purulent discharge.
    D. Prostatitis is an uncommon complication of urethritis in teens and young adults.
    E. None of the above.

64. An 18 year old male reports a one day history of burning with micturition. He is sexually active with males and females and uses a condom most of the time. He is otherwise healthy with no medical illnesses. He denies urinary frequency, urgency or penile discharge. He is afebrile and denies testicular pain. Which single investigation will most likely lead to the etiologic cause of his symptoms?

    A. Urine culture
    B. Urinalysis
    C. Testicular ultrasound
    D. Urine nucleic acid amplification test (NAAT) for gonorrhea and chlamydia
    E. Rapid antigen test for trichomoniasis

Refer to end of chapter for answers on page 468.

"Doc, I got burned . . . I think I have got the drip."

BACKGROUND

- Urethritis is defined as swelling and inflammation of the urethra.
- Symptoms may include urethral itch, tingling, dysuria, or mucoid/muco-purulent discharge.
- Patients may also be asymptomatic.
- There are multiple causes of urethritis (Table 1).
  - In young men, urethritis is most commonly due to sexually transmitted infections (STIs): *Chlamydia trachomatis* and *Neisseria gonorrhoeae* are the most prevalent pathogens.
  - Non-infectious causes are less common.
- Urinary tract infections are uncommon in older males with normal urogenital tracts.
- Untreated, urethritis may lead to strictures, epididymitis, prostatitis (rare) or Reiter's syndrome.

ASSESSMENT

HISTORY

History of Present Illness

- Inquire about testicular pain and or tenderness.
- **Epididymitis** may complicate urethritis and is usually unilateral.
- It is important to rule out **testicular torsion** as a cause of pain.
- Does the patient report perineal or rectal pain? **Prostatitis**, while less common under 35 years, should be considered.
- Has the patient used any products that could irritate the urethra such as perfumed soaps, lotions or spermicides?
- Assess for trauma, as can occur with vigorous sexual intercourse or masturbation.

Sexual History

- Get a detailed sexual history. Assess for risk factors associated with urethritis such as:
  - Prior history of an STI.
  - Multiple sexual partners.
  - Infrequent condom use.
  - Sexual practices (i.e. vaginal, insertive anal or oral intercourse).
  - Herpes and adenovirus infections may occur in the recipients of oral sex. These need to be considered in recurrent cases despite treatment.

Past Medical History

- Does the patient have a history of prior STI and if so, do they know the etiologic agent?
- Is there an underlying condition such as a urogenital tract abnormality, frequent urinary tract infections or catheterizations, HIV/AIDS, diabetes or other immunosuppressed state.

PHYSICAL

Genital Exam

- Assess for the following on exam: inguinal adenopathy, ulcers, urethral discharge, meatal edema and erythema, or inflammation of the glans penis.
- "Milk" the urethra gently down the shaft of the penis (you may ask the patient to do this) to elicit penile discharge.
- Palpate testicles for pain or enlargement. Assess for any tenderness of the epididymis.
- "Blue spot" is a harmless thrombosis of the appendix testes.

Rectal Exam

- A rectal exam is not indicated unless the patient reports anal pain or discomfort warranting further evaluation. Prostatitis is rare in teens.

STUDIES

Testing for Gonorrhea or Chlamydia

- The nucleic acid amplification test for gonorrhea and chlamydia (NAAT) has largely replaced culture or nucleic acid hybridization swabs of the urethral discharge.

Urine Culture

- Consider in cases when a UTI is suggested by history. If the patient complains of dysuria, hematuria, urgency, or nocturia; has a known urogenital tract abnormality; has a negative history of sexual activity; or if lab findings support the diagnosis (e.g. positive nitrites on urinalysis).

Urethral Discharge Analysis

- This can be done at point of care. Availability of a microscope can facilitate definitive or presumptive therapy while the patient is present in the office.
- The presence of 5 or more WBC per high power field (oil immersion) suggests urethritis.
- Noted gram negative intracellular diplococci indicates gonococcal urethritis, while their absence suggests non-gonoccocal urethritis (NGU).

Other STI Screening

- Testing for urethral pathogens other than gonorrhea and chlamydia is not routinely recommended; however, consider a herpes virus culture from suspicious urethral lesions or a rapid antigen test for trichomoniasis in cases of recurrent or persistent symptoms.
- For those with confirmed or presumed STI, offer testing for syphilis (RPR or VDRL), HIV and consider testing for hepatitis B if unimmunized.

TREATMENT

- The diagnosis of urethritis can be made clinically and/or based on laboratory confirmation.

- To diagnose urethritis, at least one of the following criteria needs to be present:
  - Urethral discharge, serous, mucopurulent or purulent.
  - Urethral discharge with 5 or more WBC per high power field (oil immersion).
  - Positive leukocyte esterase test on first-void urine or microscopic examination of first-void urine sediment demonstrating $\geq$10 WBC per high-power field.
  - If none of these criteria are present, a positive test for *N. gonorrhoeae* or *C. trachomatis.*
- All sexually active teens suspected of having urethritis should be treated empirically for gonorrhea and chlamydia infection (Table 2).
  - Many patients with negative test results respond well to empiric antibiotic therapy.
  - This may be secondary to false negative tests or infection by an organism for which testing was not done.
- Partners of teens treated empirically should be evaluated and treated.
- Clear instructions need to be provided for patients treated for an STI (Table 3).

DISPOSITION

- Patients should be reevaluated if symptoms persist or recur after completion of therapy.
- Signs of urethral inflammation or laboratory evidence of infection are required to justify retreating.
- Test of cure for gonorrhea or chlamydia is no longer recommended if a patient was treated with one of the recommended regimes; however, because of the high rate of reinfection with gonorrhea and/or chlamydia, re-testing in 3 to 6 months is recommended to determine if a new infection is present.
- Recurrent and persistent urethritis after the first episode of treatment may occur and be due to:
  - Patient non-compliance and/or re-infection from an untreated partner. If this occurs, retreat, and ensure partner(s) treatment;

  - Epididymitis or orchitis especially if there is testicular pain, tenderness or swelling;
  - Doxycycline resistant *U. urealyticum, M. genitalium* or *T. vaginalis*;
  - Enterobacter infection which can be treated with doxycycline or a floroquinolone;
  - Viral etiology confirmed by viral culture; or
  - A non-infectious cause such as perfumed soaps or products or minor trauma.
- The CDC has recommendations for the treatment of urethritis recurrences (Table 4).

What is unique about urethritis in adolescents?

- The most common cause of urethritis in males is gonorrhea and/or chlamydia infections.
- Many teens are asymptomatic and may go untreated. Hence, screening should always be considered, especially for sexually active teens in areas with a high incidence of STIs.
- In 15 to 19 year olds, gonorrheal infections are 40 times more prevalent in African–American males than Caucasian males.
- The majority of cases are not due to a urinary tract infection but rather to sexually transmitted infections. An older male diagnosed with a UTI should be worked up for urogenital tract abnormality or kidney disease.

TEST YOUR KNOWLEDGE ANSWERS

63. D. Prostatitis is uncommon in teens and young adults. Epididymitis is a more likely complication of urethritis in this patient population. UTIs, also uncommon in males, warrant further investigation for an underlying urinary tract malformation when they occur. While vigorous masturbation (especially if unlubricated) may cause urethral irritation and penile edema, this is an uncommon cause for consult (the adolescent is likely cognizant of the etiology). Although gonococcal infections in males classically presents with purulent discharge, gonorrhea and other STIs can also manifest with scant serous mucoid discharge.

64. D. Urethritis is most commonly caused by gonorrhea and/or chlamydia in sexually active teens. Urine nucleic acid amplification test (NAAT) is most likely to yield this diagnosis. Urinalysis and urine cultures are useful tests if a UTI is strongly suspected. The rapid antigen test for trichomoniasis, while not routine, can be useful in cases of persistent or recurrent urethritis. A testicular ultrasound can be useful when needing to differentiate epididymitis from testicular torsion and is indicated if the patient reports testicular pain.

Table 1. Causes of Urethritis.

Infectious	Gonococcal Urethritis (GU)	• Symptom onset usually within 2–6 days of exposure. • Symptoms are often acute, although a silent form exists. • Dysuria and urinary frequency may be present. • Urethral discharge tends to be profuse and purulent, but may be serous or mucoid. • External urethral meatus may be red and edematous.

	Non-gonococcal Urethritis (NGU)	• Symptom onset usually 1 to 3 weeks post exposure.
		• Can be due to bacteria, protozoa and viruses.
		  • Bacteria: *Chlamydia* (most common of NGU), *mycoplasma genitalium, ureaplasma* species and enteric organisms (e.g. *E. coli).*
		  • Protozoa: *Trichomonas vaginalis* (rare cause of pyuria).
		  • Viruses: Adenovirus and herpes simplex.

(*Continued*)

Table 1. (*Continued*)

	• Symptoms are often milder than gonococcal urethritis. • Urethral discharge often less profuse; may be mucoid to purulent. • Dysuria and frequency of urination may be present.
Non-Infectious	• Perfumed soaps, lotions or other topical products. • Spermicides. • Trauma from vigorous sexual intercourse or masturbation.

Table 2. Treatment Regimes for Urethritis.

Presumed or Known Organism(s)	Treatment
Etiology unknown or gonococcal urethritis. There is a high co-infection rate of chlamydia with gonorrhea, thus dual therapy is indicated for gonococcus urethritis. Oral cephalosporin is no longer recommended, thus this regime will also treat an associated oropharyngeal and or gonorrhea proctitis.	Ceftriaxone 250 mg IM × 1 dose *PLUS* Azithromycin 1 gm PO × 1 dose *OR* Doxycycline 100 mg PO BID × 7 days
Non-gonococcal urethritis. Azithromycin and doxycycline are highly effective for chlamydial urethritis; however, infections with M. *genitalium* respond better to azithromycin.	Azithromycin 1 gram PO × 1 dose *OR* Doxycycline 100 mg PO BID × 7 days Alternative: Erythromycin base 500 mg PO QID × 7 days *OR* Erythromycin ethylsuccinate 800 mg PO QID × 7 days *OR* Levofloxacin 500 mg PO QD × 7 days *OR* Ofloxacin 300 mg PO BID × 7 days

Centers for Disease Control and Prevention: Sexually Transmitted Diseases Treatment Guidelines: 2010. http://www.cdc.gov/std/treatment/2010/toc.htm. Accessed October 30 (2011).

Table 3. Patient Counseling Guide.

- Abstain from sexual intercourse for at least 7 days after treatment and until at least 7 days after present sexual partner(s) have been treated, whichever is longer.
- Patients need to inform partner(s) from at least the prior 2 months of their diagnosis and the need to be treated.
- Expedited partner therapy (EPT) can be used if necessary in heterosexual couples. EPT is not recommended for MSM.
- InSPOT is a free electronic source (www.inSPOT.org) that may be used for partner notification. It also allows for anonymous partner notification.

Table 4. Recurrent and Persistent Urethritis.

May be secondary to trichomoniasis, mycoplasma or ureaplasma infections	Retreat with initial regime if noncompliant or sex with untreated partner. Metronidazole 2 gm PO × 1 dose *OR* Tinidazole 2 gm PO × 1 dose *PLUS* Azithromycin 1 gm PO × 1 dose (if not used at initial treatment). Trichomoniasis is less common in MSMs; thus, Moxifloxacin 400 mg PO QD × 7 days may be effective against M genitalium.

Centers for Disease Control and Prevention: Sexually Transmitted Diseases Treatment Guidelines: 2010. http://www.cdc.gov/std/treatment/2010/toc.htm. Accessed October 30 (2011).

WEB REFERENCES

- Centers for Disease Control and Prevention. 'Sexually Transmitted Diseases Treatment Guidelines', 2010. MMWR2010; 59 (No. RR-12): l–110, retrieved from http://www.cdc.gov/std/treatment/2010/STD-Treatment-2010-RR5 912.pdf
- Marcell AV, Wibbelsman C, Seigel WM, and the Committee on Adolescence. 'Clinical Report: Male Adolescent Sexual and Reproductive Health Care', Pediatrics. 2011; 128(6): el658–el676, retrieved from http://pediatrics.aappublications.org/search?fulltext=adolescent+male+urethritis&submit=yes&x=O&y=O

- Plewa, MC. 'Male Urethritis in Emergency Medicine' Medscape Reference (updated May 11, 2012), retrieved from http://emedicine.medscape.com/article/778374-overview

Additional Clinician and Patient Resources:

- Puberty 101 (2012), Nonspecific Urethritis, retrieved from http://puberty 101.com/s-t-d-s/nonspecific-urethritis/
- Young Men's Health, Boston's Children's Hospital, Sexually Transmitted Diseases (STIs): General Information (updated 1/17/2013), retrieved from http://www.youngmenshealthsite.org/std-general.html

44

GENITAL WARTS: CONDYLOMA ACCUMINATA

Liana R. Clark

TEST YOUR KNOWLEDGE

65. Accurate statements about condyloma accuminata include all the following *EXCEPT*:

    A. It is a viral infection.
    B. The incubation period is 4–6 weeks after infection.
    C. There is a high risk of malignant change in these lesions.
    D. They can be worse in immunosuppresed individuals.
    E. Despite treatment, they can recur.

66. A 16 year old male requests treatment for his genital warts. All the following are important counseling points *EXCEPT*:

    A. Treatment to resolve the warts will take time.
    B. The patient should get tested for other STIs.
    C. The patient's partner should also be evaluated.
    D. The patient should have his penis and anus swabbed for high risk HPV infection.
    E. The patient is a good candidate for HPV4 vaccination.

Refer to end of chapter for answers on page 477.

A 17 year old male presents for a sports physical examination and says that he has "bumps" on his penis and scrotum.

BACKGROUND

- Condyloma acuminata, or genital warts, are generally benign raised lesions that occur following infection with low risk types of human papillomavirus (usually types 6 & 11).

ASSESSMENT

HISTORY

History of Present Illness

- Patients may report anal or vaginal irritation depending on the location of lesions.
- Lesions are usually slow growing and often occur 1–2 months after HPV infection (there is a 4–6 week incubation period).

Sexual History

- Obtain a history of sexual contact, with or without condom use.
- Multiple sexual partners increases the risk of exposure.

Contributory History

- Patients who are immunosuppressed or who smoke cigarettes are at increased risk of acquiring genital warts.

PHYSICAL

Genital Exam

- Demonstrates multiple raised warty growths on the genitalia.
  - May appear to be small cauliflower-like flesh-colored growths.
  - Non-tender and non-friable.

    - No inguinal adenopathy.
    - No urethral discharge.
- Exam can exclude other causes of genital papillomatous lesions:
    - **Pink, pearly papules of the penis**
        - One or more rows of small, flesh-colored, smooth, dome-topped to filiform papules situated circumferentially around the corona or sulcus of the glans penis.
        - Often confused with genital warts, these are benign and considered a normal anatomical variant.
    - **Ectopic sebaceous glands (Fordyce's spots)**
        - Small, painless, raised, pale, red or white spots or bumps that are 1 to 3 mm in diameter and may appear on the shaft of the penis or on the labia.
        - Common in men and women of all ages.
        - When located on the head of the penis, these are known as Tyson's glands.
        - Also a normal anatomical variant that does not require treatment.
    - **Molluscum contagiosum**
        - A viral infection of the skin that causes small raised firm papules with central umbilication.
        - Can occur anywhere on the body.
        - Caused by a DNA poxvirus called the *molluscum contagiosum virus* (MCV).
        - Often resolve within months without treatment but treatment options are available.
    - **Condyloma lata**
        - A hallmark of secondary syphilis, these are raised, rounded, highly contagious lesions that tend to occur in moist areas such as the vagina or anus.
    - **Penile and vulvar intraepithelial neoplasia**
        - Can look similar to genital warts but are exceptionally rare in adolescents.

STUDIES

Condyloma accuminata is a clinical diagnosis and laboratory studies are not necessary; however, the clinician may want to consider the following studies:

Gonorrhea and Chlamydia Testing

- May be useful to diagnose concomitant infections.

RPR Screen for Syphilis

- Can be helpful to distinguish condyloma lata from genital warts.

PAP Smear

- Universally recommended at age 21 and earlier in immunosuppressed teens (3 years after sexual debut).

SPECIAL TESTS

Immune Work-up, Including HIV Testing

- Consider when a patient presents with extensive or giant condyloma acuminata.

Darkfield Examination of Smears

- May demonstrate motile treponemes in cases of condyloma lata.

TREATMENT

- Twenty to thirty percent of women with genital warts have spontaneous resolution without therapy.
- Physician applied therapies include skin exfoliants like trichloroacetic acid (TCA), podophyllin resin, and 5-flurouracil cream. Pain and irritation are common side effects and patients have to return regularly to the clinician for follow up weekly treatments until symptoms resolve.

- Patient applied therapies includes Imiquimod and Podofilox. Patients can self treat at home, but risk pain or irritation.
- Liquid nitrogen can be used to treat genital warts.
- Topical treatment modalities may remove the visible wart, but do not necessarily eradicate the HPV DNA in the underlying epithelium; hence, there is a risk of recurrence even after treatment.
- Intralesional interferon is a less commonly used therapy.
- Surgical treatment is recommended for large, bulky warts.

What is unique about genital warts in adolescents?

- HPV vaccination confers protection to adolescents who have not already been exposed to HPV and is a recommended vaccine for both males and females early in adolescence.
- Genital warts have been shown to affect psychosocial functioning. Preventive counseling should be a component of all routine visits.

TEST YOUR KNOWLEDGE ANSWERS

65. C. Condyloma accuminata, or genital warts, are caused by low-risk HPV types 6 & 11 in most cases. These lesions have a very low risk of malignant change, in contrast to high-risk HPV types (i.e. HPV 16 & 18), known causes of cervical and anal cancer. However, since a person can be coinfected with both low-risk and high-risk types, an increased risk of malignancy in areas of undetected high-risk HPV infection cannot be ruled out. Despite treatment, condyloma accuminata can recur.
66. D. Currently, there are no commercially available screening tools for high-risk HPV infection in males. In addition, there is no treatment for subclinical disease, even if a lesion were to be found. All other answer choices are true. Despite presenting with a genital wart infection, the patient can still gain protection from the HPV4 vaccine to infections by other HPV types that he has not yet been exposed to. Vaccination should be offered.

WEB REFERENCES

- Centers for Disease Control and Prevention. 'Sexually Transmitted Diseases Treatment Guidelines', 2010. MMWR2010; 59(No. RR-12: l–110, retrieved from http://www.cdc.gov/std/treatment/2010/STD-Treatment-2010-RR5912.pdf
- Friedman L, Bell DL. 'Human Papillomavirus (HPV) Vaccine: An Updated Position Statement of the Society for Adolescent Health and Medicine', Society for Adolescent Health and Medicine (statement issues June 17, 2010), retrieved from http://www.adolescenthealth.org/AM/Template.cfm?Section=Position Statements&Template=/CM/ContentDisplay.cfm&ContentID=3225
- Kodner CM, Nasraty S. 'Management of Genital Warts', American Family Physician. 2004 Dec 15; 70(12): 2335–2342, retrieved from http://www.aafp.org/afp/2004/1215/p2335.html

Additional Clinician and Patient Resources:

- American College of Obstetricians and Gynecologists, Tool Kit for Teen Care (2nd Edition): Human Papillomavirus (2010), retrieved from http://www.acog.org/~/media/Departments/Adolescent%20Health%20Care/Teen%20Care%20Tool%20Kit/HPVirus.pdf?dmc=1&ts=20130409T1703552132
- Carusi DA. Patient Information: Genital warts in women (Beyond the Basics), last updated April 2, 2012, retrieved from http://www.uptodate.com/contents/genital-warts-in-women-beyond-the-basics
- Center for Young Women's Health, Boston's Children Hospital: Human Papillomavirus (HPV), retrieved from http://www.youngwomenshealth.org/hpv.html
- Gearhart PA. 'Human Papillomavirus', Medscape Reference, Condyloma Acuminata (updated March 4,2013), retrieved from http://emedicine.medscape.com/article/264368-overview

45

GENITAL ULCER SYNDROME (GUS)

Avril Melissa Houston

TEST YOUR KNOWLEDGE

67. Which of the following statements is true?
    A. Genital ulcers are always caused by sexually transmitted infections.
    B. Recognizing the characteristic appearance of genital ulcers is sufficient to make a diagnosis.
    C. Genital ulcers may cause dysuria and can be accompanied by constitutional symptoms.
    D. The "railroad track" or "school of fish" pattern seen on Gram stain is associated with syphilis infections.
    E. All the above.

Refer to end of chapter for answer on page 485.

"I've noticed 'bumps down there' and it burns when I use the bathroom!"

BACKGROUND

- Genital blisters, sores, or ulcers, sometimes accompanied by inguinal lymphadenopathy make their first appearance during adolescence and are often, but not always, associated with sexually transmitted infectious (STIs).
- Infections, reactions, illnesses and trauma can all cause genital ulcers (Table 1).
- Even after complete evaluation, approximately 25% of patients with genital lesions will not have a confirmed laboratory diagnosis.

ASSESSMENT

HISTORY

History of Present Illness

- Determine duration of genital lesions. How long ago did they first erupt?
- Ask the patient to describe the character and progression of genital lesions including number, appearance and associated pain.
- Lesions elsewhere? Lesions from excoriated **psoriasis** may present in the genital area.
- Has the adolescent used any new soaps, douches or lotions? **Allergic and irritant contact dermatitis** can present as genital lesions.
- Is there a history of genital trauma (i.e. scratching due to pruritis or "zipper injury").
- **Traumatic lesions** appear at the time of injury.
- Associated symptoms such as dysuria may be due to a genital lesion or suggest **urethritis.**
- Pruritis or "crawling sensation" suggests **scabies** or **pediculosis pubis.**
- A painless ulcer suggests a **primary syphilis** chancre; however, 5% of herpetic lesions are pain free.

Past Medical History

- Has the patient had genital sores in the past?
  - Recurrent painful genital lesions suggest **genital herpes simplex virus (HSV)**.
  - Recurrent oral and genital lesions, blurry vision or eye pain suggest **Behcet's disease.**
  - Weight loss and gastrointestinal symptoms suggests **granulomatous colitis.**

Medications

- Is the adolescent taking any medication? Intermittent genital ulcers associated with a medication may indicate a **fixed drug reaction** (e.g. to phenobarbitol or tetracyclines).

Sexual History

- Obtain a thorough sexual history including gender and number of sexual contacts, type of contact (manual, oral, genital, or rectal) and use of barrier protection.
- Has the patient been diagnosed with STIs and/or HIV?
- Has there been foreign travel? Unprotected sex abroad?

Review of Systems

- Constitutional symptoms (i.e. fever, myalgias, anorexia and headaches) occur with **primary HSV, primary HIV, lymphogranuloma venereum (LGV)**, and **secondary syphilis** (once the chancre has healed).

PHYSICAL

Vital Signs

- Fever raises concern for an infectious etiology.

HEENT

- Evaluate for oral ulcers and other lesions.

Genital/Anal

- Thoroughly examine the external genital and perianal areas.
- Note number and appearance of genital ulcers.
- Assess for tenderness at lesion site and associated vaginal or anal discharge (e.g. proctitis is a common presentation of LGV).

Skin

- The rash associated with secondary syphilis appears after the primary chancre has disappeared (within weeks to months), can take any form (macular or papular) and can involve the palms and soles.
- Scabies often involves the finger webs, flexor surfaces of the wrist, penis and scrotum.
- Pediculosis infection can involve pubic, perianal or thigh hair as well as eyebrows.

Lymph Nodes

- Evaluate for lymphadenopathy.
  - The "groove sign" is an inflammatory reaction of the superficial and deep inguinal nodes that can be associated with LGV or chancroid.
  - Inguinal lymphadenopathy may also accompany the syphilitic chancre.

STUDIES

As the clinical presentation of genital ulcers can vary and overlap, it is necessary to determine the etiology of a genital ulcer by diagnostic testing (Table 2).

Serologic Nontreponemal and Treponemal Tests

- Nontreponemal tests are used for screening and treponemal tests for confirmation because false positive tests can occur with infectious mononucleosis and other illnesses. Moreover, in early syphilis, the tests may be initially negative.

- Nontreponemal tests detect antibodies to cardiolipin and are not specific for treponemal infection and examples include the rapid plasma reagin (RPR) test and venereal disease research laboratory (VDRL).
- Treponemal tests detect antibodies specific to *T. pallidum* and examples include the *T. pallidum* enzyme immunoassay (EIA), *Treponema pallidum* particle agglutination (TP-PA) and the fluorescent treponemal antibody (FTA-ABS) tests.

Culture or Antigen Test for HSV

- In cases of painful or suspicious lesions.

N. gonorrhea, C. trachomatis and HIV Tests

- Any sexually active teen should be offered STI screening.

SPECIAL TESTS

Type-Specific HSV Serologic Assays

- May be useful in the following situations:
  - Recurrent or atypical genital symptoms with negative HSV culture.
  - Clinical diagnosis of HSV without laboratory confirmation.
  - A partner with genital herpes.

Darkfield Examination or Direct Immunofluorescence Tests for T. pallidum

- The best tests to confirm primary syphilis (positive when other tests are still negative) but are seldom available.

Gram Stain

- May reveal the "railroad track" or "school of fish" pattern of the Gram negative rods, *H. ducreyi.*

Culture for H. ducreyi

- Consider in settings where chancroid is prevalent or if the patient has travelled to such a region.

Biopsy or Tissue Crush Preparation

- Visualization of dark-staining Donovan bodies may be seen in cases of Granuloma inguinale.

Lymph Node Biopsy

- Rule out lymphoma.

TREATMENT

- The Centers for Disease Control and Prevention recommended medical treatment regimens are summarized in Table 3.
- Adolescents diagnosed with genital herpes should be counseled on the potential for recurrent episodes and the risks of sexual transmission even before the lesions are visible.
- Patients treated for syphilis should be counseled about the possibility of experiencing a "Jarisch-Herxheimer Reaction" which involves fever, chills, myalgias, headache and tachycardia, that can occur within 2 hours after treatment and is related to bacterial lysis.
- Patients diagnosed with primary and secondary syphilis should be reevaluated at 6 and 12 months after treatment.
- Adolescents treated for chancroid should be reevaluated in 3 to 7 days. Symptoms should improve within 3 days of treatment.
- Sexual partners should be evaluated and treated presumptively (syphilis, LGV, chancroid), offered treatment (Granuloma inguinale) or treated if symptomatic (HSV).

What is unique about GUS in adolescents?

- Self-consent for the diagnosis and treatment of adolescents with STIs is recognized in all 50 states.

- Adolescents unaware of the presence of painless lesions or concerned about privacy and confidentiality issues may delay or fail to seek medical care.
- Many adolescents self-treat genital lesions with topical medications which may also delay diagnosis and appropriate treatment.
- There are several factors that place adolescents at higher risk of acquiring genital ulcers including multiple partners and having partners with multiple partners.

TEST YOUR KNOWLEDGE ANSWER

67. C. Painful urination may be associated with ulcerative lesions on the labia and urethra. Constitutional symptoms like fever and myalgias can occur during a primary clinical infection with HSV and HIV. Genital ulcers may be associated with both infectious and non-infectious causes. Examples of non-infectious causes include fixed drug reactions and Behcet's disease. Although the physical examination may provide clues to the diagnosis, the presentation of genital ulcers can vary: it is necessary to perform diagnostic testing to confirm the etiology of a genital ulcer. Gram stain for evaluation of chancroid may reveal a "railroad track" or "school of fish" pattern, the characteristic grouping of the gram negative rods of *H. ducreyi.*

Table 1. Differential Diagnosis of Genital Ulcers.

Infectious	Herpes simplex virus (HSV)
	Syphilis
	Chancroid
	Lymphogranuloma venereum (LGV)
	Granuloma inguinale
	Scabies
	Pediculosis
Non-infectious	Fixed drug reactions
	Behcet's disease
	Granulomatous colitis
	Excoriations/Trauma
	Allergic and irritant contact dermatitis

Table 2. Etiology, Clinical Characteristics and Diagnostic Methods.*

Infection	Etiologic Agent	Clinical Characteristics			Diagnostic Methods
		Appearance	Pain	Adenopathy	
Genital Herpes	HSV-2 in most cases (HSV-1 is less common)	• Multiple, bilateral, small shallow ulcers • Proctitis, particularly in men who have sex with men (MSM)	Yes	Tender local and inguinal	• HSV cell culture • PCR (not FDA cleared) • Type-specific serologic tests
Syphilis	*Treponema pallidum*	• Papule that ulcerates to become a chancre (1–2 cm ulcer with a raised, indurated margin) • Heals spontaneously	No	Mild to moderate and regional	• Darkfield microscopy • Presumptive diagnosis made with non-treponemal tests (VDRL or RPR) AND treponemal tests (FTA-ABS) • Non-treponemal test antibody titers usually correlate with disease activity • In majority of people, a positive treponemal test will remain reactive for the rest of their life

(*Continued*)

Table 2. *(Continued)*

		Clinical Characteristics			
Infection	**Etiologic Agent**	**Appearance**	**Pain**	**Adenopathy**	**Diagnostic Methods**
Chancroid	*Haemophilus ducreyi*	• Sharply demarcated with ragged edges • Multiple lesions • Bleeds easily when scraped	Yes	Tender, suppurative and inguinal May present as fluctuant buboes	• Culture on special media • PCR (not FDA cleared)
Granuloma Inguinale	*Klebsiella granulomatis*	• Progressive ulcerative lesions • Beefy red appearance • Bleeds easily when scraped	No	No	• Visualization of Donovan bodies on tissue crush preparation or biopsy • PCR (not FDA cleared)
LGV	*Chlamydia trachomatis* L1–L3	• Self-limited ulcer or papule sometimes occurs at site of inoculation • Proctocolitis that may lead to chronic colorectal fistulas and strictures	No	Tender inguinal/ femoral	• Culture • Direct immunofluorescence • Nucleic acid detection • Complement fixation tests

Note: *In the U.S., the majority of young sexually active people presenting with genital ulcers either have genital herpes, syphilis, or rarely chancroid.

Table 3. Recommended Treatment for Diseases Characterized by Genital Ulcers.

Genital Herpes	First episode: Acyclovir 400 mg PO TID × 7–10 days OR Acyclovir 200 mg PO 5 times a day × 7–10 days OR Famciclovir 250 mg TID × 7–10 days OR Valacyclovir 1 g PO BID × 7–10 days
Syphilis*	Primary and secondary: Benzathine penicillin G 2.4 million units IM × 1
Chancroid	Azithromycin 1 gram PO × 1 OR Ceftriaxone 250 mg IM × 1 OR Ciprofloxacin 500 mg BID × 3 days OR Erythromycin base 500 mg PO TID × 7 days
Granoluma Inguinale	Doxycycline 100 mg PO BID for at least 3 weeks
LGV	Doxycycline 100 mg PO BID × 21 days

*In cases where the patient reports a chancre occurred but was not visualized or retreatment is required, it is recommended that the patient be treated with Benzathine penicillin G 2.4 million units IM once weekly for 3 weeks.

WEB REFERENCES

- Centers for Disease Control and Prevention. 'Diseases Characterized by Genital, Anal, or Perianal Ulcers (last updated January 28, 2011), retrieved from http://www.cdc.gov/std/treatment/2010/genital-ulcers.htm
- Centers for Disease Control and Prevention. 'Sexually Transmitted Diseases Treatment Guidelines', 2010. MMWR2010;59(No. RR-12):l-110, retrieved from http://www.cdc.gov/std/treatment/2010/STD-Treatment-2010-RR5912.pdf

Additional Clinician and Patient Resources:

- American Sexual Health Association, I Wanna Know: www.iwannaknow.org
- Centers for Disease Control and Prevention, Genital Herpes-CDC Fact Sheet (last updated February 11, 2013), retrieved from http://www.cdc.gov/std/Herpes/STDFact-Herpes.htm
- Centers for Disease Control and Prevention, Syphilis Information (last updated March 1, 2013), retrieved from http://www.cdc.gov/std/syphilis/default.htm
- TeenHealth Source, Herpes 101, retrieved from http://teenhealthsource.com/stisetc/herpes-
- TeensHealth from Nemours, Genital Herpes, retrieved from http://kidshealth.org/teen/infections/stds/std_herpes.html

46

CONDOMS

Mariana Kastrinakis

TEST YOUR KNOWLEDGE

68. Which of the following statements is true?

    A. The best way to avoid an STI is to simultaneously use a male and female condom.
    B. Allergic reactions to latex condoms are a minor inconvenience: frequent condom use for desensitization will solve that problem.
    C. Most adolescent girls are very interested in using the female condom.
    D. The consistent use of condoms significantly reduces the risk of acquiring HIV.
    E. All the above.

Refer to end of chapter for answer on page 494.

A 15 year old male patient, in the office for a routine physical exam, is thinking about becoming sexually active with his girlfriend who he thinks may be taking birth control pills but is not sure. "I guess we should use condoms. . ."

BACKGROUND

- Condoms are made of latex, polyurethane, lambskin or polyisoprene and they come in male and female versions. Lambskin does not protect from HIV and is scarcely used while polyurethane or polyisoprene (synthetic latex) are recommended for those with latex allergies.
- The CDC states that consistent and correct use of latex condoms is highly effective in preventing sexual transmission of HIV and **reduces** the risk of sexually transmitted infections (STIs) that are transmitted by genital fluids, such as chlamydia, gonorrhea, and trichomoniasis.
- In addition, it reduces the risk for genital human papillomavirus (HPV) infection and HPV-associated diseases (e.g. genital warts and cervical cancer) as well as genital ulcer diseases, such as genital herpes, syphilis, and chancroid, when the infected area or site of potential exposure is protected.
- Condoms are ideal as an initial form of contraception (Table 1).

ASSESSMENT

HISTORY

Sexual History

- Assess for risky sexual behaviors:
  - How old was the teen at sexual debut?
  - How many lifetime partners?
  - Use of contraception at past or present?
  - What forms of contraception has the teen used?
  - History of STIs?
  - Has the teen ever been pregnant or gotten someone else pregnant?

  - In what types of sexual activity does the teen engage (i.e. oral, vaginal or anal intercourse)?
  - Does the teen report that their partner refuses to use condoms?
- Determine if the teen has willingly made the decision to have sex. Question the teen about any "pressure" they might be experiencing from peers, partner or others and screen for potential abuse from partner.
- Does the teen identify as a sexual minority? Regardless of classification, teens who identify as homosexual may engage in heterosexual activity and vice versa.

Concerns about Past Condom Use

- Does the teen report any problems with condom use in the past? Teens who report vaginal or penile irritation to condoms may have a **latex allergy** or skin irritation from the spermicides used in many condoms. Polyurethane condoms may be a better choice.
- Has the teen used a condom in the past that broke, popped or slipped off during intercourse? Teens should be counseled on the use of back up methods such as hormonal contraception methods. If condom breakage occurred within the past 5 days, the clinician should offer Plan B to prevent unwanted pregnancy, and consider STI screening.
- What is the teen's cultural or religious beliefs about condom use? Many cultures may shy away from condom use for various reasons (e.g. many adolescent girls are reluctant to carry a condom or request that one be used for fear of being labelled a "slut").

Past Medical History

- Does the teen have a history of reproductive medical problems or menstrual disorders?
- Has the teen ever been abused, mentally, physically or sexually by current partner or anyone else?

Allergies

- Does the teen have latex allergies that would exclude use of latex condoms as a form of contraception?

Medications

- Females using intravaginal miconazole or econazole should be forewarned that these medications can cause breakdown of a latex condom rendering it ineffective.

PHYSICAL

- A physical exam should be completed *only* to address any concerns the teen may have; otherwise, a physical exam is not necessary to dispense condoms.
- The annual physical is a good opportunity for a reproductive health conversation, including condoms.

STUDIES

- Laboratory studies should be ordered as dictated by history and physical exam findings.
- STI screening and pregnancy testing can be offered to teens who engage in high risk sexual behaviors or who do not routinely use condoms for protection.

DISPOSITION

- Teens should be counseled on how to use condoms appropriately and urged to follow manufacturer's instructions:
  - Condoms should not be used if the expiration date has passed or the integrity of the packaging has been compromised.
  - Condoms should not be used if they are discolored, brittle or dry.
  - Teens should be counseled on how to place a condom on the penis. They should know to place the unrolled condom on an erect penis before penetration ensuring that the rolled up ring is on the outside. The tip of the condom should be compressed as the condom is unrolled on the penis, so that air does not get trapped inside and to prevent the condom from breaking during intercourse.
  - Water based lubrication should be used to prevent condom breakage. Oil based lubrications should not be used with latex condoms as this can weaken the condom leading to tears and breakdown.

- A new condom should be used when switching between different penetrative acts to prevent spread of infection.
- To properly remove a condom, it should be held firmly at the base of the erect penis and removed carefully, taking care not to spill semen.
- Condoms should be properly disposed. Teens should be advised to never reuse a condom.

What is unique about condom counseling and use in adolescents?

- When talking to adolescents, the clinician's goal should be to apply a NO MISSED OPPORTUNITIES approach to preventable problems. While adolescents may portray themselves as savvy and mature, they often exhibit remarkable naivete and ignorance about sexual matters.
- Ideally, teens should ask about contraception before they have started having sex; however, this is seldom the case. It is important to talk about condom use as a method of pregnancy and STI prevention at routine visits well before sexual debut.
- Clinicians can also use acute care clinic visits such as pregnancy testing with negative results or STI testing, as opportunities to review condom use as a prevention strategy.
- Condoms are an ideal method of contraception for those initiating sexual activity (Table 1).
- Teens should be encouraged to communicate about sex with each other, including discussions about contraception.
- Teens often cite discomfort or partner dislike as reasons to not use condoms. Clinicians should be prepared to address any number of concerns teens may cite as reasons to not use condoms (Table 2).
- Many teens do not use the female condom as it can be more complex to use then the male condom and requires the user to feel comfortable with touching her genitalia, with insertion, and checking a device placed within the vagina (Table 3).

TEST YOUR KNOWLEDGE ANSWER

68. D. Although condom use can not assure portection against HIV, it significantly reduces the risk of infection. The simultaneous use of male and female condoms is not recommended as it risks friction, rupture and ineffectiveness. Allergic reactions to latex can be increasingly serious with each exposure and can even lead to anaphylaxis and death. Polyurethane and polyisoprene condoms are recommended when one partner is allergic to latex. While in theory the female condom empowers young women, in practice, adolescent females have not embraced its use. Cost and manipulation may be a factor.

Table 1. What Makes a Condom Ideal as an Initial Form of Contraception?

- Safe and effective in preventing pregnancy and STIs when used correctly.
- Reversible method, free of the medication side effects seen with hormonal contraception.
- Over the counter, readily available to both males and females, and use does not require extensive planning.
- Relatively easy to use and dispose.
- Relatively inexpensive and can be carried discretely.
- The only evidence-based method that acts as a barrier to prevent both unintended pregnancy and STIs including HIV.
- Available in a variety of sizes, textures and colors to address user preferences.
- Can be available in clinicians' offices and often given to patients free of charge.
- Can help prevent premature ejaculation, a relatively common occurrence.
- Female condoms can be used for protection in anal sex.

Table 2. "We Didn't Use Condoms Because...

- I didn't think I was going to start having sex."
  - No plan
  - Lack of communication between partners
- my partner does not like how they "feel."
- I wanted sex to be "pure."
- putting them on or taking them off can interrupt sex."
- we got caught in the moment."
- they're not natural/comfortable or they're too small."
- my partner would think I'm sleeping around."
- my parents would kill me if they find them."

Table 3. Male versus Female Condom.

Male Condom	Female Condom
• Latex, polyurethane, lambskin or polyisoprene sheath • $ • One time use • Easy to use • Placement can be incorporated into foreplay	• Polyurethane sheath or pouch • Measures about 17 cm • Flexible ring at each end to keep female condom in place and keep condom from bunching up inside the vagina • $$$ • More complex and requires comfort with insertion. • Gives female more control over protection

WEB REFERENCES

- Advocates for Youth, Condom Effectiveness: http://www.advocatesforyouth.org/index.php?%20option=com_content&task=view&id=416&Itemid=177
- Advocates for Youth, Cultural competency for clinicians: http://www.advocatesforyouth.org/index.php?option=com_content&task=view&id=33&Itemid=62
- Cates, W., Steiner, M. J. (2002). "Dual Protection Against Unintended Pregnancy and Sexually Transmitted Infections: What Is the Best Contraceptive Approach?" *Sexually Transmitted Diseases* 29(3): 168–174. http://journals.lww.com/stdjournal/Fulltext/2002/03000/Dual_Protection_Against_Unintended_Pregnancy_and.7.aspx

- CDC Compendium of HIV Prevention Interventions with Evidence of Effectiveness, http://www.cdc.gov/hiv/resources/reports/hiv_compendium/index.htm (published 1999, last updated 2009), accessed July 29, 2010.
- Gallo MF, Grimes DA, Lopez LM, Schulz KF. 'Nonlatex versus latex male condoms for contraception (Review) Cochrane Database of Systematic Reviews 2006, Issue 1. Art. No.: CD003550. DOI: 10.1002/14651858.CD003550.pub2., Retrieved from http://apps.who.int/rhl/reviews/CD003550.pdf
- Kamau, Pius (August 24, 2008). "Islam, Condoms and AIDS". The Huffington Post, http://www.huffingtonpost.com/pius-kamau/islam-condoms-and-aids_b_120418.html. Accessed July 29, 2010.
- Ott MA, *et al.* 'The Trade-Off Between Hormonal Contraceptives And Condoms Among Adolescents', Perspectives on Sexual and reproductive Health. 2002 January/February;34(l), retrieved from https://www.guttmacher.org/pubs/journals/3400602.html
- Total Access Group, Chart of male versus female condoms: http://www.totalaccessgroup.com/Female-Condom-comparison_ep_83-l.html
- Walsh TL, *et al.* 'Evaluation of the Efficacy of a Nonlatex Condom: Results from a Randomized, Controlled Clinical Trial', Perspectives on Sexual and Reproductive Health, 2003 March/April;3 5(2), retrieved from http://www.guttmacher.org/pubs/journals/3507903.html

Additional Clinician and Patient Resources:

- about.com: written instructions on how to use condoms: http://contraception.about.com/od/contraceptionfailure/ht/condom.htm
- Alan Guttmacher Institute (AGI), at http://www.guttmacher.org/sections/adolescents.php multiple fact sheets on adolescent reproductive health statistics and trends in US and the World
- Association of Reproductive Health Professionals (ARHP) CORE website, has peer-reviewed, evidence-based teaching materials for professionals, free, at http://core.arhp.org/
- Centers for Disease Control and Prevention, Condom fact sheet: http://www.cdc.gov/condomeffectiveness/brief.html
- Columbia University Student Health services resources on reproductive health education, GoAskAlice at http://www.goaskalice.columbia.edu/1524.html Retrieved July 29, 2010
- Physicians for Reproductive Choice and Health website at http://prch.org/learn-about-prch, with multiple learning modules on reproductive health topics on clinicians including cases, powerpoint presentations and blog. Website accessed July 29, 2010
- Planned Parenthood, multiple reproductive health Tools for educators/providers, parents and teens, accessed July 29, 2010. at http://www.plannedparenthood.org/resources/index.htm

- Sexuality Information and Education Council of the United States (SIECUS), multiple resources on adolescent health and links, accessed July 29, 2010 at http://www.siecus.org/index.cfm?fuseaction=Page.viewPage&pageId=655&parentID=480
- Society for Adolescent Health and Medicine (SAHM), multiple resources for providers including help on maintaining confidentiality, screening questionnaires, etc a, accessed on July 29, 2010 at http://www.adolescenthealth.org/Clinical_Care_Resources/2304.htm

47

HORMONAL CONTRACEPTION

Evelyn Simpkins Evans

TEST YOUR KNOWLEDGE

69. A 16 year old confides that she is having sexual intercourse with her 17 year old boyfriend. He always uses a condom. Which of the following statements is *NOT* accurate?

   A. She should have a pregnancy test.
   B. She would benefit from starting contraception and should also be prescribed emergency contraception (EC).
   C. She needs parental permission for contraceptive treatment because of the potential for medical complications.
   D. The patient needs to be taught about potential side effects from combined hormonal therapy including the "ACHES" symptoms.
   E. She should follow up 1 month after initiating hormonal contraception.

Refer to end of chapter for answer on page 506.

You have just completed the HEEADSSS interview with a 16 year old female and she tells you that she has been having sex with one male partner for the last four months. She uses condoms intermittently and is interested in initiating a hormonal contraceptive method-she wants to know which birth control method is best for her.

BACKGROUND

- More than 95% of adolescent pregnancies are unintended.
- The Center for Disease Control's 2009 Youth Risk Behavior Survey found that 46% of teens in the United States admitted to ever having sex. Almost 40% admitted that they had not used a condom at the time of last intercourse, and almost 73% of females admitted that they had not used birth control pills or DepoProvera injection to aid in pregnancy prevention.
- Providers need to be prepared to assist young people in becoming productive and healthy adults. This includes providing information about how to prevent unplanned pregnancy and how to be protected from sexually transmitted infections (STIs).
- There are numerous contraceptive options available for adolescents (Table 1 to 3).

ASSESSMENT

HISTORY

- Perform a complete HEEADSSS assessment.

Menstrual History

- Ascertain the time of the last menstrual period and determine if menstrual periods occur monthly. If menses are not regular and periods are skipped, the examiner may need to consider causes for **secondary amenorrhea.**
- Are there concerns regarding **menorrhagia** or **dysmenorrhea?**

Sexual History

- Determine when the patient started having sex (sexual debut or coitarche), and the age of the patient's partner.
    - In more than half of the United States, a minor can consent to sex at age 16, though the range can be anywhere from 14 to 18 years old. Most U.S. experts do not believe that statutory rape laws significantly decrease adolescent pregnancy; however, it does provide protection for vulnerable teens that are possible targets for sexual exploitation.
- Is sex voluntary or coerced?
    - Involuntary sex/sexual abuse warrants further discussion and investigation.
    - Is the teen having sex for money?
        - Having sex for money might suggest **substance abuse**, or a complicated social situation such as **homelessness**.
- Is the teen having sex with males, females, or both? It is important to discuss barrier methods such as condoms for vaginal, anal, or oral sex for prevention of STIs.
- Has the teen ever been tested for STIs? Sexually active teens should have routine screening for STIs at least yearly.
- Consider patient risk factors (i.e. changing partners frequently, barrier method use) and STI prevalence in the community to determine whether more frequent screening is needed.
- When was the last time the teen had sex? How frequent are coital episodes?

Patient Concerns

- Is the patient a smoker?
- Evaluate possible concerns about excessive weight gain.
- Evaluate possible concerns about acne.
- Review methods currently being considered and why those choices are appealing.

Past Medical History

- A personal history of a clotting disorder is a contraindication to starting a patient on methods containing estrogen.
- Does the patient have medical conditions that would limit contraceptive choices such as
  - Migraine headaches?
  - Liver disease?
  - Hypertension?
- Does the patient have any medical illnesses which may affect contraceptive choices such as **sickle cell disease** or a **seizure disorder?**
- Is the patient pregnant or breastfeeding a baby under six months old?
- Is the patient ambulatory or non-ambulatory? Some immobile teens should not use a method containing estrogen as it places them at higher risk for deep vein thrombosis.
- Assess mental health status and/or developmental readiness.
  - A patient who is not able to administer methods independently may be better suited for a method that involves administration by a parent or provider, and/or a methods with less frequent administration.

Family History

- Is there a family or personal history of **clotting disorders?**
  - Estrogen inhibits antithrombin III and can predispose to clotting, making combined hormonal methods an inappropriate option for some adolescents.
  - A family history of clotting is not a contraindication to starting contraceptive methods that have estrogen; however, it might prompt the provider to look for deficiencies that predispose to clotting such as **protein C, protein** S, and **antithrombin III deficiencies.**
  - A personal history of clotting is a contraindication to estrogen methods.

Medications

- Determine if your patient is on medications that could interfere with contraceptive efficacy OR whose efficacy would be affected by hormonal therapies.
- Has there been a history of prior contraceptive use.

- Evaluate reasons for discontinuing prior contraceptive methods.

PHYSICAL

- A physical exam should be completed if appropriate to address any concerns the patient may have; otherwise, neither a physical or pelvic exam is necessary to dispense contraception.

Anthropometric Measurements

- Assess weight.
- Some contraceptive methods predispose to weight gain and may not be the best choice for a patient who is overweight or obese.
- Patients over 90 kg may not adequately absorb hormonal medicines in transdermal form and risk "escape ovulation."

Vital Signs

- Assess blood pressure at baseline and routinely while on contraception. Some hormonal methods may cause hypertension in some patients.

STUDIES

Pregnancy Test

- Should be considered in all sexually active teens.
- If positive, the provider should provide options counseling, a sensitive discussion that helps guide the patient make decisions about their future. This discussion should cover all choices including carrying a pregnancy to term and keeping the baby, carrying the pregnancy to term and adopting out, or terminating the pregnancy.
- If negative, the patient can initiate the contraceptive method of choice. Consider starting the method without waiting for the next menstrual cycle to begin. This is called Quick Start and has a lower incidence of pregnancy than waiting for menses to initiate contraception.
- Of note, if negative and the patient has had unprotected sex within the last week, the provider should repeat the pregnancy test in 1–3 weeks before initiating contraception.

SPECIAL TESTS

Protein C, Protein S, and Antithrombin III

- In patients with a personal or family history of thrombophlebitis, these tests can help rule out an underlying hypercoagulable state.

DISPOSITION

- Adolescents have a variety of contraceptive options available to them. The best method for a teen-ager is the method that she can use consistently, correctly and safely.
- Adolescents have a right to consent to contraceptive care without parental notification.
- Inform patients about common side effects to expect in the first few weeks after initiating combined hormonal therapy including nausea and headaches. These symptoms usually resolve in teens after they've been on a few cycles of contraception.
- Teach adolescents about "ACHES" symptoms when starting methods that contain estrogen. They should know to return to the clinic or emergency room as the following can indicate clot formation, infection or hypertension:
  - Abdominal pain
  - Chest pain
  - Headache
  - Eye problems (blurred vision)
  - Severe leg pain
- Provide a prescription for emergency contraception (EC), along with the prescription for a patient's chosen contraceptive method.
- EC should be used if there is known method compromise. It works best in the first 72 hours, but has been shown to be efficacious as far out as 120 hours. Inform patients that the closer to the episode of unprotected sex or method compromise, the better.

- Arrange follow up one month post method initiation to monitor progress.
  - Is the patient remembering to take the method? Methods are only as good as their use.
  - Is the patient having side effects such as breakthrough bleeding?
  - Has the patient been experiencing any of the **ACHES** symptoms?
  - Are they remembering to use a barrier method for STI prevention?

What is unique about contraception in adolescents?

- Teens often request contraceptive treatment without their parents' knowledge.
- It is not unusual for an adolescent to find out she is pregnant on her initial consultation for contraceptive services.
- Adherence to hormonal therapy may be erratic. Many teens have difficulty remembering to take pills daily and benefit from Long-Acting Reversible Contraception (LARC) such as an implantable method or an intrauterine device (IUD).
  - IUD's are recommended to nulliparous teens. They may have a slightly higher expulsion rate than older women.
- Injectable depo-provera is practical because it requires only four visits a year.
- Bone mineralization continues through adolescence and teens on depo-provera are at increased risk for low bone density. Calcium and vitamin D supplementation is recommended, especially if the diet is deficient in both. Bone density scans are not routinely advised but can be considered on an individual basis (e.g. family history of osteoporosis).
- Contraception rarely can induce depression or exacerbate migraine symptoms so teens suffering from either should be followed closely.
- Hormonal therapy has the added benefit of improving acne, dysmenorrhea and benign breast disorders.
- Obese teens and those on long-term broad spectrum antibiotics have a higher risk for contraceptive failure (likely related to induction of liver enzymes and "escape ovulation").

TEST YOUR KNOWLEDGE ANSWER

69. C. In the United States, adolescents have the right to consent to reproductive health care. A pregnancy test should be considered even if the patient does not admit to having sexual intercourse. It is a good idea to prescribe EC in case the adolescent has difficulties adhering to treatment (i.e. forgotten pills or lost patch). All patients should be instructed about potential side effects including the "ACHES" mnemonic. The risks of deep vein thrombosis or pulmonary embolism are low in otherwise healthy adolescents but when they occur, most often present in the first few months after initiating combined hormonal therapy. All smoking teens should be encouraged to stop smoking. A follow up visit one month post contraception initiation is advisable to monitor progress with method selected, ensure adherence and monitor side effects.

Table 1. Hormonal Contraceptive Methods.

Contraception	% Pregnancy Typical Use	% Pregnancy Perfect Use	Method Use	Common Side Effects	FYI
Birth Control Pills (combined)	5%	1% or less	1 pill PO QD.	Nausea, headaches (HA), hypertension, breast tenderness and cyclical weight gain.	If HA become severe, frequent or with focal neurologic symptoms, stop immediately.
Birth Control Pills (progestin only)	5%	3%	1 pill PO QD.	Bloating, constipation, increased appetite, weight gain, acne and depression.	Unforgiving method: must take at same time daily for optimal outcomes.
Hormonal Injection	1%	1%	150 mg IM Q 60–90 days.	Menstrual irregularity, weight gain, decreased bone density with long-term use, ↓ HDL, ↑ LDL, ↓ progestin effects with the SQ form.	SQ form uses smaller needle and is injected in thigh or abdomen as opposed to gluteus or deltoid (IM form); minimal drug interactions, fewer seizures, fewer sickle cell crises.
Hormonal Patch	1%	1%	1 patch Q week × 3 weeks, then patch free week and repeat.	Local skin irritation (hyperpigmentation), breast tenderness, vaginal spotting and dysmenorrhea.	Most side effects occur during first two cycles. Hyperpigmentation under patch site is reversible over time.
Vaginal Ring	Not known	1%	1 ring inserted intravaginally × 3 weeks then ring free week and repeat.	HA, nausea, breast tenderness, vaginitis, leukorrhea.	Few reported side effects.

Table 2. Long-Acting Reversible Conraception (LARC).

Contraception	% Pregnancy Typical Use	% Pregnancy Perfect Use	Method Use	Common Side Effects	FYI
Hormonal Implant: Nexplanon	1%	1%	One rod every 3 years.	Irregular vaginal bleeding, emotional lability, weight gain, depression and acne.	Return to normal menstrual cycles and fertility is rapid after removal.
Intrauterine Devices	1% or less	1% or less	LNG-IUS: one every 5 years. CopperT 380A: one every 10 years.	Irregular bleeding, cramping at time of insertion, expulsion (more common in the first year) and perforation of the uterus at time of insertion.	Device does not increase risk of upper genital tract infections; insertion process carries small transient risk in some women.

Table 3. Barrier Contraceptive Methods.

Contraception	% Pregnancy Typical Use	% Pregnancy Perfect Use	Method Use	Common Side Effects	FYI
Male Condoms	14%	3%	One each coital act.	Latex allergy in some users.	Encourage use of condom and another contraceptive method to reduce risk of pregnancy and STI.
Female Condoms	21%	5%	One each coital act.	Latex allergy in some users.	Some patients complain of squeaking noise; encourage dual method use as above.
Spermicides	26%	15%	One application each coital act.	Irritation of vulva, vagina, or penis; yeast vaginitis; bacterial vaginosis; higher rates of UTI in women.	Decreased integrity of vaginal mucosa which increases risk of STI transmission.

WEB REFERENCES

- Association of Reproductive Health Professionals: A Quick Reference Guide for Clinicians®: Choosing a Birth Control Method (Sept 2011), retrieved from http://www.arhp.org/uploadDocs/choosingqrg.pdf#search="hormonal%20contraception"
- Centers for Disease Control and Prevention, 'U.S. Medical Eligibility Criteria for Contraceptive Use, 2010'. MMWR. June 18 2010; 59(RR04): 1–6, retrieved from http://www.cdc.gov/mmwr/preview/mmwrhtml/rr5904al.htm?s_cid=rr5904al_e
- Daniels K, Mosher WD, Jones J. 'Contraceptive Methods Women Have Ever Used: United States, 1982–2010', National Health Statistics Reports. February 14, 2013; 62, retrieved from http://www.cdc.gov/nchs/data/nhsr/nhsrO62.pdf
- Ott MA, *et al.* 'The Influence of Hormonal Contraception on Mood and Sexual Interest Among Adolescents', Arch Sex Behav. 2008 August; 37(4): 605–613, retrieved from http://www.ncbi.nlm.nih.gov/pmc/articles/PMC3020653/
- Trenor CC, *et al.* 'Hormonal Contraception and Thrombotic Risk: A Multidisciplinary Approach', Pediatrics. 2011 February; 127(2): 347–357, retrieved from http://www.pediatricsdigest.mobi/content/127/2/347.full

Additional Clinician and Patient Resources:

- American College of Obstetricians and Gynecologists, FAQ Birth Control, Especially for Teens (August 2011), retrieved from http://www.acog.org/~/media/For%20Patients/faq112.pdf?dmc=1&ts=20130409T1941401917
- Association of Reproductive Health Professionals, Contraception: http://www.arhp.org/topics/contraception
- Centers for Disease Control and Prevention: http://www.cdc.gov/HealthyYouth/index.htm
- Contraceptive Technology: http://www.contraceptivetechnology.org
- Guttmacher Institute: http://wwwguttmacher.org/sections/contraception.php
- Planned Parenthood: http://www.plannedparenthood.org/health-topics/birth-control-4211.htm
- Sex, etc.: http://www.sexetc.org
- Center for Young Wornens Health, Types of Contraceptives: http://www.youngwomenshealth.org/contra_types.html

48

EMERGENCY CONTRACEPTION (EC)

*Jennifer Maehr**

TEST YOUR KNOWLEDGE

70. Hormonal EC may prevent pregnancy by doing all the following *EXCEPT*:

    A. Preventing ovulation
    B. Thickening cervical mucus
    C. Affecting movement of the sperm or ova through the uterus
    D. Preventing implantation of fertilized ovum
    E. None of the above.

71. Which of the following is the *MOST* accurate statement. Ulipristal, or "ella,"

    A. Is licensed for medical abortions.
    B. Is effective up to 120 hours after unprotected sexual intercourse to prevent pregnancy.
    C. Can be administered more than one time in a given menstrual cycle.
    D. Causes a large percentage of teens to experience nausea and vomiting when given as EC.
    E. None of the above.

Refer to end of chapter for answers on page 516.
*The author would like to acknowledge Jessica Burns, RN, MSN/MPH and Alison Smith, RN, MSN/ MPH for their contributions to this chapter.

Your 16 year old patient is sexually active and not consistently using condoms. She hesitantly reports that her last sexual encounter was 2 nights ago and a condom was not used. She is not on hormonal birth control and does not want to be pregnant.

BACKGROUND

- EC is a method of birth control that a woman can use to prevent pregnancy, either immediately or soon AFTER unprotected or questionably protected sexual intercourse.
- There are currently several types of EC including hormonal contraceptive pills, oral selective progesterone receptor modulators, and copper bearing intrauterine devices that have been approved for use as EC (Table 1).
- All methods approved as EC that are used correctly do not interrupt an established pregnancy, defined by medical authorities as beginning with implantation; therefore, EC methods are not abortifacient (Table 2).
- Oral methods of EC are often referred to as "the morning after pill" and will be the focus of this chapter.
  - Plan B is a progestin only form of EC that is associated with fewer side effects and better pregnancy prevention (Table 3).

ASSESSMENT

HISTORY

History of Present Illness

- Determine when the teen last had sex. If within the past 5 days, EC can be offered.
- Assess the teen's current birth control methods. Does she primarily use condoms? Is she on any form of hormonal contraception? Failure of these methods is a common reason patients present for EC.
- Did the teen have unprotected sexual intercourse more than 5 days ago? If so, there is a possibility that she may be **pregnant.**

- Does the patient have any vaginal irritation or discharge which may indicate an underlying **sexually transmitted infection (STI)**?

PHYSICAL

- A physical exam should be completed to address any concerns the patient may have; otherwise, a physical or pelvic exam is not necessary to dispense EC.

STUDIES

Pregnancy Test

- A pregnancy test is *NOT* required before taking a progestin-only EC; however, if the patient is in the clinic, obtaining a rapid pregnancy test is quick and easy. If prescribing ella, a pregnancy test is mandatory.
- If negative, it reassures the patient that she is not already pregnant and if positive, it allows the clinic visit to focus on the newly diagnosed pregnancy.
- Teens should obtain a pregnancy test if they do not get their period by 3 to 4 weeks after taking the EC.

Wet Prep (optional)

- If the capability exists (microscope and materials available) consider swabbing vaginal specimen to rule out vaginitis if the patient reports symptoms of vaginal discharge or irritation.

HIV and STI Testing (optional)

- If a teen presents soon after unprotected intercourse, it may be too soon for STI testing to detect exposure; however, consider universal testing on all sexually active teens.

TREATMENT

- EC should be offered when a teen does not want a pregnancy to result from a sexual interaction that occurred in the past 5 days or 120 hours.

- Some clinics like to use protocols and/or consent forms to ensure that proper screening is performed and the teen understands the risks and benefits of the medication. This is usually not necessary.
- Clinics and private offices that see a large volume of teens should consider having EC on site to dispense directly to teens.
- If not available on-site, clinicians should know where teens can go to get EC, which pharmacies carry EC and the approximate cost of the medication.

- Offer preventive counseling.

  - Offer condoms and STI/HIV testing.
  - Discuss starting a regular method of birth control if the patient is not already on one or changing to a different method if the current method is not working out well.
  - Hormonal birth control with the patch, pill or vaginal ring can be started the day after taking a progestin-only EC. Depo-provera can be given immediately.

- EC may be prescribed over the phone with counseling.

  - Clinicians should discuss the importance of regular condom use or abstinence to prevent pregnancy and STIs/HIV.
  - The patient should be encouraged to return to clinic within 3 weeks for STI/HIV testing and to discuss family planning.
  - A pregnancy test may be considered at follow up if needed.

- If the patient vomits within 1–2 hours of taking the EC, consider a repeat dose.
- If the patient was raped, refer to a sexual assault treatment center for appropriate assessment, treatment and counseling.
- Be familiar with your state laws on minor consent and reproductive health services as they vary by jurisdiction. EC may be available over the counter to adolescents 17 years old and above.

DISPOSITION

- Parental consent is not required before prescribing, dispensing or administering EC to teens.

  - However, the teen may want the parent to be involved or may agree to a request by the clinician to include a parent in the discussion.
  - Parental involvement should not occur if it will be detrimental to the teen or if the teen is against it.
  - Dispensing or prescribing EC can remain confidential between the teen and the provider. Providers are encouraged to obtain the consent of the teen before releasing information about reproductive health and family planning to a parent or guardian.

- Communicate clearly with the teen about EC.
  - Remember this is the teen's decision.
  - Remain non-judgmental and do not push the teen into taking EC or discourage its use based on personal rather than medical opinions.
  - Have EC patient education fact sheets in clinic (Table 4).
  - Clinicians should review the most common side effects of EC: nausea, abdominal pain, headache and possible alteration in the next menstrual period.

What is unique about EC and adolescents?

- In the United States, almost 1 million teens or close to 10% of all 15 to 19 year old females become pregnant each year. Most of these pregnancies are not planned.
- Teens may fail to use condoms consistently or correctly.
- Adolescent females may start having sex before they are on a consistent method of contraception and may also not use birth control perfectly.
- Some teens are more likely to engage in risky sexual behaviors that result in unintended pregnancies due to their lack of knowledge about or access to birth control; difficulty negotiating condom use; and underlying issues such as past sexual abuse or assault, mental health conditions, and substance use and abuse.
- Adolescents may not know about EC or other forms of birth control or may have misconceptions about EC that need to be dispelled before prescribing (Table 5).
- Education on EC and other forms of birth control should be a part of anticipatory guidance for all adolescents, females and males, during clinic visits.

- EC is an important tool to safely and effectively prevent unintended pregnancies and reduce abortion rates.

TEST YOUR KNOWLEDGE ANSWERS

70. D. Hormonal EC works to prevent pregnancy by preventing ovulation, thickening cervical mucus and affecting the movement of sperm and/or ova through the reproductive tract. While in theory, Plan B could prevent implantation of a fertilized ovum, there is no scientific evidence that this is the case.
71. B. Ulipristal is a selective progesterone reuptake modulator (SPRM) as is mifipristone, also known as RU-486, which is a well known abortifacient. But unlike Mifipristone, ulipristal, or "ella," is not an abortifacient and instead acts by preventing fertilization. It is effective up to 120 hours after unprotected sexual intercourse. Ulipristol should only be administered once during a given menstrual cycle until further safety studies are completed. Some women may experience side effects such as headaches, nausea and abdominal pain but the majority of women do not experience any side effects after its use.

Table 1. EC Timeline.

"Yuzpe" Method	1974	• Off label use of a two-dose burst of oral contraceptive pills containing both estrogen and progesterone, first described by Dr. Albert Yuzpe. • If taken within 72 hours of unprotected sex, reduced risk of pregnancy by approximately 50% to 80%. • High dose of estrogen associated with nausea and vomiting, experienced by approximately 50% and 20% of women, respectively; as a result, anti-emetics were frequently given.
Plan B	1999	A progestin only form of EC available in the U.S.
	2006	The FDA approved over-the-counter (OTC) sales of Plan B to adults, ages 18 and over.
	2009	• The FDA approved a generic form of Plan B, Next Choice, and lowered the age of OTC sales of both to 17 years of age for men and women. • In some states, Plan B and Next Choice are available OTC for teens younger than 17 and teens of any age can be prescribed EC.
Ulipristal Acetate	2010	• A selective progesterone receptor modulator (SPRM), became available in the U.S. under the trade name "Ella" (Table 6). • Its benefits over Plan B are that it is more effective in the prevention of pregnancy and more efficacious in obese adolescents; however, it is associated with some contraindications and precautions.

Table 2. Progestin-Only EC: Mechanism of Action.

EC does...	• Prevent ovulation • Thicken cervical mucus • Have possible effect on the movement of sperm and ova through the uterus
EC does not...	• Prevent implantation • Harm an established pregnancy • Cause an abortion

Table 3. Progestin-Only EC: Levonorgestrel Facts.

Dispensed as...	• Two 0.75 mg tablets or • One 1.5 mg tablet
Available as...	• Plan B • Plan B One Step • Next Choice (generic)
Efficacy	• Approved for up to 72 hours after intercourse. • May be effective for up to 120 hours or 5 days after unprotected intercourse. • Most effective if taken as soon after unprotected intercourse. • If taken within 24 hours of unprotected sex, reduces risk of pregnancy by 95%. • If taken within 3 days of unproteted sex, reduces risk by up to 80%.

Table 4. EC Educational Fact Sheet.

- EC needs to be taken within 120 hours of unprotected sex — the sooner the better!
- Taking EC is a responsible decision if someone does not want to become pregnant after unprotected sex.
- EC is safe and will not harm an existing pregnancy, will not cause an abortion and will not prevent future pregnancies.
- EC may cause some side effects which are normally very mild such as nausea, headache, or stomach pain, and the next period may come earlier or later or be heavier or lighter in flow than normal.
- If you do not get your period in 3 to 4 weeks after taking EC then you should get a pregnancy test.
- EC does not protect from STIs and HIV — using condoms or not having sex at all are the best ways to protect yourself. Get tested for STIs/HIV at least once a year!
- If you are going to continue to be sexually active, being on a regular form of birth control is recommended to prevent future pregnancies.

Table 5. Common EC Misconceptions.

- It's the abortion pill.
- It will prevent future pregnancies.
- It has bad side effects and will make me sick.
- People will judge me and think badly of me if I take EC.
- If I am pregnant, it will hurt the baby.
- My parents will find out.
- Parents misperceive that EC encourages risky sexual behavior.

Table 6. Ulipristal Acetate Facts.

Is a...	• Selective progesterone receptor modulator (SPRM) with agonist, antagonist or partial agonist effects at the progesterone receptor • Synthetic steroid derived from 19-norprogesterone
Dispensed as...	• 30 mg tablet
Available as...	• "Ella"
Mechanism of action...	• Inhibit or delay ovulation by suppressing growth of follicles and inhibiting follicle rupture • MAY (but unproven) alter endometrial lining, which may inhibit implantation of trophoblast; however, this is considered unlikely at this low dose
Efficacy...	• Works up to 5 days after it is taken
Is not...	• Mifepristone (RU-486) which is chemically different although also a SPRM
Side effects...	• Headaches (18–19%) • Nausea (12–13%) • Abdominal pain (8–15%) • Dysmenorrhea (7–13%) • Fatigue (6%) • Dizziness (5%)
Contraindications...	• Don't use more than once in a menstrual cycle until further safety studies are done • Known or suspected pregnancy (test for pregnancy before administering) • Breastfeeding • Hepatic impairment • Severe asthma insufficiently controlled by glucocorticoids • Rare hereditary problems of galactose intolerance, Lapp Lactose deficiency or glucose-galactose malabsorption
Medication interactions...	• Reduced efficacy if taken with medications that increase gastric pH such as antacids, proton pump inhibitors or H2 receptor antagonists • Reduced plasma concentrations if taken with CYP3A4 inducer such as rifampicin, phenytoin, phenobarbital, carbamazepine, ritonavir, or St John's wort/*Hypericum perforatum*
versus Plan B...	• Recent studies suggest this form of EC is better in preventing pregnancy • The risk of pregnancy increases as body mass index increases regardless of form of EC used; studies suggest ulipristal may be more efficacious than Plan B in obese or overweight women

WEB REFERENCES

- Access to emergency contraception. Committee Opnion No. 542. American College of Obstetricians and Gynecologists. Obstet Gynecol 2012; 120: 1250–1253, retrieved from http://www.acog.org/Resources_And_Publications/Committee_Opinions/Committee_on_Health_Care_for_Underserved_Women/Access_to_Emergency Contraception
- Committee on Adolescence. 'American Academy of Pediatrics Policy Statement on EC', Pediatrics. 2012 Dec 1; 130(6): 1174-1182, retrieved from http://pediatrics.aappublications.org/content/130/6/1174.full?sid=88f35506-8609-4469-b94e-66b47fd56ba7
- Gold MA, Sucato GS, Conard LA, Hillard PJA. 'Provision of emergency contraception to adolescents: Position paper of the society of adolescent medicine', Journal of Adolescent Health. 2004 July; 35(l): 66–70, retrieved from http://www.jahonline.org/article/S1054-139X(04)00120-X/fulltext
- Guttmacher Institute State Policies in Brief: Emergency Contraception (2013), retrieved from http://www.guttmacher.org/statecenter/spibs/spib_EC.pdf

Additional Clinician and Patient Resources:

- International Consortium for Emergency Contraception (includes Country to country information including availability): http://www.cecinfo.org/what-is-ec/general-information/
- Plan B Website: http://www.planbonestep.com
- The Emergency Contraception Website by the Office of Population Research at Princeton University and by the Association of Reproductive Health Professionals: http://ec.princeton.edu/
- To find an EC provider:
  - http://ec.princeton.edu/providers/
  - 1-888-NOT-2-LATE (1-888-668-2528)
- For information on "ella":
  - http://www.fda.gov/NewsEvents/Newsroom/PressAnnouncements/ucm222428.htm
  - http://www.plannedparenthood.org/files/PPFA/fact-ella-EC.pdf
  - http://ec.princeton.edu/news/Glasier%202010%20-%20UPA.pdf
- For information about the legal aspects of reproductive health services (including EC), see the following links:
  - Center for Adolescent Health and the Law: http://www.cahl.org
  - Guttmacher Institute: http://www.guttmacher.org/index.html

49

TEEN PREGNANCY AND OPTIONS COUNSELING

Karen Soren

TEST YOUR KNOWLEDGE

72. Which one of the following statements is true?
    A. Most teens do not use contraception at first intercourse.
    B. Three quarters of teens ages 15–19 years are sexually active.
    C. Teen mothers have the same risk of having a premature baby as older mothers do.
    D. Teens present later for prenatal care than older women.
    E. All the above.
73. Which one of the following statements is true?
    A. In most U.S. states, adolescents need parental consent to start oral contraceptives.
    B. In most U.S. states, a 15 year old can consent for prenatal care.
    C. In all U.S. states, an adolescent requires parental consent to access abortion services.
    D. Adolescent access to prenatal care has worsened over the past decade.
    E. All the above.

Refer to end of chapter for answers on page 531.

A mother brings her 15 year old daughter to your office. The teen is complaining of four days of nausea, intermittent vomiting and dizziness. Mom suspects a "stomach virus" but when the adolescent is questioned alone, she reveals that her last menstrual period was 8 weeks ago…

BACKGROUND

- Every year, approximately 700,000–900,000 U.S. adolescents become pregnant.
- Four out of five teen pregnancies are unintended and 1/3 result in abortion.
- 59% of pregnancies among 15–19 year olds end in live births.

RISK FACTORS

- Developmental (curiosity, experimentation) and behavioral (impulsivity) factors as well as a sense of invulnerability.
- Limited access to contraceptive services.
- Decreased adherence to contraceptive regimens.
- Lack, or limited knowledge, of reproductive health care rights and fear of disclosure to parents.

ASSESSMENT

HISTORY

- Always consider pregnancy:
  - Only a minority of pregnant teens present with the chief complaint of suspected pregnancy.
  - Many present with vague complaints such as nausea, weight gain, fatigue and back pain.
  - If a teen presents with vague symptoms, it may be helpful to ask: "Is there any chance that you may be pregnant?"

Sexual History

- It is important to ask questions during both routine and sick adolescent visits.
- If a teen is sexually active, elicit date of last unprotected intercourse.

Menstrual History

- Determine the date of last menstrual period (LMP), asking specifically about the first day of menses.
- Most pregnant teens will report a "late period," many do not keep track of their periods, and others have irregular periods at baseline.
- Some teens may mistake implantation bleeding (usually of shorter duration than regular menses) for normal menses.
- Pregnancy can be a cause of secondary amenorrhea among adolescents who deny having had sexual intercourse.

Medications

- Teens on hormonal therapy (i.e. depo-provera, combined contraceptive pills, etc.) may have amenorrhea or spotting, lower abdominal cramping, breast tenderness or weight changes.
- Some medicines (i.e. anti-seizure medications and rifampin) can decrease the effectiveness of hormonal contraception. It is important to screen for pregnancy if there is a concern.

Review of Systems

- Presenting symptoms of pregnancy are varied and extensive but can include:
    - Nausea and/or vomiting
    - Fatigue, dizziness and syncope
    - Increased appetite and weight gain
    - Breast tenderness
    - Back pain
    - Mild pelvic cramping. Teens report: "It feels like my period is coming, but nothing happens."

  - Lower abdominal pressure or pain
  - Urinary frequency

- Abdominal discomfort and urinary frequency can be present with **urinary tract infections** and can occur concurrently with pregnancy.
- **Pseudocyesis**, the false belief that one is pregnant, is rare in adolescents, although many teens with late periods who are NOT pregnant can report "feeling pregnant."

PHYSICAL

Vital Signs

- If there is a history of persistent nausea and vomiting (hyperemesis gravidarum), check hydration status (tachycardia, dry mucus membranes).

Breasts

- If breast discomfort is a presenting symptom, a breast exam will usually reveal diffuse fullness and mild tenderness, without focal lesions.

Abdomen

- Abdominal exam is usually unremarkable in early pregnancy; however, teens can present in their second and third trimesters, so check for "lower abdominal mass" and determine fundal height (Table 1).

Pelvic Exam

- A speculum and/or a bimanual exam are important in a teen who presents with symptoms of an **ectopic pregnancy**, such as lower abdominal pain (usually unilateral), vaginal spotting or bleeding.
- A bimanual exam can help determine the stage of gestation and can direct options counseling.

Skin

- **Melasma or chloasma**, or increased facial hyperpigmentation, can occur as a result of the hormonal changes of pregnancy which lead to an increase in melanin production.

STUDIES

Urine Human Chorionic Gonadotropin (Qualitative Urine hCG)

- Most offices can run a urine pregnancy test.
- There are now many low-cost highly sensitive tests available that are easy to use and give positive results in less than a few minutes.
- Most urine tests turn positive around 10 to 14 days after conception, when the concentration of hCG reaches between 20 and 50 mlU/ml.

Serum Pregnancy Tests (Quantitative)

- Usually positive 3–4 days after conception (at 1 to 5 mlU/ml of hCG).

STI Screening: Urine for Gonorrhea and Chlamydia

- Chlamydia is a common cause of 1st term spontaneous abortions.

Pelvic Ultrasound

- Can help determine if a pregnancy is intrauterine and viable.
- Can date a pregnancy, especially if the last menstrual period is unknown, there is irregular menstrual bleeding, or if the adolescent was using hormonal contraception.
- Consider if an ectopic pregnancy is in the differential diagnosis (the adolescent will present with a positive pregnancy test, pain, spotting and/or vaginal bleeding).

Transvaginal Ultrasound

- Preferred early in pregnancy and can detect the:
  - Gestational sac at 4.5 to 5 weeks of gestation
  - Yolk sac at 5 weeks of gestation
  - Heartbeat at 5.5 to 6 weeks of gestation

TREATMENT

Before obtaining a pregnancy test, it can be helpful to ask a possibly pregnant teen: "If you are pregnant, what will you do? Who will you tell?"

- The majority of adolescent pregnancies (82%) are unplanned.
- Teens trying to conceive will be happy with the diagnosis.
- Others, having suspected a pregnancy, had a positive test at home and present to the clinician for confirmation and options counseling.
- Some teens become extremely distraught when told they are pregnant and it is helpful to be prepared in such circumstances. If available, a social worker, health educator or psychologist can provide additional counseling in these cases.
- A follow up visit scheduled soon after diagnosis can also be helpful to discuss options or aid in the disclosure process to a partner or family member.

Once a Pregnancy is Established,

Determine gestation:

- You can use the LMP to give a rough guideline of gestation.
- Perform a pelvic examination if dates are uncertain or there are concerning symptoms.
- Obtain an ultrasound if gestational age is uncertain, you cannot do an examination or if the exam is unreliable, especially if the teen is considering termination.

Rule out ectopic pregnancy.

- Consider if the teen presents with pain and/or spotting or bleeding.
- Refer to the emergency room for urgent gynecologic assessment if ectopic pregnancy is suspected.
- If uncertain, obtain a serum hCG and ultrasound and consider urgent assessment.

DISPOSITION

Options Counseling:

- Multiple factors affect a teen's decision about whether to continue a pregnancy to term including personal belief system, family and peer support, relationship with the father of the pregnancy, education level and financial status.

- Counsel about the options: continuing the pregnancy to term (this usually implies the teen will raise the child, often with family or partner support), keeping the pregnancy and giving the child up for adoption (few teens do this) and accessing abortion services.
- If you do not feel comfortable doing options counseling, refer your patient to someone who can, such as a colleague, social worker or an agency that specializes in young women's reproductive health care services.

Working with the Adolescent and her Family:

- Privately discuss the diagnosis of pregnancy with the teen, provide options counseling, and then assess next steps.
- The teen may need support at this visit; if possible, involve a social worker.
- Often, the teen will not be ready to make a decision about the pregnancy at the initial visit, especially if she has not anticipated the diagnosis.
- Determine who the pregnant teen will tell about the pregnancy (i.e. boyfriend, parent(s), sister or friend).
- If the teen asks you to help tell a parent, be there as a supporting professional. Depending on the family's beliefs, you can guide the conversation and answer questions about available options.
- If she chooses not to tell her parent(s) about the pregnancy, by law, you have to respect her confidentiality. However, if she does not keep her follow-up appointments, you should counsel that confidentiality may be broken if she poses a threat to herself or others.
- Other exceptions to maintaining confidentiality include the scenarios where the pregnancy is the result of sexual abuse, or if the teen has significant developmental delay.

If the Teen Chooses to Continue the Pregnancy to Term:

- Refer for prenatal care and encourage the teen to make a timely appointment-the sooner the initial evaluation, the lower the rate of maternal and fetal complications.
- Review medications being taken and stop those that are teratogenic; consider replacing with safer alternatives.
- Prescribe prenatal vitamins with at least 800 micrograms of folic acid.
- Provide anti-smoking and substance abuse counseling.

- Counsel about eliminating or limiting caffeine from the diet.
- Counsel about maintaining a healthy, well-balanced nutrition plan.
- Screen for sexually transmitted infections including HIV.
- Refer for genetic counseling if the patient is high-risk (has a chronic disease or family history of genetic disorders).

Adolescent Abortion:

- In the United States, laws regarding minors' access to abortion services vary.
- Currently, 36 states require some form of parental involvement for an abortion, either parental notification or consent.
- Few states require the involvement of two parents.
- States requiring parental involvement do have an alternative process in which a minor may seek a judicial bypass to obtain an abortion without parental involvement.
- In many states, minors are permitted to seek an abortion under medical emergency circumstances or in cases of abuse, neglect, incest or assault.
- Access to abortion services varies by region in the United States.
- An adolescent who lives in or near a metropolitan area may be able to access abortion services more easily than an adolescent who lives in a rural area.

Medical Abortion:

- A medical abortion can be performed when gestation is less than 9 weeks.
- Mifepristone, is given in the office and is used to end the pregnancy.
- A second medication, misoprostol, is usually taken by the patient at home after the office visit. It can be swallowed, placed inside the cheek to dissolve, or placed inside the vagina.
- The misoprostol causes bleeding and contractions, resulting in shedding of the uterine lining and expulsion of the pregnancy.

Surgical Abortion:

- Surgical abortion refers to methods that involve instrumentation to end the pregnancy.
- Most first trimester (up to 13 weeks) abortions are done via suction and curettage, a minor surgical procedure sometimes referred to as dilation and curettage.

- Abortions performed after the first trimester (14–24 weeks) are usually done by dilation and evacuation; some may be done as 2-day procedures.

Follow-up:

- If the teen needs time to think about her pregnancy decision, make sure to schedule her for follow up, to ensure that she does not ignore the issue.
- Many providers choose to see the teen for a post-termination follow-up visit.
- Make sure to address contraception, either at this visit or at the post-abortion visit.

What is unique about pregnancy during adolescence?

- Many pregnant teens have no symptoms at all! Adolescents' bodies are changing, and many teens do not even know what is normal for them.
- Teens who are pregnant, especially young ones, may be in denial about the possibility of pregnancy.
- Teens may not feel comfortable sharing news of their pregnancy with family members. The clinician's role is often to help facilitate that discussion, as a supporting, nonjudgmental professional.

TEST YOUR KNOWLEDGE ANSWERS

72. D. Several studies have shown that pregnant teens present later for prenatal care than older women. Of particular concern, pregnant pre-teens and young teens enroll even later in prenatal care than older adolescents. In the United States, most sexually experienced teenagers report using a condom at first intercourse (66% of females and 71% of males), and 94% of adolescent females report having used a condom sometime during their lifetime. In 2007, surveys showed that 47.8% of adolescents ages 15–19 reported having had sex at least once. The average age of sexual debut was age 17, with 13% of teenagers reporting having sex by the age of 15. By 19 years, 7 in 10 adolescents report having engaged in sexual intercourse. Teen mothers experience a higher incidence of pregnancy-induced hypertension, preeclampsia, preterm birth, and anemia than

older mothers. In addition to being more likely to be born premature, infants of teen mothers have a higher risk of low birth weight.

73. B. In most states, a teen is able to consent for prenatal care and care for their child. Currently, 26 states and the District of Columbia have laws that explicitly state that minors may consent to contraceptive services, and in all states, minors may consent to services for screening and treatment of sexually transmitted infections. Teen access to abortion services varies by state. Presently, 34 states require parental notification or consent for abortion, although a judicial bypass is possible if a teen does not want her parents to know. Access to prenatal health care services has improved for teens in the United States in the last two decades, with a notable decrease in the rates of late or no prenatal care when Medicaid expanded funding for pregnant women.

Table 1. Dating Gestation by Physical Examination

Date of Gestation	Fundal Height on Abdominal Examination	Size of Uterus on Pelvic Examination
6–8 weeks		Small pear
8–10 weeks		Orange
10–12 weeks		Grapefruit
Over 12 weeks	At the pubic symphysis	
16 weeks	Midway between pubic symphysis and umbilicus	
20 weeks	At the umbilicus	

WEB REFERENCES

- Center for Disease Control and Prevention. 'Vital Signs: Repeat Births Among Teens-United States, 2007–2010', MMWR 2013 April 5; 62(13): 249–255, retrieved from http://www.cdc.gov/mmwr/preview/mmwrhtml/mm6213a4.htm?scid=mm6213a4w
- Guttmacher Institute, Facts on American Teens Sexual and Reproductive Health, retrieved from: http://www.guttmacher.org/pubs/FB-ATSRH.html

Additional Clinician and Patient Resources:

- American Congress of Obstetricians and Gynecologists, Tool Kit for Teen Care (2nd Edition): Pregnancy Options (2009), retrieved from http://www.acog.org/~/media/Departments/Adolescent%20Health%20Care/Teen%20Care%20Tool%20Kit/PregnancyOptions.pdf?dmc=l&ts=20130409T2113430052
- Center for Young Women's Health, Boston Children's Hospital. Teen Pregnancy (last updated 6/4/2010), retrieved from http://www.youngwomenshealth.org/pregnancy.html
- Centers for Disease Control and Prevention, Teen Pregnancy, retrieved from http://www.cdc.gov/TeenPregnancy/
- healthychildren.org, Teen Pregnancy (last updated 1/2/2013), retrieved from http://www.healthychildren.org/English/ages-stages/teen/dating-sex/Pages/Teenage-Pregnancy.aspx
- National Adolescent and Young Adult Health Information Center: http://nahic.ucsf.edu/
- Planned Parenthood, Info for Teens: Pregnancy, retrieved from http:// www.plannedparenthood.org/info-for-teens/pregnancy-33811.asp
- Physicians for Reproductive Choice and Health: www.prch.org
- Young Men's Health, Boston Children's Hospital, Becoming a Father (last updated 6/28/2010), retrieved from http://www.youngmenshealthsite.org/teen_fatherhood.html

SECTION IV

URGENT CARE

50

HEAT EXHAUSTION AND HEAT STROKE

Noel V. Pesce

TEST YOUR KNOWLEDGE

74. What are the first signs of heat exhaustion?
    A. Dizziness, muscle cramps, sweeting and nausea.
    B. Headaches followed by syncope.
    C. Tachycardia followed by seizures.
    D. A and B
    E. All the above

75. What can be done to prevent heat exhaustion or heat stroke?
    A. Stay hydrated with ice cold beers.
    B. Wear tight fitting clothing.
    C. Avoid strenuous activity during a hot and humid day.
    D. Take a daily antihistamine.
    E. Apply sun tan lotion 20 minutes before sun exposure.

Refer to end of chapter for answers on page 544.

Heat Exhaustion

A 16 year old athlete just started training for the upcoming football season on an especially hot day with a reported high of 98°F and relative humidity of 60%. One hour into practice, he complains of dizziness and is sweating profusely. He only took one water break and now complains of muscle cramps and extreme fatigue.

BACKGROUND

- Heat exhaustion is a state in which the body overheats due to weather with high temperatures (with or without high humidity) and strenuous physical activity.
- Impaired cooling mechanisms lead to a raised core body temperature not exceeding 104°F.
- Although preventable, heat exhaustion can progress to life threatening heat stroke.

RISK FACTORS

- **Hot humid weather:** sweat is unable to evaporate appropriately to cool the body.
- **Dehydration.**
- **Alcohol use** can adversely affect temperature regulation.
- **Overdressing.**
- **Medications** such as beta blockers, diuretics and antihistamines.
- **Illicit drugs** such as ecstasy and cocaine.
- **Obesity:** increased fat retains heat.
- **Sudden temperature changes:** inadequate time to acclimatize to higher temperatures.

ASSESSMENT

<u>HISTORY</u>

History of Present Illness

- Ascertain onset and duration of symptoms. These may present acutely or develop gradually, presenting several days after heat exposure.

- Rule out viral or bacterial infections. Were there symptoms before exposure to heat?

Medications

- Obtain a history of over-the-counter and prescription medications: antipsychotics, tranquilizers, diuretics, beta blockers, and antihistamines.
- Ask about illicit drug use: ecstasy, amphetamines and cocaine can result in hyperthermia.

Review of Systems

The teen may be disoriented at presentation and unable to answer questions. Red flags for heat exhaustion include:

- heavy sweating
- dizziness
- fatigue
- muscle cramps
- nausea
- headaches
- dark colored urine

PHYSICAL

Vital signs

- Elevated body temperature, tachycardia with weak pulse and low standing blood pressure are consistent with heat exhaustion.

Skin

- May be cool and moist with noticeable goose bumps in heat.

STUDIES

- Laboratory tests are not necessary unless indicated by a history and exam that are not consistent with the diagnosis.
- Consider alcohol and drug testing if the teen appears altered.

TREATMENT

It is important to recognize the symptoms of heat exhaustion and begin treatment on the field. Provide emergent care if the teen is disoriented, confused or if seizures occur.

On the field:

- Rest in a cool place (i.e. air-conditioned building or shaded area).
- Drink cool fluids that are caffeine or alcohol free.
- Apply cool water to the skin.
- Spray the body with cool water, soak in a cool bath, pond or stream, or apply damp sheets to the body.
- Loosen or remove excess clothing.

In the emergency room:

- The primary aim is to lower the core body temperature. This can be accomplished via:
  - Cold water immersion
  - Misting the skin
  - Use of fans, ice packs or cooling blankets
- Fluid resuscitation via intravenous hydration may be required.

PREVENTION

- Educate coaches and athletes of the dangers of heat exhaustion and key prevention techniques.
- Avoid strenuous activity in the heat: perform only low intensity exercise if there are plans to be active more than 15 minutes.
- Avoid hot spots (i.e. sitting in a parked car).
- Give the body time to acclimate to the heat. Up to 2 weeks may be necessary (Table 1).
- Seek a cooler environment when the weather gets hot.
- Stay hydrated: athletes should drink plenty of fluids before sports participation and at regularly scheduled intervals during activity.

- Wear loose fitting, lightweight, light-colored clothing limited to a single layer, especially since athletes often wear additional protective equipment.
- Avoid sunburn by covering up and using sunscreen.
- Use caution when taking certain medications: vasoconstrictors, beta blockers, diuretics, antidepressants, antipsychotics and amphetamines can affect the ability to stay hydrated.

Heat Stroke

BACKGROUND

- A life-threatening medical condition in which the brain's cooling system stops working and the internal body temperature rises to the point where brain damage or damage to other internal organs may result.
- Occurs with the escalation of heat cramps and heat exhaustion. Core body temperatures may reach 104°F (40°C) or greater.
- Extreme environmental conditions can lead to ***nonexertional heatstroke.***
- Strenuous activity can lead to ***exertional heatstroke.***

RISK FACTORS

- **Increased exposure to heat:** lack of air conditioning and increased time spent outdoors on hot, humid days.
- **Poor hydration:** decreased fluid intake and/or alcohol use.
- **Poor temperature regulation:** impaired ability to sweat, intolerance to hot weather and excess clothing that prohibit sweat evaporation.
- **Medications:** such as vasoconstrictors, beta blockers, diuretics, antidepressants, antipsychotics, stimulants and sympathomimetics (e.g. decongestants).
- **Obesity:** increased fat retains heat.
- **Underlying medical conditions** such as cardiovascular disease.

ASSESSMENT

HISTORY

History of Present Illness

As with heat exhaustion, teens may be disoriented and unable to provide appropriate history. Red flags for diagnosis include the following signs and symptoms:

- Lack of sweating
- Flushed skin
- Muscle cramps
- Weakness
- Headache
- Dizziness
- Neurological Symptoms: seizures, loss of consciousness, hallucinations, confusion and difficulty speaking

- What was the teen doing before onset of symptoms?

PHYSICAL

Vital Signs

- High body temperature (104°F or higher), tachypnea and tachycardia with a strong pulse may be present.
- If untreated or if urgent medical care is delayed, the teen may develop hemodynamic shock (very low blood pressure, blue lips and nails, cool and clammy skin), organ and/or brain damage from edema and death.

STUDIES

Electrolytes and Blood Gases

- Assess for kidney function and CNS damage.
- Send creatine phosphokinase (CPK) to check for rhabdomyolysis.

Urinalysis

- Assess urine color as dark urine may reflect kidney damage or muscle breakdown.

- A "positive blood" result on dipstick may indicate myoglobinuria or hemoglobinuria. Further testing is necessary to differentiate.
- Specific gravity indicates the degree of dehydration.
- Dehydration will often present with abnormal urinary sediment.

TREATMENT

- This is a medical emergency requiring immediate medical attention.
- Depending on the level of cognition and extent of injury, CPR may be warranted with aggressive IV hydration, especially if rhabdomyolysis is also suspected.
- Goal is to rapidly cool the body to prevent or reduce damage to the brain or other vital organs.
    - Immerse in cold water (this can restrict access to body for IV insertion or CPR).
    - Initiate evaporation cooling techniques: mist the body with cool water and then fan with warm air to evaporate the water on the skin.
    - Pack with ice and use cooling blankets.
    - Administer muscle relaxants to stop the body from shivering.
- Take steps to prevent heat exhaustion (refer to prior section on Heat Exhaustion).

What is unique about heat exhaustion and heat stroke in adolescents?

- Heat illness during practice or competition is a leading cause of disability and death among U.S. high school athletes.
- These are preventable conditions that most commonly occur in August during preseason practice and football players are most at risk.
- Adolescents are less likely to complain during sports, out of concern that they will appear weak, so it is often up to coaches to ensure that athletes are safe on the field.
- Primary prevention strategies involve implementation of acclimatizing periods as well as proper hydration before, during, and after strenuous activity.
- The National Athletic Trainers' Association recommends a 14-day acclimatization period.

- It is recommended that athletes consume 200–300 mL every 10–20 minutes during exercise to ensure appropriate fluid replacement.
- Secondary prevention strategies are vital to prevent the progression of heat illness. This involves removal from activity, rehydration and various cooling techniques.

TEST YOUR KNOWLEDGE ANSWERS

74. A. On a hot day, a patient who presents with dizziness, muscle cramps, sweating and nausea may have heat exhaustion. These early signs should not be ignored and treatment should be initiated immediately.
75. C. The best strategy to prevent heat illness is to avoid strenuous activity during hot and humid days. Hydration should be with water or sports drinks. Alcohol leads to dehydration. Clothing should be loose and light in weight and color. Medications that have anticholinergic effects can interfere with the body's thermoregulatory actions and increase the risk of heat stroke. Sun block, not sun tan lotion, prevents sunburns.

Table 1. Acclimating to the heat.*

Intensity	Low intensity physical activity if lasting more than 15 minutes.
Fluids	Athletes should drink plenty of fluids before practice and at regular beverage breaks.
Clothing	Limit to single layer of light-colored, lightweight material. Consider limiting protective equipment as well

*For specific guidelines, refer to the seven key recommendations for a 14-day heat-acclimatization period from the National Athletic Trainers' Association.

WEB REFERENCES

- Armstrong LE, *et al.* 'Position Stand: Exertional Heat Illness during Training and Competition', American College of Sports Medicine. Medicine & Science in Sports & Exercise. 2007: 556–572, retrieved from http://esef.com.ar/Material%20did%C3%A1ctico/Salud%20y%20condicion%20fisica/0307.pdf

- Centers for Disease Control and Prevention. 'Heat Illness Among High School Athletes-United States, 2005–2009', MMWR. 2010 August 20; 59(32): 1009–1013, retrieved from http://www.cdc.gov/mmwr/preview/mmwrhtml/mm5932al.htm?s_cid=mm5932al_w
- Council On Sports Medicine and Fitness and Council on School Health. 'Policy Statement: Climatic Heat Stress and Exercising Children and Adolescents', Pediatrics. 2011 August 8; 128(3): e741–e747, retrieved from http://www.pediatricsdigest.mobi/content/128/3/e741.full
- Howe AS, Boden BR. 'Heat-Related Illness in Athletes', The American Journal of Sports Medicine. 2007; 35(8): 1384–1395, retrieved from https://pedclerk.uchicago.edu/sites/pedclerk.uchicago.edu/files/uploads/heat.pdf
- National Athletic Trainers' Association: Preseason Heat Acclimitization Guidelines for Secondary School Athletics, retrieved from http://www.nata.org/health-issues/heat-acclimatization

Additional Clinician And Patient Resources:

- Emedicine Health, Heat Exhaustion and Heat Stroke, retrieved from http://www.emedicinehealth.com/heat_exhaustion_and_heat_stroke/article_em.htm
- Heat Index: http://www.newnan.cc/weather/charts.html
- Mayo Clinic, Heat Exhaustion (updated August 12, 2010), retrieved from http://www.mayoclinic.com/health/heat-exhaustion/DS01046

51

SYNCOPE

Rick Place

TEST YOUR KNOWLEDGE

76. Most adolescents with syncope, that is not obviously otherwise explainable (e.g. standing in church on a hot day), should get

    A. An EKG
    B. A CT scan of the brain
    C. An EEG
    D. A CBC
    E. None of the above

77. Which of the following conditions is the *MOST* common cause of syncope in adolescents?

    A. Brugada syndrome
    B. Wolff-Parkison White
    C. Prolonged QT interval
    D. Hypertrophic cardiomyopathy
    E. None of the above

Refer to end of chapter for answers on page 554.

A 14 year old girl presents to the office after a fainting episode. She had myalgias and a low grade fever the evening before. After getting up in the morning, she walked out of her bedroom and passed out in the hallway.

BACKGROUND

- Syncope, or fainting, is defined as a transient loss of consciousness (LOC) with a lifetime risk approaching 50%.
- While syncope is an uncommon event in childhood, it becomes much more common in the teen years; the incidence during adolescence may exceed 10%.
- Syncope is rarely serious but there are circumstances where syncope may be a sentinel event pointing to an underlying life-threatening problem that if unrecognized, could result in sudden death.
- Families are often very concerned as the perceived risk of a serious underlying cause is high.
- There are many different causes of syncope but the predominant cause is neurocardiogenic (Table 1).
- Inappropriate emphasis is often placed on the central nervous system, most likely because the symptomatic expression of syncope is neurologic, but CNS causes of syncope are uncommon, particularly in adolescence.
- Syncope results from a decrease in cerebral perfusion. This can be the result of a rhythm disturbance (i.e. tachycardia, bradycardia) or profoundly decreased peripheral vascular resistance (hypotension).

ASSESSMENT

HISTORY

History of Present Illness

- The presence of premonitory symptoms (dizziness, visual changes, nausea, slight diaphoresis and/or weakness) prior to the syncopal event helps distinguish **benign neurocardiogenic syncope** from potentially lethal **cardiac syncope.**

- Determine the circumstances or context of the event: syncope while getting blood drawn is very different from syncope during exercise.
- Determine the patient's position at the time of syncopal event: syncope while sitting or supine is of greater concern than fainting that occurs after rising from a seated position or prolonged standing.
- The sensation of palpitations prior to the event is neither sensitive nor specific but should be asked. Did the patient experience shortness of breath, or other symptoms that suggest **hyperventilation syndrome** (i.e. dizziness, tingling or coldness of hands/feet/mouth, fast heart beat)?
- Observation can often distinguish between common myoclonic jerks experienced with the syncopal and seizure activity. The convincing absence of a postictal period is an important consideration. If not seen, a description by a reliable witness can be helpful.

Past Medical History

- A history of previous syncopal episode and resultant evaluation should be explored.
- Does the patient have a known medical condition that could explain the syncopal episode?
- Ask adolescent females about date of last menstrual period (pregnant?) and assess details of menstrual history including severity of flow and duration of bleeding to determine amount of monthly menstrual blood loss.
- Other causes of possible chronic blood loss should be noted (e.g. inflammatory bowel disease or other hematologic conditions).

Family History

- Family history is important: families may not be aware of a genetic disorder, but sudden death at a relatively young age of any close family is of great concern.

Medications

- Assess current medication use as many drugs cause **prolonged QT** and may place certain patients at risk of malignant **arrhythmias.**

Review of Systems

- Concurrent medical conditions such as a gastroenteritis may predispose patients to dehydration and orthostatic instability.
- **Febrile infectious illnesses** such as influenza, hepatitis, infectious mononucleosis, etc. can all induce fainting.
- A thorough review of symptoms may suggest less common precipitating conditions.

PHYSICAL

A complete physical exam is mandatory to assess the presence of suspected or unsuspected underlying **systemic conditions** contributing to the syncopal episode, e.g. influenza, deyhydration, anorexia nervosa, etc.

Vital Signs

- Relative (or more pronounced) bradycardia or tachycardia should be noted.
- Orthostatic blood pressures are neither sensitive nor specific and are not routinely recommended. This value may be more useful if measured when a patient is symptomatic (e.g. dizzy) during the test.

General Appearance

- Is the patient healthy appearing? Cachectic (**anorexia**)? Pale (**anemia**)? Chronically ill appearing? Most adolescents with **vasovagal syncope** will appear normal.

HEENT

- Examination of the **conjunctiva** for pallor may be useful for identifying the presence of **anemia**.

Cardiac Exam

- The presence of murmurs may suggest critical conditions such as **aortic stenosis** or **idiopathic hypertrophic cardiomyopathy**.

- The murmur will *increase* in intensity for maneuvers that *decrease* ventricular blood volume, i.e. straining, Valsalva maneuver or standing (decreases preload or blood return).
- The murmur will *decrease* with maneuvers that *increase* ventricular blood volume, i.e. squatting (increases afterload).
- These changes occur because increased blood volume "stents" and reduces the outflow obstruction to some degree, decreasing the intensity of the murmur.

Neurologic Exam

- A thorough exam is important to exclude a neurologic etiology (and the need for neuroimaging).

STUDIES

Laboratory testing is NOT routinely indicated for the majority of syncopal episodes.

Rapid Serum Glucose

- Consider testing, especially in diabetic patients.

Complete Blood Count

- Can confirm anemia based on history and exam, and may determine the need for transfusion.

Basic Metabolic Panel

- Is frequently a part of a standard blood "screen" but is not useful in the primary evaluation of syncope.
- It may have a role in the context of an underlying systemic illness (e.g. renal insufficiency, Addison's disease).

Toxicology Screen

- These studies are expensive and rarely yield valuable and actionable information unless abuse is a specific concern.

Urine Pregnancy Test

- Should always be a consideration in the adolescent female.

Electrocardiography (EKG)

- An EKG is THE critical test in the patient with syncope.
- Seeing the offending rhythm is extremely unlikely, but tell-tale signs may exist.
- Evidence of a **prolonged QT interval** should be assessed in every patient.
- An unusual QRS axis or a delta wave (precordial lead V4) may suggest the presence of an accessory conduction pathway (e.g. **Wolff-Parkinson-White Syndrome**).
- Evidence of ventricular hypertrophy and repolarization abnormalities may be found in **hypertrophic cardiomyopathy**
- **Brugada syndrome** is diagnosed by a characteristic EKG pattern in the precordial leads that confirm that the adolescent is at risk for sudden death.

Electroencephalogram (EEG)

- Consider when there is uncertainty about distinguishing the myoclonic jerks commonly associated with syncopal events from a seizure disorder.

SPECIAL TESTS

Imaging studies are generally NOT indicated in syncope.

Echocardiogram (Echo)

- Indicated in teens with evidence of ventricular hypertrophy on screening EKG, with an abnormal exam (i.e. murmur) or concerning history (e.g. exertional syncope).
- If there is concern for cardiomyopathy or valvular abnormalities.

Continuous Holter Monitor

- Can be placed to assess for intermittent arrhythmias that may not be otherwise identified.

Tilt Table Studies

- May be performed in adolescents with recurrent vasovagal or postural syncopal episodes.
- Some individuals have an exaggerated response to postural changes.

The decision to conduct an Echo, Holter or Tilt table study are generally made in coordination with the cardiology consultant.

Computerized Tomography (or rarely MRJ) of the head

- May be indicated if a neurologic etiology is suspected (for instance, if seizure activity accompanies the syncopal event).
- CT may be indicated if there is significant head trauma associated with the syncopal event.

DISPOSITION

- The vast majority of syncopal episodes in adolescents are benign vasovagal or orthostatic events that can be confidently diagnosed on history and physical. In the absence of recurrent events, these do not require referral to a sub-specialist.
- Cardiology consultation is warranted for patients with recurrent syncope or those with concerning historical features, such as an abnormal physical examination or EKG.
- After initial evaluation, exercise restriction may be indicated before cardiology consultation in patients who are thought to be at risk for cardiac syncope.
- Neurology consultation is generally unnecessary but may be indicated if there is a concern that the event may be seizure related.
- Unlike adults, admission for adolescents is generally unnecessary since continuous cardiac monitoring is rarely indicated.
- Exceptions to this are possible, e.g. a run of ventricular tachycardia on EKG or recurrent syncopal events in a single day.

What is unique about syncope in adolescents?

- Syncope is a very common event.
- The vast majority of syncopal episodes in adolescents are benign and are not cardiac in nature, in contrast to older patients in whom ischemic heart disease may manifest as syncope or sudden death.
- Adolescents are rarely at risk for uncommon but life-threatening conditions. A careful history and physical exam and focused diagnostic testing will identify these patients.

TEST YOUR KNOWLEDGE ANSWERS

76. A. The predominant cause of syncope is neurocardiogenic or vasovagal and tests are not required. However, when the cause is unclear, an EKG is THE critical test for patients with syncope because it could identify a rare cause, such as prolonged QT interval, Brugada syndrome, etc. Imaging studies and EEG are generally not indicated unless a neurologic etiology is suspected, such as concomitant seizures, severe headaches or abnormal findings on neurologic exam.
77. E. Vasovagal syncope is by far the most common cause of syncope.

Table 1. Causes of Syncope in Adolescents.

	Common Causes
Neurocardiogenic or Vasovagal Syncope	Most common cause of syncope in adolescents. Vagally medicated event in which profound parasympathetic activity from the vagus nerve leads to bradycardia and/or hypotension. Reflex may be induced by distressing emotional situations (e.g. blood draws, sudden fright), prolonged standing or fasting. Generally preceded by symptoms of low cerebral blood flow: dizziness, visual changes (dimming of vision, spots), weakness or possibly nausea.
Orthostatic Hypotension	Similar to vasovagal syncope, a condition in which the body fails to adjust to changes in body posture. Normally, the fall in blood pressure when an individual changes position from sitting/ lying to standing is rapidly compensated; this may not happen with postural hypotension. Things that might lead to orthostatic hypotension include fever, prolonged sitting with sudden standing, or a dysfunctional autonomic nervous system.
Postural Orthostatic Tachycardia Syndrome (POTS)	A condition that may result in persistent near-syncopal symptoms or syncope.
	Cardiac Causes
Primary Arrhythmia	Far less common than neurocardiogenic syncope and chronic fatigue.
Prolonged QT Syndrome	Predisposes patients to ventricular tachycardia/fibrillation May result from a genetic channelopathy or medication side effect.
Brugada Syndrome	A heritable channelopathy with a distinctive EKG pattern, predisposing patients to polymorphic ventricular tachycardia.
Catecholaminergic Polymorphous Ventricular Tachycardia	Induced by exercise and another potential cause of syncope or sudden death in this age group.
Wolff-Parkinson-White	Abnormal electrical pathway of the heart that may lead to tachycardia and rarely syncope.
Bradycardia	Less common cause of syncope than the tachyarrhythmias noted above (e.g. anorexia nervosa or heart block).

(*Continued*)

Table 1. (*Continued*)

The most common causes of sudden death in adolescence are arrhythmogenic and the result of (previously unrecognized) structural heart disease.	
Hypertrophic Cardiomyopathy (formerly IHSS) & Anomalous Coronary Artery Insertion	Can lead to ischemia-induced ventricular tachycardia and ventricular fibrillation.
Arrhythmogenic Right Ventricular Dysplasia/ Cardiomyopathy	A rare condition in which myocytes of the right ventricle are replaced by adipose and fibrous tissue.
	Neurologic causes of syncope are uncommon
Basilar Migraine	Presumably from transient brainstem ischemia.
Seizure	Myoclonic jerks are commonly associated with syncopal events and may be difficult to confidently differentiate from seizures based on history alone.
Subarachnoid hemorrhage	The concurrent presence of severe headache may suggest this exceedingly rare cause of isolated syncope.
Miscellaneous Causes	Hyperventilation Conversion Reaction

WEB REFERENCES

- ACC Expert Consensus Document. 'Tilt Table Testing for Assessing Syncope', Journal of American College of Cardiology. 1996 July; 28(l): 263–275, retrieved from http://cardiosource.org/~/media/Images/ACC/Science%20and%20Ouality/Practice%20Guidelines/t/tilt.ashx?w_nav=Search&WT.oss=syncope%20in%20adolescence&WT.oss_r=153&
- Driscoll DJ, *et al.* 'Syncope in Children and Adolescents', Journal of the American College of Cardiology. 1997; 29(5): 1039–1045, retrieved from http://content.onlinejacc.org/article.aspx?articleid=1121664
- McLeod KA. 'Dizziness and syncope in adolescence', Heart. 2001; 86: 350–354, retrieved from http://www.ncbi.nlm.nih.gov/pmc/articles/PMC1729890/pdf/v086p00350.pdf

- Ritter S, *et al.* 'What is the Yield of Screening Echocardiography in Pediatric Syncope', Pediatrics. 2000; 105(5): e58, retrieved from http://www.pediatricsdigest.mobi/content/105/5/e58.full
- Strieper MJ, Auld DO, Hulse JE, Campbell RM. 'Evaluation of Recurrent Pediatric Syncope: Role of Tilt Table Testing', Pediatrics. 1994;93(4):660-662, retrieved from http://pediatrics.aappublications.org/content/93/4/660.abstract
- Wieling W, Ganzeboom KS, Saul JP. 'Reflex syncope in children and adolescents', Heart. 2004 September; 90(9): 1094–1100, retrieved from http://www.ncbi.nlm.nih.gov/pmc/articles/PMC1768435/

Additional Clinician and Patient Resources:

- Children's Memorial Hospital, Initial Workup for Syncope in Children by Sabrina Tsao: http://www.childrensmemorial.org/ce/online/article.aspx?articleID=153
- DukeHealth.org, Advice from Doctors on When Children Faint (last updated on 9/21/2011), retrieved from www.dukehealth.org/health_library/advice_from_doctors/your_childs_health/fainting
- Healthy Children.org, Dizziness and Fainting Spells (last updated 2/27/2013), retrieved from http://www.healthychildren.org

52

CONCUSSION AND POST CONCUSSION SYNDROME

Michael A. Lee

TEST YOUR KNOWLEDGE

78. A 17 year old football running back has a helmet-to-helmet collision to the front of his head with loss of consciousness lasting 5 seconds, retrograde amnesia of 15 minutes and post-traumatic amnesia lasting 30 minutes. This concussion would be classified as a

    A. Mild concussion
    B. Moderate or severe concussion
    C. Grade 1 concussion
    D. Grade 2 or 3 concussion
    E. Concussion

79. Concussion recovery occurs in 80% of the cases within:

    A. 24 hours.
    B. 1 to 3 days.
    C. 1 to 3 weeks.
    D. 1 to 3 months.
    E. 6 months.

Refer to end of chapter for answers on page 574.

"Doctor, my daughter fell from the top of her cheerleading team's pyramid. After the fall, she was dazed. This happened last week and she still has a headache, although it is getting better. Can you clear her? She really wants to get back to practice."

BACKGROUND

- Preteens and adolescents suffer concussions at alarming rates and many go unreported.
- Recently, the public and the medical community have become more aware of the significance and long-term complications of concussions.
- In the past, different guidelines were used and no one guideline or grading system was optimal. Patients were often told to take it easy for a few days and then to return to play.
- Now every concussion is managed individually.
- International concussion conferences in Vienna, Prague and Zurich as well as recent research have changed concepts about concussions such as:
    - Minor head injuries, frequently called bell-ringers or dings, are in fact concussions.
    - Relatively minor head injuries take longer to heal than previously believed.
    - Concussions can occur without loss of consciousness, vomiting or other symptoms.
    - Headache, dizziness, fogginess, poor attention span and unusual behavior are often the only signs of concussions.
    - Cognitive activity, particularly intense or over extended time, can have the same effect on prolonging concussion symptoms and slowing recovery as does physical exertion.
    - The management of ostensibly minor head injuries has changed dramatically. *Restricting mental exertion and physical exertion until asymptomatic and then gradually increasing each is the cornerstone of this new treatment strategy.*

RISK FACTORS

- Not wearing protective equipment.
- Being "taken by surprise."
- Velocity impact.
- Continuing to play after a head injury.
- Being allowed to return to sports too soon before full recovery.

ASSESSMENT

HISTORY

- Assess for symptoms that can occur after a concussion:

Headache:

- Headaches are the most common symptom reported by concussed patients.
- Headaches initially present on awakening and are described as dull and achy but became throbbing with cognitive or physical exertion, light or noise.
- Some patients describe their headaches as feeling pressure.
- Occasionally patients do not report headaches but report lightheadedness as their main concussion symptom.

Sleep Problems:

- Patients may feel tired and want to sleep during the first 24–48 hours, with increased sleep need persisting for several days.
- Patients may have difficulty falling asleep during the 2nd or 3rd week and require melatonin to help regulate sleep cycles.
- Limiting naps after the first two days helps solve this problem.

Feeling "Foggy and Slowed Down":

- This symptom is difficult for patients to understand or describe.
- Teens may feel that their brain is functioning like a dial-up connection to the internet instead of broad band (DSL) or that their brain is like a computer infected with a virus.
- Patients who do not report this symptom after their concussion usually recover rapidly (in less than a week).

- This symptom usually resolves one to two days before the headache disappears and serves as an indicator of when patients will recover.

Lightheadedness and Nausea:

- Patients often confuse lightheadedness with dizziness.
- They feel lightheaded during positional changes (not present before the concussion) or when the headache becomes severe.
- Both lightheadedness and nausea occur when the headache increases after physical or cognitive over-exertion (reading, computer use, text-messaging, etc.).

Dizziness:

- A less common symptom but significant if present.
- It is important to distinguish dizziness from lightheadedness as the patient may have sustained cochlear damage which possibly requires vestibular rehabilitation therapy.
- Spinning movements should be avoided. Teens have reported that their symptoms worsen after riding on spinning carnival rides and they may have a marked increase in symptoms after having chiropractic adjustments to their necks.

Balance Problems:

- Initially, patients may have difficulty with gait (ataxia) or experience balance problems.
- Teens report that their balance is off and that they are unsteady and bump into objects.
- This clinical phenomenon involves proprioception which is the ability to sense where one's body or body part is in relation to the environment.
- These symptoms usually resolve quickly in most patients.

Light and Noise Sensitivity:

- Light, whether from sunlight, bright fluorescent light or from car headlights at night can cause worsening headaches.
- This is usually seen with injuries involving the back of the head.

- Headaches may intensify if exposed to excess noise at home, school or in movie theaters.

Concentration and Memory Loss:

- After experiencing a concussion, many patients are unable to read a paragraph or page of text without an increase in the severity of their headaches.
- Computer use for even five to 10 minutes markedly increases headaches.
- Cognitive concentration increases symptoms and patients report having trouble focusing.
- Some patients cannot remember what was said a few minutes before, or are unable to select the correct word to use in a conversation. They may also lose track of what they were saying mid-sentence.
- Some have difficulty remembering where they put things.
- Working memory and prospective memory are also frequently challenged functions.

No Symptoms:

- There are patients with documented loss of consciousness who have no symptoms following their concussions and yet may take one to two weeks to recover as determined by ImPACT (neuro-cognitive) testing.

PHYSICAL

- A complete neurologic exam should be performed following a concussion.
- A musculoskeletal exam should also be completed as indicated by the nature of injury.

HEENT

- Assess for horizontal nystagmus.
- *Rapid lateral eye and/or head movements (saccades)* leading to complaints of lightheadedness is the most common positive physical finding.
- This finding usually does not resolve until the patient is almost fully recovered (it usually goes away when the sensation of feeling foggy and slow resolves).

Neck

- *Any patient who sustains a concussion should be evaluated for an associated neck injury.*
- Assess for trapezius (upper and/or mid) muscle spasm and tenderness and for loss of range of motion.

Neurologic Exam

- Patients may experience balance problems.
- Patients may have an abnormal Romberg test (unable to balance with one foot in front of the other with eyes closed), have difficulty walking a straight line or walking on their heels.
- Balance difficulties usually resolve rapidly after a few days.

STUDIES

Computerized Tomography Scans and MRIs

- CT scans and MRIs of the head are usually normal in patients with concussions and are not necessary unless the patient exhibits worsening symptoms.

Neurocognitive Testing

- *Decisions to return to play should never be based on neurocognitive testing alone.*
- Neurocognitive testing offers objective evidence about the athlete's brain function.
- When used in conjunction with the history, physical exam and imaging studies, testing can better determine when an athlete is able to return to play.
- There are a variety of tests available such as Headminder, Cogstate, ANAM, ImPACT, etc.
- The most widely used test is ImPACT (Immediate Post-Concussion Assessment and Cognitive Testing) which is presently used by the NFL, NHL, professional baseball, auto racing, international rugby, and many colleges and high schools throughout the US.

Neurocognitive testing with ImPACT

- ImPACT provides objective data to help determine an athlete's injury status. It is a computerized test developed by researchers at the University of Pittsburgh Medical Center and accounts for individual differences in cognitive ability and symptom reporting through baseline testing.
- It can be used without baseline testing because of the large data base that has been accumulated on normal individuals, broken down by age and sex.
- At this time, it is only available for athletes over 11 or 12 years old.
- A comparison of ImPACT testing with fMRI demonstrated that the ImPACT test returns to normal at the same time the fMRI becomes normal. This further validates its use as a tool to manage concussions since there is a clinical correlation between the assessment and functional neuroimaging.
- Normal neurocognitive testing plus the resolution of symptoms and normal physical findings are the determinant variables considered when a concussed patient can return to normal activities and contact sports.
    - Concussion symptoms should have resolved with no significant difference from the baseline test.
    - The ImPACT test results should be normal and the patient should be treatment or medication-free before being allowed to return to contact sports.
    - Extremely low ImPACT test composite scores (low single digits and 1st percentile or less) on all parameters of the test are prognostic indicators that patients might develop post-concussion syndrome.
    - Decreasing serial ImPACT test scores indicate patients not complying with activity restrictions.
- Cognitive fatigue can also be determined through the ImPACT test.
    - Most unrecovered patients develop a worsening headache *while taking the test* (usually 15 minutes into the test).
    - A worsening headache or developing a headache further into the testing or *after taking the test,* is more typical of those patients who are closer to full recovery.

TREATMENT

- Marked by several phases including an initial rest period ("cocoon therapy"), followed by cognitive therapy (before return to school), then a monitored return to school period, culminating in clearance for return to play.
- To help patients recover rapidly, the following protocol has been found to resolve symptoms:

Initial Cocoon Therapy

- Place patients on "cocoon therapy" immediately after the concussion.
  - The patient should sleep in a darkened room for the first 24 to 48 hours and remain isolated from stimulation.
  - Patients are usually willing because they are often tired after their concussion.
- To minimize increased metabolic demands on the injured vulnerable brain cells as well as avoid depleting cerebral-vascular efficiency, student-athletes should not participate in the following activities: school, reading, computer use, videogames, text-messaging, physical exercise, hot tubs, attending team practices or games and socializing with friends.
- Any activity that causes the headache or symptoms to worsen should be discontinued immediately.
  - Attending movies may cause a marked increase in symptoms if the student-athlete has trouble with light or noise.
  - Light sensitive teens should wear sunglasses. Noise should be kept to a minimum.
- After the first couple of days, brief periods (initially 10 to 15 minutes set by a timer) may be spent listening to books-on-tape and if tolerated, TV movies (not cartoons) may be watched.
  - Movies should be watched at 10 to 15 minute intervals, gradually increasing intervals as tolerated.
  - Parents can also read the student's schoolwork to them at 15 minute intervals.
- When this protocol is adhered to, most patients become headache free in five days. Cessation of symptoms can also be achieved in some patients who had their symptoms for a few weeks.

- When patients report lightheadedness and nausea with worsening headaches, they are likely overdoing their activities.
- *The cornerstone of concussion management should be to prevent progression of headaches to those that are throbbing in nature.*
- This protocol does not work for all patients (i.e. those with multiple hits to the head).

Cognitive Exercise Protocol Before to Return to School

- No school initially.
- Concussed adolescents should not return to school until their headaches and other symptoms resolve.
- On the first day that no symptoms or headaches are present, patients may read and use the computer in gradually increasing increments for the 24 hours before they return to school. This helps ensure tolerance to the level of activity they will have to endure in school.
- Advise teens to begin by reading a couple of pages, followed by a break, then doubling the amount of reading every 10 to 15 minutes.
- Teens may alternate reading with computer use (no video game play) starting with 10 minutes and gradually adding 10 minutes.
- When teens report no symptoms with cognitive exercise (an hour on the computer or 1-2 hours doing homework), they can be allowed to attend school with modifications if needed, gradually increasing the amount of time they spend at school as tolerated.
- Guidelines for returning to school should be followed (Table 1).

Monitoring Upon Return to School

- Attending school presents a major problem for student-athletes suffering from a concussion whether it is at the high school or college level.
- Returning the student-athlete to school is the highest priority and is associated with low risks once symptoms have disappeared.
- A school nurse, guidance counselor, certified athletic trainer, athletic staff member, psychologist and/or social worker should be made aware of the student-athlete's injury and should work as a team to coordinate accommodations. This will ensure a smooth transition to activity during an otherwise difficult period.

- Teachers and professors often believe that student-athletes are malingering and may be less understanding when student-athletes are excused from tests, or need extra time for tests and turning in papers.
- Team coaches may fail to understand the severity of the injury and may want their athlete, especially star athletes, to return to play before they are fully recovered.
- Coaches may be unsympathetic to injured student-athlete needs and may be unaware of *Second Impact Syndrome* or more common risks of re-injury with prolonged recovery.
- The absence of visible signs of injury, such as a cast, brace or bandage, contributes to misunderstandings by coaches and others.
- Exercise, whether it is physical or mental, will usually increase a concussed teen's symptoms such as headaches, dizziness, nausea and lightheadedness.

Successful Return to School

<u>Gradual Return</u>

- Teens may return to school for gradually increasing intervals when they can tolerate at least an hour of thinking.
- Rest periods may be necessary when teens first return to school.
- Some teens may require a later start time to allow a longer sleep period at night.
- Teens should be driven to school to avoid noise on the bus or walking to school.
- Teens may attend classes unless they develop symptoms (usually a headache). If they become symptomatic in a class (usually after 15 minutes) they should be allowed to close their eyes or put their head down on the desk for 10 minutes OR go to the nurse's office, lie down, and skip the next period to rest.
- If symptoms occur again in the next period, even after rest, they should return home.
- Initially, math, chemistry and foreign language classes may need to be avoided since they seem to cause more symptoms than other classes.
- If the teen can only attend school part-time, core subjects (English, History, Science and Language) can be taken while non-core classes should be avoided.

Papers, Projects and Homework

- Term papers and projects may need to be delayed and spaced out. Extensions for work should be given.
- Extra time for homework may be necessary.
- Preprinted class notes or copies of classmate's notes are often helpful.
- Audio-text may be helpful for teens with reading difficulty due to their symptoms.
- Having someone read their school work to them may be of benefit. Some teens may need tutors to help them with schoolwork, including test preparation and organization.

Taking Tests

- Most teens are so symptomatic in the early post-injury phase they are unable to take tests.
- If they do attempt to take tests before they have sufficiently recovered, they may become dizzy and nauseous or manifest other post-concussion signs and symptoms that negatively affect their performance.
- If the teen has taken any tests during the time he/she is recovering and received poor test scores, it is appropriate to ask that these grades be voided or discounted.
- SAT, ACT, AP, and GRE tests may need to be postponed and some teens may need to obtain permission for extra time while taking these examinations.
- Final exams may need to be delayed until school breaks, the next semester or the summer.
- When teens return to school, they should take tests after catching up on missed work.
- Teens may require un-timed tests due to their decreased processing speed.
- Tests may need to be spaced out and limited to no more than one per day.
- Tests need to be taken in a quiet place, free of distraction. This is because some post-concussion teens have ADHD-like characteristics such as distractibility or difficulty with concentration and sustained attention.
- Occasionally oral tests or open book tests may be necessary.
- Written responses to multiple choice questions may be helpful to some students.

Exemptions

- Unfortunately, some teens have prolonged symptoms and will need to miss an extended period of school during recovery.
- Teachers should take this into account when assigning grades.
- Possible solutions for this problem include: exempting teens from tests, especially if they have done well previously, or assigning grades for that duration, based on previous work.

Physical Accommodations

Elevators

- Initially, teens should not walk up stairs if there are elevators in the school.
- An elevator pass should be given unless the teen becomes lightheaded or dizzy when riding the elevator.

Noise

- If noise is not well tolerated, teens should be excused from music class.
- It is recommended that teens sit in a quiet spot during lunch (not in the noisy cafeteria) and should avoid assemblies, school dances or sports events.
- It may also be helpful for these teens to leave class a few minutes early to get to the next class and avoid hallway noise between classes.
- Construction noise at school may also increase symptoms.

Light

- Problematic for teens, especially those with injuries to the back of the head.
- Increased symptoms may be caused by bright fluorescent lights, smartboards or movies watched in a dark room.
- Sunglasses may need to be worn in and out of school.
- Teens may have difficulty driving at night due to the glare of headlights.
- Activities with strobe lights should be avoided.

Preferential Seating

- Teens who develop ADHD-type symptoms following their concussions are advised to sit in the front of classrooms and away from windows and doors to avoid distractions.

Gym Class and Team Sports

- Initially, both should be avoided.
- Attending a team's practice or game can increase symptoms due to the noise, light and rough-playing with friends.
- Teens might sustain another head injury.
- As they recover, they may attend, but not participate in, practice and games as long as symptoms do not worsen.

Recovery and Return to Play

- Once in school full time AND symptom free for 24 hours, teens may start the return-to-play exercise program as recommended by the Zurich International Concussion Conference. This is usually a 5 day process.
- Athletes are allowed to start an exercise program when they are off pain medications, are symptom free and have normal neurocognitive test results (if available).
- They may walk the first day, jog the following day and run the third day.
- When these steps are completed without symptoms, they may practice sport specific drills with their team and then full participation, including contact, is allowed.
- Some athletes who have missed many weeks of play may need reconditioning.
- Note: Patients can develop a recurrence of their symptoms if they exercise (especially sprinting) before they are reconditioned.

Post-Concussion Syndrome

BACKGROUND

- **Post-Concussion Syndrome (PCS)** or **Complex Concussion** (newer terminology) is used to describe patients who experience concussion symptoms lasting longer than three weeks.
- These patients occasionally require months or more than one year to recover.
- PCS symptoms can be divided into four categories with some overlap (Figure 1).

TREATMENT

- If the teen experiences PCS, treatment strategies are available to help ease their symptoms (Table 2) with the goal of returning to normal function as soon as possible.

Vestibular Therapy

- A small group of patients who have dizziness (not lightheadedness) may require specific vestibular therapy to aid recovery.
- These patients generally take much longer to recover, often several months.
- The physical therapist doing the rehabilitation will need to do therapy gradually as overdoing it will markedly increase the symptoms for the next day or two.

Eye Convergence Difficulty

- Some patients with concussions develop difficulty with eye convergence.
- Usually resolves over a few weeks but some may need to use reading or prism glasses.
- Uncorrected, headaches may occur with reading.

Neurocognitive Testing

- Great strides have been made in treating PCS but much still remains unknown.

- After a few months of having difficulty with concentration and memory, some patients may need to be referred for comprehensive neurocognitive testing.
  - This can help find areas of cognitive weakness so that appropriate school modifications can be made.
  - While neurocognitive testing is probably the best tool available to help manage a concussion at this time, newer modalities may be found that will replace it.

DISPOSITION

- About 20% of teens with concussions develop PCS with symptoms that last over a month.
- 504 plans should be considered for some teens with more severe symptoms and home tutoring or home schooling may need to be considered in teens who cannot tolerate the active school environment during their recovery.
- School guidance counselors can work with clinicians to help expedite these accommodations.
- Some teens may develop depression either as a result of the injury or because they are unable to attend school and participate in sports.
  - They may become irritable and more emotional than usual.
  - Support for this problem may be addressed by the psychologist, guidance counselor or social worker on the school staff.

What is unique about concussions in adolescents?

- Younger patients may be more sensitive to concussions because their brain cells are still growing and are therefore more vulnerable to trauma.
- Females have more difficulty with concussions than males, likely due to weaker neck muscles and subsequent inability to stabilize their heads after sustaining a blow.
- While most clinicians do not allow concussed adolescents to return to physical exertion after sustaining a concussion, many are allowed to return to school with the caveat: "if your symptoms increase you need to discontinue the activity."

- This is difficult for most adolescents to follow once they are in school attending classes and socializing with their friends.
- To prevent worsening symptoms and prolonged recovery, both mental and physical exertion is not recommended during the early stages of recovery.

- Adolescents often resist treatment recommendations:
  - They may want to attend school before they are ready out of fear that they will miss necessary work and get too far behind.
  - They often want to socialize with friends and participate in their usual activities.
  - If they have a part-time job, they may also want to continue their usual work schedule.

TEST YOUR KNOWLEDGE ANSWERS

78. E. Since the last International Conference on Concussions held in Zurich in 2008 all concussions are no longer graded. A concussion is a concussion unless the symptoms last longer than 3 weeks. If this occurs, patients are said to have post-concussion syndrome and they often need medications and modifications to school. Concussion duration has turned out to be far more important than the initial symptoms of concussions in predicting outcome, which is why the severity of a concussion is initially unknown.
79. C. While some athletes may recover in less than a week, others may take more than a month to fully recover: 40% of adolescent concussions resolve in 1 week, 60% in 2 weeks and 80% by 3 weeks. 20% of adolescents with concussions take longer than 3 weeks to recover. Patients who experience concussion symptoms longer than 3 weeks suffer from post-concussion syndrome (PCS) and require further evaluation.

Table 1. Guidelines for Return to School: Clinician and School Roles.

Physician	• Before returning to school, the clinician should write a letter listing school modifications based on the teen's injury and recovery. • Letter should describe injury and the specific modifications that will need to be made to the school day. • All letters should indicate that the teen may have difficulty concentrating, with their memory (working and short term), and processing speed, all of which can negatively affect learning and performance. "Overusing" the brain may negatively affect recovery. • This letter ensures that all parties involved are informed that the teen is not malingering.
School Contact/ School Nurse	• Will serve as the liaison between teachers, athletic trainers and coaches to facilitate modifications recommended by the clinician. • If no school nurse or athletic trainer is available, the teen's guidance counselor may be the clinician's contact person at school.

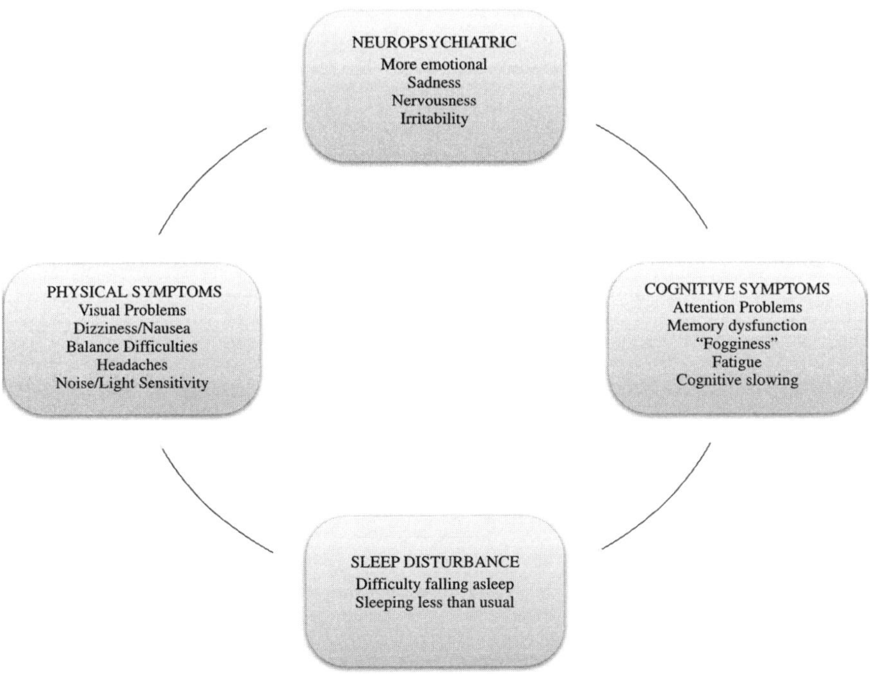

Figure 1 Factor Analysis, Post-Concussion Symptom Scale. Printed with permission. Copyright © 2012 by IMPACT Applications, Inc. All rights reserved.

Table 2. Post-Concussion Syndrome Symptoms and Treatment.

Somatic	• Headaches are the most common. • Medications that have traditionally been used to treat these patients include Amitriptyline (Elavil), Nortryptilene, Topamax and Inderal.
Cognitive	• Difficulty with concentration and memory. • Patients with no previous history of Attention-Deficit Hyperactivity Disorder (ADHD) may develop ADHD-like symptoms after their concussions. This raises the possibility that concussions may have a causal relationship with ADHD in some patients. • Usually they respond well to the use of Attention Deficit Disorder (ADD) medications such as Dextroamphetamine/Amphetamine (Adderall), Lisdexamfetamine (Vyvanse), Atomoxetine (Strattera) or Guanfacine (Intuniv). • Patients with no previous history of Attention-Deficit Hyperactivity Disorder (ADHD) may develop ADHD-like symptoms after their concussions. This raises the possibility that concussions may have a causal relationship with ADHD in some patients. • A small subset of these patients, who describe themselves as "feeling like they are in a cloud," can be treated with Amantadine.
Sleep Disturbances	• Melatonin may be used to help teens fall asleep. • After three to four weeks, if headaches are associated with difficulty falling asleep, Elavil can be helpful. • Trazodone can also be used in more refractory patients.
Emotionality	• Some patients may require mental health referrals for their symptoms and benefit from psychopharmocologic therapy.

WEB REFERENCES

- Centers for Disease Control and Prevention, Heads Up: Concussion in Youth Sports (last updated May 29, 2012), retrieved from www.cdc.gov/ConcussionInYouthSports
- Duff MC. (2009, July 14). Management of Sports-Related Concussion in Children and Adolescents. The ASHA Leader. Retrieved from http://www.asha.org/Publications/leader/2009/090714/f090714a/
- Grady ME. 'Concussion in the Adolescent Athlete', Curr Probl Pediatri Adolesc Health Care. August 2010; 40: 154–169, retrieved from http://web.eccrsd.us/christy/public/Athletic_Training/Concussion_Research_files/concussion%20in%20the%20adolescent%20athlete%20Grady.pdf

- Hall RCW, Hall RCW and Chapman MJ. 'Definition, Diagnosis, and Forensic Implications of Postconcussional Syndrome', Psychosomatics. 2005 May-June; 46(3): 195–202, retrieved from http://drryanhall.com/Articles/postconcussion syndrome.pdf
- Halstead ME and Walter KD. 'Sport-Related Concussion in Children and Adolescents', Pediatrics. 2010; 126(3): 597–615, retrieved from http://pediatrics.aappublications.org/content/126/3/597.full
- Lee MA. 'Adolescent Concussions-Management Recommendations (A Practical Approach)', Sports Med. 2006: 1–4, retrieved from https://www.csms.org/upload/files/sportsmed/Spring 2006.pdf
- Lee MA and Fine B. 'Adolescent Concussions', Connecticut Medicine. March 2010; 74(3): 149–156, retrieved from http://www.connecticutconcussiontaskforce.org/leefine.pdf
- Lee MA and Perriello VA. 'Adolescent Concussions-Management Guidelines for Schools', retrieved from http://www.sportsconcussion.com/pdf/management/Adolescent%20Concussions%20Management%20Guidelines%20for%20Schools.pdf
- McCrory P, *et al.* 'Consensus Statement on Concussion in Sport: the 3rd International Conference on Concussion in Sport held in Zurich, November 2008', British Journal of Sports Medicine. 2009; 43(Suppl I): i76–i84, retrieved from http://bjsm.bmj.com/content/43/Suppl_1/i76.full.pdf
- Scorza KA, Raleigh MF, O'Connor FG. 'Current Concepts in Concussion: Evaluation and Management', American Family Physician. 2012 Jan 15; 85(2): 123–132, retrieved from http://www.aafp.org/afp/2012/0115/pl23.html

Additional Clinician and Patient Resources:

- Brain Injury Association of America: http://www.biausa.org/
- Centers for Disease Control and Prevention, Concussion in Sports and Play: Get the Facts (last updated 10/6/2011), retrieved from http://www.cdc.gov/concussion/sports/facts.html
- Connecticut Concussion Task Force, links for parents and student athletes on identifying a concussion: http://www.connecticutconcussiontaskforce.org
- Think First: National Injury Prevention Foundation, Concussion: A Force to be Reckoned With!: http://www.thinkfirst.org/Concussion.asp

53

ACUTE CHEST PAIN

Dana Kornfeld and
Rick Place

TEST YOUR KNOWLEDGE

80. A 17 year old male presents with a one day history of fever, malaise and chest pain, most intense while supine and relieved with leaning forward and breathing shallowly. On exam, you detect a pericardial friction rub, distant heart sounds and pulsus paradoxus. You recommend:

    A. Immediate cardiac consultation with EKG and ECHO
    B. An x-ray and starting antibiotics immediately
    C. Initiate steroids and refer to cardiology
    D. All the above
    E. None of the above

81. A 16 year old female presents with an intermittent midsternal burning sensation in her chest, worse when lying supine but not worsened with exercise. The patient drinks 3 cups of coffee a day and is a smoker. She is stressed by a demanding school and extracurricular schedule. Physical exam is benign. The next *BEST* step is:

    A. Initiate NSAIDS therapy
    B. Obtain an EKG and echocardiography
    C. Initiate a proton pump inhibitor or antacid
    D. Refer the patient to psychiatry
    E. None of the above

Refer to end of chapter for answers on page 591.

A tall and thin 15 year old presents for his annual physical. Upon review of systems, he comments that he has been getting sharp chest pains lasting for no more than few seconds over the past couple of weeks.

BACKGROUND

- Chest pain is a relatively common condition in adolescents and is the second most common reason for pediatric cardiology referrals.
- There are many causes of chest pain in adolescence (Table 1); fortunately, most are benign: musculoskeletal, anxiety related or idiopathic.
- Serious etiologies of chest pain are uncommon in teens. Features most concerning for serious underlying conditions include younger age, exertional onset and associated syncope.
- The best approach when evaluating adolescent chest pain is to consider etiology by system. Serious causes of acute chest pain tend to be either cardiac or pulmonary but problems in other systems should also be considered (Table 1).
- Many teens complain of "heart pain" emphasizing the underlying concern and misperception that all chest pain represents a risk of coronary artery disease and subsequent myocardial infarction. Heart attacks are exceedingly rare in teens and young adults; however, uncommon causes of cardiac chest pain do exist and must be identified.
- Although chest pain is rarely an emergency in adolescents, it can be frightening to the teen, especially when there is a family history of heart disease.

ASSESSMENT

HISTORY

History of Present Illness

- Onset of symptoms: Any initiating events such as trauma or heavy exertion?
- Weight lifting and pain that increases with movement suggests **muscle strain.**
- Consider **fractured rib** or **pneumothorax** with history of trauma.
- Location of pain.

- Quality of pain (e.g. tight, stabbing, burning, sharp or dull).
- Stabbing pain of brief duration that occurs with inspiration is consistent with **precordial catch syndrome** (irritation or "pinching" of the parietal pleura).
- Sudden, unbearable, ripping or tearing sensation is seen with **aortic dissection.**
- Timing of pain: continuous (versus intermittent) pain suggests a more serious etiology.
- Duration: fleeting chest pain, worse with deep breathing or bending forward, suggests a **"stitch"** (benign condition of uncertain etiology).
- Does the pain affect normal activity or routine (i.e. school attendance)?
- Pain associations: Does pain worsen in certain positions or with activity?
- Pain increasing with breathing, cough or movement suggests pleural or chest wall etiology such as can occur with **pleurodynia** or **pericarditis.**
- Pleurodynia can be associated with fever in infections such as coxsackie B.
- Pleuritic pain that is relieved by sitting up, leaning forward and taking shallow respirations is consistent with **acute pericarditis.**
- Radiation of pain down the arm, to the jaw or shoulder or a sensation of tightness suggests **coronary artery disease.**
- For seriously ill teens presenting with acute chest pain, it is important for the clinician to focus on pulmonary and cardiac etiologies:

Pulmonary Etiologies

- Chest pain that varies with respiration suggests pleuritic irritation that can be associated with **pleurisy/pleuritis, pleural effusion, pericarditis, pneumonia** and rarely **pulmonary embolism (PE).**
- Cough and fever, with or without shortness of breath or chest discomfort, are frequent findings in **pneumonia** or more commonly in **acute bronchitis** (generally a nonbacterial process).
- Shortness of breath and chest pressure with exertion may be harbingers of cardiac disease, but are more commonly symptoms of undiagnosed **exercise-induced asthma (EIA).**
- **Spontaneous pneumothorax,** a relatively common condition that usually affects tall, thin males, is abrupt in onset, sharp and pleuritic and often unilateral; however, pain can rapidly become dull, low-grade, and constant, and even disappear.

Cardiac Etiologies

- Dyspnea or shortness of breath (to be distinguished from shortness of breath secondary to the pain itself) may be present in conditions associated with impaired oxygen exchange (hypoxemia) or impaired cardiac output (**i.e. myocarditis, pericardial tamponade, cardiomyopathy** or **congestive heart failure**).
- Anterior, substernal chest pain in a very tall, thin male with other Marfanoid features should prompt consideration of **aortic pathology/dissection,** particularly if the pain radiates to the back.
- Associated symptoms such as syncope or severe dizziness suggest concurrent **cardiac arrhythmia,** found in conditions such as **hypertrophic cardiomyopathy** (HCM formerly idiopathic hypertrophic subaortic stenosis).
- Patients may perceive palpitations or **supraventricular tachycardia** (SVT) as chest pain.
- **Pneumomediastinum** may occur in the context of an acute asthma attack in younger children, but can also occur with deep inhalation while smoking marijuana.

Other Urgent Causes of Chest Pain

- Severe pain after intense vomiting may be associated with **Boerhaave syndrome** (esophageal rupture). This is rapidly followed by shock.
- Chest pain associated with unilateral leg pain, lower extremity edema or in patients with risk factors for venous thromboembolism such as recent immobilization from trauma, oral contraceptives, recent abortion, pregnancy, or a family history of thrombophilia, may be the only clue to **PE.**

Past Medical History

- Past episodes of anxiety, hyperventilation and vague somatic complaints are common in patients with functional chest pain.
- While ischemic chest pain is rare in adolescents, a history of **Kawasaki disease** in a patient with vague, anterior chest discomfort should prompt this consideration.

- A medical history of HIV, other primary/secondary immunodeficiency or pulmonary infection, may predispose patients to **infectious esophagitis** from herpes simplex virus or candida albicans.
- Asthma may complicate with **pneumomediastinum.**
- A history of severe **hypercholesterolemia** should raise suspicion for atherosclerosis/ishemia.
- Patient's with **Marfan's syndrome** may present with aortic dissection or pneumothorax.
- Patient's with sickle cell anemia can present with chest crisis.

Family History

- Is there a family history of HCM, Marfan's syndrome, autoimmune disease or premature heart disease to which the patient may be predisposed.

Medications

- Reports of a pill getting stuck on attempts to swallow suggests **pill esophagitis** (chemical irritation of the esophagus from certain medications, especially if ingested with less fluid).

Social History

- Use of tobacco, alcohol, caffeine or drugs of abuse such as methamphetamines, cocaine, and dextromethorphan can cause cardiac ischemia with acute chest pain.
- Evaluate for anxiety, school phobia, or depression, which can all coexist.
- Inquire about recent (or anniversary) cardiac events in the patient's family.

Review of Systems

- Ascertain any associated symptoms such as fever, respiratory distress, lightheadedness, joint pain or rashes.
- Chest pain associated with fever can occur in **bronchitis, pneumonia, rheumatic disease, or osteomyelitis**.
- Coughing, wheezing or difficulty breathing suggests **asthma** or **pneumonia**.
- Pain exacerbated by respiration and reproducible on exam is consistent with **costochondritis** or **Tietze syndrome.**
- Reflux, hoarseness, sour taste in mouth, association with meals or alleviation with antacids suggests **reflux esophagitis** or **peptic ulcer disease.**

- Chest pain associated with rashes and joint pain is suggestive of a rheumatic condition such as **systemic lupus erythematosis** (SLE), which can present with pleural effusions.
- Presence of stress or anxiety may cause hyperventilation, palpitations and pain.
- Night sweats or weight loss can be seen with a **thoracic tumor.**
- Acute onset of chest pain with dyspnea can occur with **pneumothorax.**
- Acute onset of dyspnea and chest pain suggest **PE**. Risk factors are oral birth control pills, immobilization, obesity and family history.
- A burning pain sensation following a neurodermatome may be the prodrome of a herpes zoster outbreak.

PHYSICAL

The most common physical exam finding in an adolescent complaining of chest pain is a normal exam.

Vital Signs

- Fever can be seen with **pneumonia, bronchitis, pleurodynia** or SLE.
- Tachypnea is associated with **pneumonia, asthma exacerbation, PE or congestive heart failure**.
- Tachycardia consistent with **anxiety, heart arrhythmias or failure, infection, asthma, PE, or stimulant drug/cocaine use.**
- Elevated blood pressure can be associated with heart disease such as **aortic stenosis** or stimulant drug/cocaine use.

General Appearance

- Severe distress might be seen in **tension pneumothorax, flail chest, myocarditis or myocardial infarction.**
- Nasal flaring and/or retractions of chest wall muscles is consistent with respiratory exertion as can occur during an **asthma exacerbation.**
- Note body habitus: **aortic dissection** or **spontaneous pneumothorax** often occur in tall, thin males.

Chest Wall

- Palpate the ribs, looking for rib fractures or bruising caused by **direct trauma.**
- Palpate the anterior chest, ribs and sternum assessing for costochondral or costosternal pain such as seen with **costochondritis.**
- Pain with palpation and swelling at the upper costochondral junctions suggests **Tietze syndrome.**
- Tenderness or pain over breast tissue is associated with **gynecomastia.**
- Acute pain on palpation of lower ribs suggests **slipping rib syndrome.**
- Rarely, pain with palpation of the ribs can be associated with metastatic disease to the bone in an ill appearing teen.

Lung

- Wheezing is associated with **exercise induced asthma** or **acute asthma exacerbation.** A more nuanced variance is a subtle or mild increase in the expiratory phase of the respiratory cycle.
- Diminished air exchange (i.e. somewhat distant or "quiet" normal breath sounds) and a prolonged expiratory phase may be associated with relatively severe compromise.
- Focal decreases in breath sounds are typically found when there is an insulating medium between the chest wall and the lung, e.g. **pulmonary effusion** or **pneumothorax.**
- Increased breath sounds are heard in conditions that increase the transmission of sound, such as the focal pulmonary consolidation of **bacterial pneumonia.** This finding is often associated with egophony ("e" to "a" changes heard on auscultation).
- Crackles (rales) are often incorrectly attributed to pneumonia. While focal rales can indeed be associated with **pneumonia,** this physical exam finding is neither *sensitive* (always there) nor *specific* to pneumonia. Crackles are found in other conditions such as **acute bronchitis,** acute **asthma exacerbation** (from mucous) or **congestive failure** with pulmonary edema.
- Rhonchi are long, low-pitched breath sounds frequently confused with wheezing. These are more commonly associated with partial occlusion of the large bronchi (often from mucous) rather than bronchoconstriction of the smaller airways.

- A pleural rub typically varies with the respiratory cycle, but in a regular fashion. It is secondary to pleural inflammation and may be found in **pleurisy, pleuritis** (from connective tissue disease), or secondary to a peripheral **PE.**

Heart

- Tachycardia and irregularity can be heard with **SVT** or other dysrhythmias.
- Murmurs may be consistent with **mitral valve prolapse** (**MVP**), **HCM, or pulmonic or aortic stenosis.**
- **Pericarditis** is suggested by the constellation of a pericardial friction rub, distant heart sounds and pulsus paradoxus.
- Hammon's crunch is a well-described finding in which crackles vary with the cardiac cycle and is considered pathognomonic for **pneumomediastinum.**

Skin

- Vesicular rash with dermatomal distribution is characteristic of **herpes zoster** (note: chest pain or parasthesias precede the rash).

STUDIES

The two most common and useful tests are the electrocardiogram and chest radiograph.

Electrocardiogram (EKG)

- The literature suggests a low yield in the evaluation of nonspecific chest pain but there are several important reasons to maintain a low threshold in obtaining this test:
  - Cardiac chest pain may present in a very nonspecific manner and the diagnosis may depend upon EKG findings (e.g. myocarditis or arrythmias such as SVT.
  - For many adolescents (and their parents), the main concern is not the chest pain but rather the possibility that the chest pain is of cardiac etiology. An EKG will frequently provide conclusive relief.
  - The test is relatively inexpensive and noninvasive.

Key findings of the EKG:

- *ST elevation* suggests myocardial injury:
  - If focal and found with reciprocating ST depression elsewhere, consider **coronary occlusion.** It may also be early, not yet generalized, **pericarditis.**
  - If diffuse, it may identify **pericarditis.**
- *ST depression* suggests the presence of **myocardial strain.**
- Ventricular hypertrophy (LVH/RVH), particularly in the context of exertional chest pain points to the possibility of **cardiomyopathy.**
- Coronary artery disease related to Kawasaki's disease, aberrant left coronary artery, aortic stenosis or HCM may also cause EKG changes.

Chest X-Ray (CXR)

- The yield is low but any questionable findings may justify obtaining this low-risk, inexpensive study.
- Can identify many conditions such as **spontaneous pneumothorax/mediastinum, pneumonia, rib fractures, pleural effusion, thoracic mass, cardiomegaly** and **pericardial effusion.**
- A normal CXR (particularly in association with a normal EKG) can be very reassuring.

Complete Blood Count

- **Leukocytosis** may help to establish infectious processes such as **bacterial pneumonia** versus **acute bronchitis, or sterile pleural effusion** versus **empyema.**

Erythrocyte Sedimentation Rate (ESR) or C-Reactive Protein

- Can help discriminate an inflammatory from a noninflammatory process.

SPECIAL TESTS

Pulmonary Function Tests

- May be useful for confirming the diagnosis of exercise inducted asthma.

Drug Screen

- May be useful for identifying the presence of cocaine but should be obtained with the permission or knowledge of the adolescent patient if possible.
- The typical drug screen is not the same as a **comprehensive drug screen** (an expensive, low yield test) and will not identify most drugs of abuse, such as dextromethorphan.

Cardiac Enzymes, Specifically Serum Troponin

- Sensitive for the identification of myocardial injury.
- An elevation does not necessarily imply intracoronary thrombosis (i.e. acute myocardial infarction) and may be precipitated by anything that produces myocardial injury, such as cocaine, pericarditis, or myocarditis.
- The value and sensitivity of a serum troponin for the identification of cardiac injury is time-dependent. This test does not achieve full sensitivity for 8–12 hours *after* myocardial injury. Even a patient with an acute myocardial infarction may therefore have a completely normal troponin if the test is drawn early enough after the onset of symptoms.

D-Dimer

- A screening test for PE in the low risk patient. Most adolescents without specific risk factors would fall in this category.
- This test is sensitive for thromboembolism and has a high negative predictive value that is useful to *exclude* the possibility of PE in low risk patients.
- The test is not very *specific:* an elevated value does *not* indicate a high probability of pulmonary thromboembolism. An elevated test mandates further diagnostic study to detect or exclude the presence of a PE (e.g. CT scan).

Echocardiography

- May be indicated to assess for pericarditis, aortic stenosis, HCM or mitral valve prolapse.

CT Scan

- Can identify congenital pulmonary blebs responsible for **spontaneous pneumothorax.**
- With contrast, is the initial study of choice for **PE** in the high-risk patient (either because of clinical features or an elevated d-dimer).
- CT with angiography is also often the initial study for identification of **aortic dissection.**

V/Q Scan

- Has largely been supplanted by CT scan for the identification of **PE** due to significant problems with sensitivity and specificity. It is still useful in patients with contrast allergies.

Coronary Angiography

- May be acutely employed for patients with evidence of **acute myocardial injury/infarction.**
- Can identify coronary occlusion and congenital coronary abnormalities.

Endoscopy

- Used for the evaluation of **severe esophagitis** or **peptic ulcer disease**.

DISPOSITION

- Most teens with chest pain can be managed by their primary care physician.
- The vast majority of adolescents with chest pain do not have identifiable pathology, particularly in the context of a normal EKG and CXR. These teens can be followed clinically and their pain generally resolves within days.
- Treatment should be directed toward the cause of the chest pain:
  - Relaxation techniques, paper bag rebreathing and counseling for **psychogenic cause** or **hyperventilation**.
  - Analgesics for musculoskeletal pain as with **costochondritis** or **pleurodynia.**

  - H2 blocker or proton pump inhibitor for **ulcer/gastritis.**
  - Antibiotics for **pneumonia.**
  - Anticoagulation for **PE.**
  - Emergent care including chest tube placement for **pneumothorax,** unless small enough that it may resolve spontaneously.
- Occasionally, more serious causes of chest pain may require referral to a specialist.
  - Emergent causes require immediate evaluation in the emergency room.
  - Refer to a cardiologist if cardiac etiology is suspected.
  - In cases of severe pulmonary disease, referral to pulmonary medicine may be warranted.

What is unique about chest pain in adolescents?

- Chest pain in adolescents is usually benign.
- Nevertheless, clinicians should not dismiss adolescents with chest pain because significant disease is "unlikely." Avoid "anchoring" on benign diagnoses that may not be fully supported by clinical data and "premature diagnostic closure" which can lead to failure to pursue important clues.
- Teens are often involved in sports and intense exercise that predisposes them to musculoskeletal injury, especially if not optimally fit ("weekend athletes").
- Adolescents are more prone to accidents and trauma causing injury to the chest. On occasion, this may occur in fights or circumstances that teens may prefer to hide.
- Stressors make teens more susceptible to muscular tension and psychogenic chest pain.
- Teens may be exposed to illicit drugs such as methamphetamines and cocaine that can increase the risk of cardiac ischemia.
- Healthy adolescents generally have significant "physiologic reserve" and the typical symptoms of disease may be muted (e.g. an adolescent with a large PE may not have tachycardia or shortness of breath, unlike their adult counterparts).

TEST YOUR KNOWLEDGE ANSWERS

80. A. This patient is presenting with signs of acute pericarditis, an inflammation of the pericardial space. EKG and echocardiography are indicated for diagnosis. Viral infection is the most common cause of pericarditis in adolescents. Viruses implicated include coxsackie, echovirus, adenovirus, influenza, parainfluenza and Ebstein Barr Virus. Purulent pericarditis from bacterial infection can occasionally be seen. Also consider collagen vascular diseases such as lupus. Although antibiotics would be indicated if this patient had bacterial pericarditis, a definitive diagnosis needs to be established.
81. C. This patient has esophagitis caused by gastroesophageal reflux. The patient's use of caffeine and cigarettes increases the risk of this disorder. This can also occur from chemical irritation of the esophageal mucosa by certain medications especially when swallowed with too little fluid. NSAIDS would be used to treat costochondritis or other causes of musculoskeletal pain. NSAIDS are contraindicated in esophagitis. This patient does not have a history or physical exam findings consistent with a cardiac or psychiatric disorder.

Table 1. Differential Diagnosis of Acute Chest Pain in Adolescents.

Cardiac	Hypertrophic Cardiomyopathy
	Coronary Artery Thrombosis
	Coronary Arteritis (Kawasaki)
	Accelerated Atherosclerosis (Familial)
	Abnormal Coronary Anatomy
	Coronary Vasospasm (Idiopathic; Drugs)
	Myocardial Ischemia/Infarct
	Pericarditis (Myocarditis Less Common)
	Mitral Valve Prolapse
	Aortic Dissection
Pulmonary	Pulmonary Embolism
	Pneumothorax (Pneumomediastinum)
	Pneumonia/Bronchitis
	Acute Chest Syndrome (Sickle Cell Disease)
	Exercise-Induced Asthma
	Pleural Effusion
	Pleurisy (Pleuritis/Pleurodynia)
Gastrointestinal	Esophagitis
	Achalasia
	Gastroesophageal Reflux
	Peptic Ulcer Disease
	Infectious Esophagitis
	Boerhaave Syndrome (Rupture)
	Foreign Body
	"Pill Esophagitis"
Musculoskeletal	Nonspecific Musculoskeletal Chest Pain
	Intercostal Muscle Strain
	Costochondritis
	Precordial Catch
	Slipping Rib Syndrome
	Myositis
	Rib Fracture
	Breast Pain
Functional	Psychogenic Chest Pain
	Hyperventilation Syndrome
	Panic Disorder
Dermatologic	Herpes Zoster

WEB REFERENCES

- American International Health Alliance, Chest Pain: Clinical Practice Guideline for Primary Health Care Physicians, pp. 31–32, retrieved from http://www.aiha.com/en/resourcelibrary/products/curricula/pdf/cpg%20chest%20pain%20en.pdf
- Lane JR, Ben-Shachar G. 'Myocardial Infarction in Healthy Adolescents', Pediatrics. 2007; 120(4): e938–e943, retrieved from http://pediatrics.aappublications.org/content/120/4/e938.full?sid=96b41265-7316-4ef8-931b-0cbd613afl7b
- Leung AKC, Robson WLM, Cho H. 'Chest pain in children', Canadian Family Physician. 1996 June; 42: 1156–1164, retrieved from http://www.ncbi.nlm.nih.gov/pmc/articles/PMC2146478/pdf/canfamphys00076-0114.pdf
- Reddy SRV and Singh HR. 'Chest Pain in Children and Adolescents', Pediatrics in Review. 2010 January I; 31(l): el–e9, retrieved from http://pedsinreview.aappublications.org/content/31/1/el.full

Additional Clinician and Patient Resources:

- Cincinnati Children's Health Topics, Chest Pain: http://www.cincinnatichildrens.org/health/c/chest/
- Dukehealth.org. Advice from doctors, Chest Pain in Children and Adolescents: http://www.dukehealth.org/health_library/advice_from_doctors/your_childs_health/chest_pain_in_children
- Mayo Clinic: Costochondritis: http://www.mayoclinic.com/health/costochondritis/%20DS00626
- Mayo Clinic: Pericarditis: http://www.mayoclinic.com/health/pericarditis/DS00505
- Pubmed Health, Pericarditis (last reviewed June 4, 2012), retrieved from http://www.ncbi.nlm.nih.gov/pubmedhealth/PMH0001234/
- Shiel WC. emedicinehealth, Costochondritis: http://www.emedicinehealth.com/costochondritis/article_em.htm
- University of British Columbia, Approach to Pediatric Chest Pain: http://learnpediatrics.com/body-%20systems/cardiology/approach-to-pediatric-chest-pain/

54

ACUTE ABDOMINAL PAIN

Rick Place

TEST YOUR KNOWLEDGE

82. In teens with acute abdominal pain, which of the following diagnoses is more likely to have an atypical presentation?

    A. Acute appendicitis
    B. Biliary colic
    C. Ectopic pregnancy
    D. Pyelonephritis
    E. All may present atypically

Refer to end of chapter for answer on page 606.

A 15 year old female presents with two days of throbbing right lower quadrant pain, vomiting and low-grade fever.

BACKGROUND

- Acute abdominal pain is one of the most common adolescent complaints at urgent visits.
- For the clinician, the priority is to discriminate a surgical condition from a nonsurgical one.
- While nonsurgical causes of abdominal pain can be quite serious, surgical conditions usually require more timely identification and management.
- There are more organs packed into the abdomen than anywhere else in the body. Their proximity and similar neurological innervation can make distinguishing between them based on history and physical quite challenging.

ASSESSMENT

HISTORY

History of Present illness

Pain Location

- Critical when evaluating abdominal pain. For instance, **biliary colic** is more likely to be perceived in the right upper quadrant (RUQ) than the left lower quadrant (LLQ).
- Pain may be perceived in adjacent areas. Neurologic innervation is variable and often overlaps, and visceral (internal) sensation is usually vague and poorly localized.
- In some patients, the organ (e.g. the appendix) may be mildly displaced internally from the typical individual and produce atypical symptoms.
- **Biliary colic** and **pancreatitis** may be centered in the epigastric region and improperly ascribed to gastritis.
- Pain with **pyelonephritis** may sometimes be perceived more anterior than posterior.

- A **kidney stone** at the ureterovesicular junction may be perceived anteriorly in the RLQ or LLQ, with mild tenderness on exam.
- **Ovarian** pathology is relatively easy to identify when localized to the LLQ, but is often perceived in the RLQ, suprapubic or lower pelvic region.
- Intestinal complaints (**small bowel obstruction** (**SBO**) or **early appendicitis**) are often perceived in the periumbilical region.

Pain Severity

- Can help to rapidly identify serious conditions.
- The most severe pain is often found in conditions with tubular dilatation (e.g. **biliary colic, renal colic**, or **intestinal obstruction from small bowel obstruction or severe constipation, intestinal cramping from enteritis**). These patients often fail to find relief with repositioning or any other intervention.

Pain Duration

- Acute surgical conditions are generally of shorter duration (i.e. hours) while chronic causes of abdominal discomfort may last days to weeks. This is due to the rapid and progressive nature of these conditions.
- Intermittent discomfort of a moderately severe, colicky nature suggests tubular dilatation (e.g. **kidney stone, biliary colic** or **constipation**).
- **Crohn's disease** is occasionally confused with **appendicitis**; it may present as persistent low grade RLQ pain whereas acute appendicitis has a more rapid tempo and shorter duration.

Pain Migration

- Appendiceal pain (i.e. visceral pain) is poorly localized and may be initially perceived as periumbilical since afferent fibers enter the spinal cord around T10.
- With inflammation of local somatic tissues, the pain is perceived more focally in the RLQ (if that is where the appendix is located).

Pain Radiation

- Is similar to migration in that different locations can be perceived as painful based on variable neurologic innervation of visceral organs.

- Pain radiating to the upper right or mid-back suggests **biliary colic** or **pancreatitis.**
- **Ovarian** (or fallopian) pathology and **renal colic** may also be perceived in the back.
- Rarely, post-traumatic **splenic** or **liver laceration** may be perceived in the corresponding shoulder region. This is known as *Kehr's sign.*
- **Testicular torsion** may present as lower abdominal pain and many consider a testicular exam a critical part of a thorough evaluation of abdominal pain.

Associated Symptoms

- Fever may be present in **acute appendicitis, gastroenteritis** or **pyelonephritis.**
- Vomiting suggests **acute gastroenteritis**, but may also be associated with almost any abdominal condition including **renal colic, ovarian pathology, acute appendicitis, pancreatitis** or **hepatitis**.

Past Medical History

- Deposition of hemoglobin degradation products in the gall bladder may lead to **gallstones** and **biliary obstruction** in teens with sickle cell disease and other hemolytic anemias.
- Teens with mononucleosis who develop LUQ pain may have a **"ruptured" spleen.**
- Adolescents with a diagnosis of polycystic ovarian syndrome (PCOS) are at increased risk of a **ruptured ovarian cyst.**

Past Surgical History

- A history of abdominal surgery years before (e.g. for acute appendicitis) provides context for a teen with severe abdominal pain and vomiting (i.e. **adhesions causing SBO**).

Medications

- Certain drugs used in the treatment of HIV predispose patients to **pancreatitis, hepatitis**, or **kidney stones.**

- Many drugs can cause significant **hepatitis**, including unrecognized suicidal attempts with **acetaminophen ingestion**. Identification of acetaminophen overdose in the hepatitis phase is very concerning.

Social History

- Sexually active teens may be diagnosed with **pelvic inflammatory disease (PID)**, **ectopic pregnancy** and other pregnancy related complaints. These conditions are also frequently found in teens who deny sexual activity.
- Likewise, being sexually active should not inappropriately focus the diagnostic process on these conditions. Premature diagnosis of conditions such as PID may preclude an accurate diagnosis of other conditions such as ovarian torsion, complications of pregnancy, or even acute appendicitis, leading to serious diagnostic mistakes and delay of care.

PHYSICAL

Chest and lung exam should be performed if appropriate but a well performed abdomen exam can help narrow the differential.

Vital Signs

- Fever, tachycardia and low blood pressure may all indicate more serious underlying pathology warranting emergent evaluation and treatment.

Abdomen

Discern the presence or absence of tenderness.

- **Ovarian pathology** is typically very tender while **renal colic** typically presents with severe pain that by far outweigh tenderness.
- **Gastritis** and **pancreatitis** are perceived as epigastric pain, but the latter is more tender.
- Similarly, severe colic from intestinal cramping in **enteritis** will far outweigh tenderness on exam. The same may be true of **diabetic ketoacidosis**.

Determine the location of tenderness.

- Focal RUQ tenderness in the presence of vomiting and radiation to the right back suggests **biliary colic**, but **acute appendicitis** (atypical location) may provide a similar exam.
- **Hepatitis** and occasionally right **pyelonephritis** may have features of RUQ tenderness, as does **Fitz-Hugh Curtis** (perihepatitis or inflammation *around* the liver from ascending chlamydia or gonorrhea infection).
- Epigastric or LUQ tenderness suggests **pancreatitis, gastritis**, or **severe fecal impaction.**
- RLQ tenderness is a key finding with **acute appendicitis** but can also occur with other conditions including: **ovarian pathology (torsion, cyst, mittelschmerz, tubo-ovarian abscess), Crohn's disease, mesenteric adenitis** (in the context of gastroenteritis), **kidney stone** and **pyelonephritis.**
- LLQ tenderness is uncommon and suggests **ovarian pathology** or constipation.
- **Intestinal disorders (impaction, bowel obstruction)** present with periumbilical or generalized abdominal tenderness.
- Guarding occurs when patients tighten their abdominal muscles in response to palpation.
  - Guarding implies a significant degree of inflammation below the exam site.
  - It may be "voluntary" or "involuntary," but such a designation is of limited value.
  - Rebound pain occurs when the clinician presses down on the abdomen, then suddenly releases pressure, resulting in significant distress from the patient.
    - The finding is neither sensitive nor specific, even when performed by experienced clinicians, but is of clinical importance as it implies **peritonitis.**
    - **Peritonitis** from a **ruptured appendix** presents with increased RLQ pain severity, guarding and rebound tenderness.
  - The presence or absence of bowel sounds may be helpful. High-pitched bowel sounds suggest **intestinal obstruction** while the absence of bowel sounds suggest **intestinal ileus.**

- Costovertebral angle tenderness with percussion may be found with **dilatation of the renal capsule, ureteral obstruction (stone)** or **pyelonephritis**.

Digital Rectal

- Of limited routine value but can provide information about the presence of blood (guaiac testing), hard stool (**constipation**) and localization of pain (**appendicitis**).

Pelvic Exam

- Its value as a mandatory part of every abdominal evaluation has been questioned, particularly with the availability of current laboratory and imaging techniques; however, there are times when a speculum and/or bimanual exam can provide important information.
- A speculum exam can assess the presence or absence of cervical discharge, determine vaginal anatomy, and evaluate for products of conception with threatened miscarriages.
- A bimanual exam can localize pain to the genital tract and detect masses.
- Cervical motion tenderness may be seen with *any* cause of peritoneal irritation but tends to be a marker for **PID** in the presence of vaginal discharge.

STUDIES

Urine Beta-hCG

- Mandatory with serious abdominal complaints in any adolescent female who has started menses, regardless of reported sexual history.

Complete Blood Count (CBC)

- Of value in the context of clinical picture and rarely useful as an isolated test.

- Can provide information on the severity of the condition, for example, leukocytosis with biliary colic or acute pancreatitis suggests more severe illness.
- Leukocytosis also lacks specificity and can be part of a stress response (e.g. kidney stones).
- A normal white count does not exclude acute appendicitis.

Lipase and Amylase

- Tests for **acute pancreatitis**; however, amylase lacks specificity and lipase is preferred.

Liver Function Tests

- Note: Cellular enzymes are released with hepatic injury; they are not a test of function.
- *Elevated transaminases (AST, ALT).*
  - Indicate hepatocellular injury, while the presence of an elevated **alkaline phosphatase** suggests hepatobiliary disease. When accompanied by elevated bilirubin, it suggests obstruction of the biliary tree.
- *Coagulation profile (PT, PTT, INR).*
  - True test of liver function that provides information on the severity of liver dysfunction.

Basic Metabolic Panel (electrolytes, BUN, creatinine, glucose)

- Provides basic information on hydration status as well as renal function.
- Occasionally, a high glucose may identify unsuspected **diabetic ketoacidosis** as the cause of diffuse abdominal pain and vomiting.

Urinalysis

- The presence of nitrites and leukocyte esterase on the dipstick and/or WBCs on the microscopy suggest urinary tract infection (kidney or bladder).
- Beware "anchoring" on equivocal results (e.g. 10 WBC per HPF): local irritation of the ureter (e.g. acute appendicitis) may produce mild pyuria and a poorly collected clean catch specimen, contaminated by vaginal secretions, can be misleading.

SPECIAL TESTS

Stool Studies

- Should be sent when there is a history of blood or mucus in the stool.
- **Stool Cultures:** Each lab has a different "standard" culture set. For instance, the lab may routinely assess for salmonella, shigella, and campylobacter but yersinia and *E. coli* 07:H157 may need to be ordered separately.
- **Ova and parasites** are rarely indicated for acute abdominal pain unless there has been recent travel outside the U.S.
- ***H. pylori*** antigen can be positive in peptic ulcer disease.
- **Calprotectin** is positive in granulomatous colitis.
- **Fecal leukocytes**, of limited sensitivity and specificity, generally need not be ordered.

Abdominal Flat Plate and Upright

- Is of limited value despite widespread use.
- This study may be diagnostic for **small (or large) bowel obstruction**.
- Frequently ordered to diagnose **constipation** but should not be relied upon exclusively to make the diagnosis nor is it a substitute for a proper physical exam (i.e. rectal).

Pelvic Ultrasound

- Most radiologists will not perform transvaginal studies in virginal adolescents; therefore, a pelvic sonogram is frequently transabdominal (a less optimal study) and requires a full bladder for adequate evaluation of the genital tract.
- *All patients who present with acute abdominal pain with a positive pregnancy test must have a pelvic ultrasound to exclude ectopic pregnancy.*
  - The most common ultrasonographic finding in **ectopic pregnancy** is an empty uterus.
  - Sometimes there is no visible ectopic pregnancy and that can be attributed to a completed miscarriage.
- A pelvic ultrasound can confirm **ovarian cysts**.
  - A **ruptured cyst** may only have indirect evidence (i.e. free fluid in the pelvis).

- An **ovarian torsion** is a high-risk, time-dependent condition. A study ordered for the identification of ovarian cysts should also include a request for *doppler studies* to evaluate for ovarian torsion.

- Pelvic sonography is also useful to evaluate for the presence of **tubo-ovarian abscess** in a patient with a probable diagnosis of either severe or indolent smoldering **PID**.

Limited Abdominal Ultrasound

- Is becoming the study of choice **for acute appendicitis.**
- Highly sensitive but importantly, negative studies can exclude acute appendicitis.
- Positive findings may require follow up with a CT scan.
- Can also evaluate for **biliary obstruction** by identifying a dilated gall bladder and/or common bile duct.
- Mandatory in the presence of acute pancreatitis to exclude **gallstone pancreatitis.**

Computerized Tomography of the Abdomen/Pelvis

- There is concern regarding radiation exposure; however, the long-term significance remains uncertain and controversial.
- Presentations of acute abdominal pain can be confusing and diagnosis can be difficult. A CT scan can aid by excluding serious pathology such as **intestinal perforation, intussusception, epiploic appendicitis, internal intestinal hernias** and **malrotation**.
- CT is the study of choice to diagnose **acute appendicitis**, particularly in the presence of an equivocal ultrasound or when there is concern of a **perforated** or **retrocecal appendicitis.**
- At times, CT scan for appendicitis may establish an alternative diagnosis such as **ovarian cyst, RLL pneumonia, pyelonephritis** or **Crohn's disease.**
- Non-contrast CT is the study of choice to identify **obstructing kidney stones.**

HIDA Scan

- Consider if **biliary colic** is suspected but unproven by sonography.

Endoscopy

- Necessary to diagnose **gastritis** and/or **duodenitis**.

Colonoscopy

- Biopsy can confirm the diagnosis of **inflammatory bowel disease** (IBD).

DISPOSITION

- Therapeutic strategies depend on the underlying etiology.
- Adolescents with acute abdominal pain represent a high-risk group: difficulty in identifying significant pathology does not indicate the absence of significant pathology.
- Mild or atypical presentations may escape immediate detection, but symptoms will often persist or progress.
- Close and timely follow up is mandatory. "Follow up in 2–3 days" is not appropriate as this may result in delay in diagnosis and treatment. "Follow up in 12–24 hours" may be more appropriate, with instructions to present to the emergency department if symptoms progress.
- With time, acute abdominal pain can become subacute or chronic and the diagnostic algorithm is necessarily different, often involving specialty care.

What is unique about acute abdominal pain in adolescents?

- Adolescents with acute abdominal conditions usually do not present "differently" than other age groups; however, adolescents have emotional or psychological overlay that may make interpretation of their symptoms challenging. The safest approach is to take the adolescent's complaints at face value to provide optimal care.
- Teens can present with "adult" disorders, such as gallbladder disease, that may not be considered by clinicians more familiar with pediatric disorders. Therefore maintaining a broad differential is important.
- Teens may be reluctant to disclose information for fear of embarrassment or recourse and may be reluctant to talk about rectal bleeding, scrotal pain, vaginal discharge or bleeding, or sexual activities, especially in an acute

setting. It is important to conduct the history in private without parents/legal guardians present.

TEST YOUR KNOWLEDGE ANSWER

82. E. All the above may present atypically. Biliary colic, though usually presenting with right subcostal pain radiating to the shoulder, can also present as chest or epigastric pain. An appendix in an atypical location (e.g. retrocecal) can mimic biliary colic by inducing vomiting, right upper quadrant tenderness and radiation to the right back. Ectopic pregnancy may initially present only as vaginal bleeding without abdominal pain. Pyelonephritis may sometimes be perceived to be more anterior than posterior.

WEB REFERENCES

- Armstrong FD. 'Analgesia for Children with Acute Abdominal Pain: A Cautious Move to Improved Pain Management', Pediatrics 2005; 116(4): 1018, retrieved from http://pediatrics.aappublications.org/content/ll6/4/1018.2.full.pdf+html
- Flasar MH, Goldberg E. 'Acute Abdominal Pain', Med Clin Am. 2006. 90: 481–503, retrieved from http:// medicina . iztacala.unam.mx / medicina / Acute % 20 Abdominal%20Pain.pdf
- Leung AKC, Sigalet DL. 'Acute Abdominal Pain in Children', American Family Physician. 2003 Jun l; 67(ll): 2321–2327, retrieved from http://www.aafp.org/afp/2003/0601/p2321.html

55

HEMATEMESIS

Leslie A. Hayes

TEST YOUR KNOWLEDGE

83. Which one of the following is *MOST* likely to present with an episode of massive hematemesis?

    A. Esophagitis
    B. Mallory Weiss tears
    C. Dieulafoy's lesion
    D. Peptic Ulcer Disease (PUD)
    E. All the above.

Refer to end of chapter for answer on page 614.

"My daughter told me that she vomited blood twice in the last two months!"

BACKGROUND

- Hematemesis is defined as vomiting bright red blood or coffee ground-like material (blood that has been denatured by gastric acid).
- When hematemesis occurs, an upper gastrointestinal bleed (i.e. a bleeding site proximal to the ligament of Treitz) is inferred.
- The causes of hematemesis are outlined in Table 1.

ASSESSMENT

HISTORY

History of Present Illness

- Determine color and consistency of blood to ascertain the source of bleeding along the GI tract. Bright red blood is consistent with an upper GI bleed while dark coffee ground appearing blood implies lower GI tract source.
- Ascertain the time of onset of hematemesis and the amount of blood that was vomited (specks or flecks, streaks, spoonful or cupful) as well as the frequency of the bleeding.
- A massive hemorrhage may be due to **Dieulafoy's lesion**, a pin-point ulcerated arterial lesion in the fundus of the stomach, often associated with melena.
- Following trauma, right upper quadrant pain and jaundice associated with massive hemorrhage indicates **hemobilia**.

Dietary History

- Determine if it is really blood. A detailed dietary history can determine if substances that contain red food coloring (i.e. Kool-Aid®, candy, liquid acetaminophen/ibuprofen, cough medicines, cereal, Jell-O®, red beets or fruit juices) were ingested.

Medications

- Continuous use of non-steroidal anti-inflammatory drugs (NSAIDs) or corticosteroids suggests **peptic ulcer disease (PUD) or gastritis.**

Past Medical History

- A detailed medical history may elicit an underlying bleeding disorder. Ask about **renal disease, cardiac problems** and **coagulopathies** such as hemophilia, thrombocytopenia or other platelet dysfunctions.
- Diseases such as sepsis, acidosis, sickle cell anemia, cystic fibrosis, systemic lupus erythematosus, and severe hypoglycemia are associated with **secondary ulcer disease.**

Review of Systems

- Determine if the bleeding site is within the GI tract. A history of sore throat, nose-picking, epistaxis, recent dental work, tonsillectomy, or other types of trauma to the nose, mouth or neck suggest **swallowed blood.**
- Ask about dizziness, syncope, lethargy, shortness of breath and chest pains.
- Recent onset of jaundice, easy bruising, and change in stool color indicate **liver disease.**
- Weight loss, abdominal pain, heartburn, swallowing difficulty, binging and purging, and changes in menstrual period may suggest an **eating disorder.**

Social History

- Episodes of forceful vomiting suggests **Mallory-Weiss tears** that can occur with **bulimia** or **alcohol abuse.**
- Ingestion of a corrosive substance, medication or foreign body that may have lodged in the esophagus or stomach suggests of **esophagitis** or **gastritis.**
- Be alert for red flags on detailed psychosocial history that may suggest **gastritis** secondary to **alcohol ingestion.**
- **Munchausen/Munchausen-by-proxy syndrome** should be considered when there are discrepancies in history, physical and laboratory findings.

PHYSICAL

Vital Signs

- Assess vitals for hemodynamic stability: check pulse, heart rate, blood pressure and capillary refill.
- Document orthostatic blood pressures.

Anthropometric Measurements

- Measure height and weight and plot on a growth chart to compare to previous measurements. Poor growth and/or weight loss suggests an underlying chronic disease.

HEENT

- Examine nares and oropharynx for potential bleeding sites.
- Erosion of teeth enamel suggests self-induced vomiting seen in **bulimia.**

Cardiac

- Auscultate the patient's heart and listen to the abdomen for a venous hum.

Abdomen

- Percuss the liver and spleen to assess for hepatosplenomegaly and check for ascites.

Anal

- Examine the rectum to check for hemorrhoids, anal fissures or trauma.

Skin

- Note the color of skin, conjunctiva and mucosa to assess for jaundice or pallor.
- Evaluate the patient's skin for petechiae, purpura, bruising, ecchymosis or prominent abdominal vasculature (caput medusae, spider angiomas).
- Scars on the patient's knuckles (Russell's sign) suggest self-induced vomiting.

STUDIES

Nasogastric (NG) Lavage

- Is recommended for patients with a history or physical examination that indicates a significant bleeding episode.
- Is performed to remove particulate matter, blood and clots.
- Will facilitate visualization if endoscopy is deemed necessary.
- Blood or coffee-ground material present in the NG aspirate suggests an upper gastrointestinal bleed.
- The absence of blood in the NG aspirate suggests either no active upper gastrointestinal bleed or a closed pylorus.
- The presence of bilious fluid and no blood in the NG aspirate suggests no active upper gastrointestinal bleeding and an open pylorus.
- Repeated bloody gastric aspirates suggest a significant or ongoing bleed.

Gastroccult®

- Can detect gastric occult blood in emesis (as small as 300 mcg/dL of hemoglobin).

Complete Blood Count

- Leukopenia and thrombocytopenia can be seen with sepsis or hypersplenism due to portal hypertension.
- In an acute bleeding episode, there may be a delay before the hematocrit registers the magnitude of the anemia.
- Chronic mucosal bleeding can cause a low mean corpuscular volume (MCV) and hypochromic, microcytic anemia.

Coagulation Studies

- Prothrombin time (PT) is prolonged in patients with liver disease, related to decreases in vitamin K dependent and independent clotting factors.
- Activated Partial Thromboplastin Time (aPTT) is prolonged with a deficiency or inhibition of any clotting factor except factor VII.

SPECIAL TESTS

Liver Function Tests

Alanine aminotransferase (ALT, SGPT)
- Increases with damage to hepatocytes as can occur with drug or toxin use, as well as with hepatocellular inflammation.

Aspartate aminotransferase (AST, SGOT)
- Also increases with injury to the hepatocytes.
- It is a less specific test than ALT.

Alkaline phosphatase (AP)
- Increases in cholestatic disease.
- Isoenzyme will determine the source of cholestatis.

γ-Glutamytransferase (GGT)
- Is a more specific marker for cholestasis than alkaline phosphatase.

Conjugated/direct bilirubin
- Taken up by the liver and converted enzymatically to a more water-soluble form.
- Can be elevated compared to unconjugated/indirect bilirubin.

Albumin
- Abnormal levels can represent chronic impairment of hepatic synthetic function.

Ammonia
- Removal is impaired in patients with chronic liver disease.

Blood Urea Nitrogen/Creatinine Ratio

- A value greater than 30 may indicate resorption of blood due to an upper gastrointestinal bleed without renal disease.

Helicobacter pylori Antibody

- The stool antigen test, in suspected cases of PUD, is preferred to the H. pylori antigen blood-test.

Type and Cross-Match

- Whenever a blood transfusion is anticipated.

Endoscopy

- For visualization and biopsies.
- May need to be done emergently in a patient with active bleeding to identify the source.

Angiography

- Reserved for those with active bleeding when visualization by the endoscope is difficult.

Tagged Red Blood Cell Scan

- Also reserved for the patient with active bleeding.

TREATMENT

Treatment will depend on etiology:

- Refer to a gastroenterologist for endoscopy to identify and potentially treat the bleeding.
- Acid suppression to treat mucosal lesions.
- Treat underlying chronic illnesses that may predispose patient to have hematemesis.
- Determine the potential for rebleeding and provide therapeutic interventions if necessary.

DISPOSITION

- History and physical findings often dictate the patient's workup and disposition.
- Hospitalize the patient whenever there is a persistent or recurrent bleeding episode(s) and/or the patient is hemodynamically compromised. If unstable, a PICU admission is warranted.

What is unique about hematemesis in adolescents?

- Bleeding is self limited for most causes of hematemesis.

- Teens may not understand appropriate medication dosing (i.e. NSAIDs) or the medical consequences of medication misuse or alcohol abuse. Educating teens is an important part of routine assessments.
- Chronic illnesses like cystic fibrosis, liver disease, and purging eating disorders are more likely to be the underlying cause of hematemesis in adolescents than in children.
- Adherence to prescribed medications (i.e. acid suppressors) is often difficult for adolescents and they may present with rebleeding episodes.
- Mental health referrals should be considered in adolescents who abuse alcohol or self induce emesis.

TEST YOUR KNOWLEDGE ANSWER

83. C. Dieulafoy's lesion is an unusual cause of GI bleeding. Massive hemorrhage occurs from a pinpoint non-ulcerated arterial lesion usually located high in the fundus of the stomach. Its characteristic presentation is massive hematemesis. The management of this type of bleeding is the same as it would be for any patient with a significant GI bleed. Acute GI bleeding is the major clinical presentation for Mallory Weiss tears. A history of epigastric pain or pain in the back may also accompany the bleeding. A patient will often give a history of non-bloody vomiting or retching before the onset of hematemesis. The blood loss that occurs with a Mallory Weiss tear is usually small and self-limited although a more severe hemorrhage can rarely occur. Bleeding from Mallory Weiss tears stops spontaneously in 80%–90% of patients, and less than 5% of patients will rebleed. PUD is a common cause of GI bleeding in adolescents that usually stops spontaneously and rarely rebleeds. Bleeding due to esophagitis is mostly occult and not acute. A teen with an underlying coagulopathy or extensive ulcerative disease is very likely to have a clinically obvious bleed, but is seldom massive.

Table 1. Etiology of Upper Gastrointestinal Bleeds in Adolescents.

Common Causes	**Less Common Causes**
Gastritis	
Mallory-Weiss Tears	
Peptic Ulcer Disease (PUD)	Hemobilia
Stress Ulcers	Dieulafoy's Lesion
Esophagitis	
Esophageal Varices	

WEB RESOURCES

- The American College of Gastroenterology, Clinical Guidelines: http://gi.org/clinical-guidelines/clinical-guidelines-sortable-list/
- Gold BD, *et al.* 'Medical Position Statement: The North American Society for Gastroenterology and Nutrition, Helicobacter pylori Infection in Children: Recommendations for Diagnosis and Treatment', Journal of Gastroenterology and Nutrition. 2000 Novemebr; 31: 490–497, retrieved from http://naspghansite.wms.cdgsolutions.com/user-assets/Documents/pdf/PositionPapers/00005176_200011000_00007.pdf
- Pediatric Education.org. Case on "What Causes Gastrointestinal Bleeding?" (May 3, 2010): http://www.pediatriceducation.org/2010/05/03/
- Squires RH, Colletti RB. 'Indications for Pediatric Gastrointestinal Endoscopy: A Medical Position Statement of the American Society for Pediatric Gastroenterology and Nutrition', Journal of Pediatric Gastroenterology and Nutrition. 1996; 23: 107–110, retrieved from http://www.naspgn.org/endoscopy.htm
- Wilson, D. Chapter 85 Hematemesis, Melena and Hematochezia. National Center for Biotechnology Information, Clinical Methods, 3rd edition (1990), retrieved from http://www.ncbi.nlm.nih.gov/books/NBK411/

Additional Clinician and Patient Resources:

- The Helicobacter Foundation: www.helico.com

56

BLOODY STOOLS: MELENA AND HEMATOCHEZIA

Leslie A. Hayes

TEST YOUR KNOWLEDGE QUESTION

84. What is the *MOST* commonly described initial symptom at presentation in adolescents with inflammatory bowel disease (IBD), though not specific for IBD?

    A. Abdominal pain
    B. Diarrhea
    C. Rectal bleeding or hematochezia
    D. Weight loss
    E. Delayed puberty

Refer to end of chapter for answer on page 624.

Your 17 year old female patient presents with 6–7 episodes of bloody diarrhea per day associated with dizziness and weakness.

BACKGROUND

- Melena, the passage of dark, tarry stools, occurs when blood remains in the gastrointestinal tract for a long time and is due to the breakdown of blood to hematin and other heme components by bacteria.
- Bleeding that occurs in the upper gastrointestinal tract and the proximal small bowel can produce melena.
- A small bleed from the ascending colon can also produce dark, tarrry stools.
- Hematochezia, the passage of bright red stools per rectum, usually suggests a lower gastrointestinal bleed; however, a massive rapid bleed from the upper gastrointestinal area can also cause hematochezia.
- Table 1 lists possible causes of melena and hematochezia in adolescents.

ASSESSMENT

HISTORY

History of Present Illness

- Determine the color and consistency of the blood seen by the patient:
  - Black tarry stools suggests an upper GI bleed.
  - Maroon-colored stools suggest a **Meckel's diverticulum.**
  - "Currant jelly" stools are seen with **intussusception.**
- Determine if the blood is mixed with the stool, covering the stool, only on the toilet paper or dripping into the toilet bowl. Blood streaked stools are common with **hemorrhoids.**
- Assess if the bleeding is associated with pain or is painless.
- Determine the duration and amount of bleeding. **Meckel's diverticulum** is usually associated with rapid bleeding.
- Ascertain if there has been a change in bowel habits (i.e. **constipation** or diarrhea).

Dietary History

- Inquire about the recent ingestion of substances that could change the color of stool (i.e. Pepto-Bismol®, iron supplements, spinach, beets or gelatin).

Medications

- Chronic use of aspirin, ibuprofen or other NSAIDs may contribute to mucosal irritation and **ulcer disease.**
- A recent course of antibiotics may be associated with **pseudomembranous colitis.**

Past Medical History

- A recent history of bleeding associated with dysenteric symptoms suggests **infectious enterocolitis.**
- A history of liver disease may indicate portal hypertension and can be associated with **esophageal varices.**

Family History

- A family history significant for polyps can indicate an **inherited polyposis disorder.**

Social History

- A sexual history that reveals anal intercourse should raise concern for **anorectal trauma** (e.g. lacerations, tears, fissures, infection).
- A substance abuse history that is significant for alcohol ingestion and/or a recent episode of forceful vomiting suggests **Mallory Weiss tears.**

Review of Systems

- History of iritis, oral lesions, weight loss, abdominal pain, diarrhea, skin rashes, musculoskeletal complaints and/or rectal bleeding suggest **inflammatory bowel disease** (IBD).
- Growth failure and decreased caloric intake suggest **Crohn's disease** (CD) while bloody stools with mucous suggests **ulcerative colitis** (UC).
- Fatigue with pallor can be the result of anemia due to blood loss from bleeding.

- Palpable purpura with colicky abdominal pain, arthralgia or arthritis and GI bleeding suggests **Henoch-Schönlein purpura** (HSP), which can be associated with **intussception.**
- A history of bloody diarrhea associated with rapidly progressing anemia, thrombocytopenia and acute renal injury suggest **hemolytic uremic syndrome** (HUS).

PHYSICAL

Vital Signs

- Assess vital signs such as pulse and blood pressure for hemodynamic stability.

Anthropometric Measurements

- Measure height and weight and plot on the appropriate growth chart.
- Poor weight gain and pubertal delay may suggest underlying chronic disease.

HEENT

- Inspect the nares and mouth for potential sites of bleeding.

Abdomen

- Inspect for ascites or abnormal venous patterns, both signs of **portal hypertension.**
- Palpate for pain, masses or hepatosplenomegaly.

Genital Exam

- Inspect the female genitalia for potential sites of bleeding that may be misinterpreted as coming from the rectum.

Anal Exam

- Check for hemorrhoids, fissures, anal tags, warts, ulcers or vesicular lesions, polyps, abscesses and fistulae, all of which can cause rectal bleeding.

STUDIES

Complete Blood Count (CBC)

- Anemia can be seen with chronic illnesses like **IBD.**
- Leukocytosis can be seen with infectious processes.
- Thrombocytopenia occurs with bleeding diatheses or **HUS.**
- Leukopenia and thrombocytopenia can be seen with sepsis or hypersplenism due to **portal hypertension.**

Comprehensive Metabolic Panel

- Hypoalbuminemia can be seen in cases of **colitis.**
- Total protein should be checked in suspected **CD.**
- Aminotransferases are elevated with hepatocyte damage.
- Alkaline phosphatase is increased in cholestatic disease.
- Bilirubin increases with cholestatic disease.

Coagulation Studies

- Prothrombin time (PT) is prolonged in patients with liver disease.
- Activated Partial Thromboplastin Time (aPTT) is prolonged with a deficiency or inhibition of any clotting factor except factor VII.

Erythrocyte Sedimentation Rate and C-Reactive Protein

- Elevations suggest an inflammatory process.

Stool Studies

- *Guaiac tests* for occult blood in stool can be performed in office.
- Red meats, iron supplements, and peroxidase-containing vegetables like turnips, horseradish, broccoli, cauliflower and cantaloupe, can produce false-positive results on guaiac tests.
- Consider ova and parasites, and cultures for Salmonella, Shigella, Campylobacter, Yersinia, E.coli 0157:H7, and C. difficile, if there is a high index of suspicion.

- Consider cultures for *C. difficile* in immunosuppressed patients or those who are on prolonged courses of antibiotics.
- *Fecal calprotectin* is highly sensitive to detect granulomatous bowel disease.

Type and Cross Match

- Indicated with a history of significant blood loss when transfusion may be needed.

SPECIAL TESTS

Gastric Lavage

- Is used to differentiate an upper from lower GI bleed.
- A bloody aspirate suggests an upper GI bleed while a non-bloody aspirate suggests that the bleeding is from a source other than the upper GI tract.
- A bile colored aspirate suggests sampling of the duodenum but does not exclude an upper GI bleed.
- Blood can act as a cathartic and cause rapid transit through the gut preventing stools from becoming melanotic.

Anti-Saccharomyces Cerevisiae Antibodies (ASCA)

- This antibody is found in 40–80 percent of individuals with CD and tends to identify disease of the terminal ileum and cecum.

Perinuclear Antineutrophil Cytoplasmic Antibodies (P-ANCA)

- Detected in 60–80% of individuals with UC and closely associated with colonic disease.

Anti OmpC Antibodies

- Can detect patients not detected by ASCA or P-ANCA.

Anti CBir1

- Antibody found in approximately 50% of individuals with CD.

Endoscopy

- Can be diagnostic and therapeutic.

Barium Enema

- Not recommended in acute settings as it can interfere with visibility during other tests.

Colonoscopy

- Procedure of choice.
- Not recommended acutely because of poor visibility due to the presence of stool and blood as well as the high risk of perforation.
- There are also adverse effects associated with cleansing the colon in the acute setting.

Upper GI Series with Small Bowel Follow Through

- Recommended in cases where IBD is suspected.

Meckel's Scan

- High affinity for gastric mucosa.

Scintigraphy

- Uses labeled RBCs or leukocytes to locate site of bleeding.

Visceral Angiography

- When the site of bleeding cannot be localized with other studies.

DISPOSITION

- Reassure the adolescent and parent that most cases of bloody stools resolve spontaneously without recurrence.
- Referral to a pediatric gastroenterologist is essential to establish a definitive diagnosis.
- Once an etiology is found, the adolescent should be counseled about the importance of medication compliance and follow up when indicated.
- A mental health counselor can assist in addressing issues related to a specific diagnosis (such as the psychological impact of sexual assault, chronic illness and long term medication use).

- Nutritional counseling is often needed when significant weight loss has occurred, in cases of inadequate weight gain or with poor eating habits.

What is unique about melena or hematochezia in adolescent?

- Chronic illness has life changing implications as it impacts various aspects of an adolescent's psychosocial development and function.
- IBD is the most common chronic illness to cause bloody stools in adolescents. The median age at diagnosis is 15 years old.
- Self esteem issues can be significant for the teen diagnosed with a chronic illness like IBD and these teens should be followed closely.

TEST YOUR KNOWLEDGE ANSWER

84. A. Abdominal pain is the most commonly described symptom at presentation. Determining whether the pain is due to inflammatory bowel disease (IBD) or another cause may be difficult. When the pain is described as localized, persistent, chronic and severe it may lead a clinician to suspect IBD. By contrast, a history of diffuse intermittent or periumbilical pain suggests functional abdominal pain. The amount of rectal bleeding at presentation varies. Rectal bleeding is more common in adolescents with ulcerative colitis (UC) than those with Crohn's disease (CD). Up to half of children and adolescents with IBD present with only minimal intermittent hematochezia. Weight loss is more common in CD than in UC. Undernutrition occurs to a greater degree in CD than UC and is an important factor for weight loss. Many adolescents with IBD present with diarrhea. The diarrhea is often associated with gross blood when the colon is involved. When the inflammatory process is isolated to the small bowel, diarrhea may be the only presenting symptom. Pubertal delay can be prolonged in patients with IBD. Delay at the onset of puberty is more commonly seen in patients with CD. In patients with frequent relapses, the duration of puberty can be prolonged.

Table 1. Differential Diagnosis of Bloody Stools.

Melena	Hematochezia
Inflammatory Bowel Disease (IBD)	IBD
Peptic Ulcer Disease (PUD)	Infectious Diarrhea
Mallory Weiss Tear	Hemorrhoids
Meckel's Diverticulum	Fissures, Tears
Esophageal Varices	Polyps
	Henoch Schonlein Purpura (HSP)
	Hemolytic Uremic Syndrome (HUS)
	Vascular Lesions
	Lymphonodular Hyperplasia
	Colon Cancer

WEB REFERENCES

- The American College of Gastroenterology, Clinical Guidelines: http://gi.org/clinical-guidelines/clinical-guidelines-sortable-list/
- Pediatric Education.org. Case on "What Causes Gastrointestinal Bleeding?" (May 3, 2010): http://www.pediatriceducation.org/2010/05/03/
- Wilson, D. Chapter 85 Hematemesis, Melena and Hematochezia. National Center for Biotechnology Information, Clinical Methods, 3rd edition (1990), retrieved from http://www.ncbi.nlm.nih.gov/books/NBK411/

Additional Clinician and Patient Resources:

- Johns Hopkins Children's Center, Gastrointestinal Bleeding or Blood in the Stool: http://www.hopkinschildrens.org/blood-in-stool.aspx
- MedicineNet.com, Rectal Bleeding (Blood in Stool, Hematochezia (reviewed 4/25/2012), http://www.medicinenet.com/rectal_bleeding/article.htm
- Web MD, Digestive Disorders Health Center: Blood in Stool: http://www.webmd.com/digestive-disorders/blood-in-stool

57

SCROTAL PATHOLOGY: PAIN AND MASSES

David S. Reitman

TEST YOUR KNOWLEDGE

85. A 15 year old male presents for his annual sports examination. On review of systems, he mentions that over the past year he occasionally feels a "heavy ache" in his left testicle. On physical examination, the patient has Tanner 4 pubic hair and genital development. You palpate a worm-like structure superior to the left testicle. This structure is visible without Valsalva. The right testicle is normal but larger than the left testicle. Which of the following would be the *MOST* reasonable next step in the management of this patient?

    A. Referral to urology
    B. Urgent referral to the emergency department
    C. Scrotal ultrasound
    D. Semen analysis
    E. Reassurance and follow-up when he turns 18 years.

86. A 17 year-old male presents complaining about pain in the groin that began last night. He admits to sexual activity with a new partner (occasionally without condoms) but denies trauma to the area. On physical examination he has Tanner 5 male genitalia. The right hemiscrotum is warm and red to the touch and the testicle tender. Superior and posterior

Refer to end of chapter for answers on pages 636.

to the testicle is a fluctuant area which is exquisitely tender to palpation. The cremaster reflex is intact bilaterally. The *MOST* likely diagnosis is:

A. Testicular torsion
B. Epididymitis
C. Incarcerated hernia
D. Testicular seminoma
E. Spermatocele.

Scrotal Pain

A 16 year old patient presents to clinic with the following complaint: "I was having some soreness in my balls and when I checked it out, I noticed a lump."

BACKGROUND

- Males start noticing changes in their genitalia during puberty, and become concerned when they experience any mild discomfort or perceive an abnormality in their penis and/or scrotum.
- While most of these complaints are benign in nature, clinicians should recognize situations that require more urgent diagnosis and treatment.
- Causes of mild scrotal tenderness include varicocele, orchitis, testicular tumor, spermatocele and "blue balls."
- More severe pain and tenderness occurs following trauma, epididymitis, incarcerated hernia and testicular torsion.

ASSESSMENT

HISTORY

History of Present Illness

Pain characteristics:

- Assess the quality of pain or discomfort: A dull ache can be present with **varicoceles** and **testicular tumors.** Sharp, intense pain suggests **testicular torsion** or an **incarcerated hernia**.
- Determine if the pain began suddenly (as in **torsion**) or started insidiously and then worsened (as in **epididymitis**).
- How long have symptoms been present? Is it an acute issue that developed over hours or more longstanding, becoming more noticeable over weeks or months?
- Determine pain location. Early in its presentation, **epididymitis** frequently produces pain in the epididymis itself.
- Determine if the pain is worsened with certain activities such as urinating, sexual intercourse, or ejaculating. Consider infectious etiology with these symptoms.

- Is there a history of trauma to the scrotum?
- Excessive or forceful masturbation or sexual activity can also lead to genital discomfort.
- Prolonged sexual stimulation without ejaculation may lead to **testicular vasocongestion (a.k.a. "blue balls")**.

Review of Systems

- The presence of fever or other systemic symptoms such as chills, should raise the suspicion of infectious causes such as **epididymitis** or **orchitis.**
- If the patient also complains of blood in urine, consider **renal stones** which may present with back pain radiating to the testicle.

Social History

- History of sexual activity raises the suspicion of infectious etiologies such as **epididymitis** or **prostatitis.**

PHYSICAL

Vital Signs

- Assess vital signs for fever, tachycardia and elevated blood pressure which suggest underlying infectious etiology.

Abdomen

- With the patient lying supine, palpate the abdomen for signs of tenderness.
- Frequently, testicular pathology may have referred pain to the abdomen.

Genital

- Examine the inguinal lymph nodes. Enlarged, tender inguinal lymph nodes are frequently seen with infectious causes of testicular pain such as **epididymitis.**

- Inspect the scrotum and phallus.
  - Reddened and swollen scrotal skin can suggest **epididymitis.**
  - Examine the urethral meatus for penile discharge and/or erythema that would further suggest **urethritis.**
  - A small, blue dot seen on the anterosuperior aspect of the testicle suggests a harmless **torsion of the appendix testes.**
- Examine the skin of the scrotum and phallus for signs of piercing or recent tattoos which can cause **scrotal cellulitis.**
- Palpate the testicles and assess for mass and localized tenderness.
  - **Epididymitis** will present with warmth and tenderness to palpation posterior-laterally to the testicles.
  - A hard mass, fixed onto the testicle must raise the clinical suspicion for **testicular cancer.**
  - **Testicular torsion** should be suspected if palpation causes severe pain (with or without swelling).
  - An area surrounding the vas deferens that feels like a "bag of worms" suggests a **varicocele.**
- Assess the cremasteric reflex (lightly scratching the medial upper thigh on both sides) to see that the testicles rise in response. Absence of the cremaster reflex suggests a **testicular torsion.**
- A painful mass protruding through the inguinal canal may be an incarcerated hernia. Place the bell of the stethoscope over the mass to assess for bowel sounds.

Digital Rectal

- Can be performed to assess for prostate tenderness.
- The prostate should have a 2.5 cm diameter and feel smooth and rubbery to touch.
- A boggy, tender prostate suggests a diagnosis of **prostatitis.**

An entirely normal examination should prompt the clinician to look for causes of referred pain, such as **renal stones, appendicitis or neuropathic pain.**

STUDIES

Urine Culture and Urinalysis

- Leukocytosis can be seen with epididymitis.

Gonorrhea and Chlamydia Cultures or DNA Testing

- Should be considered in all sexually active teens.

Ultrasound with Doppler Flow

- Consider urgently if a torsion is suspected: a delay can compromise the testicle's viability.
- Twisting of the spermatic artery, accompanied by decreased blood flow suggests **testicular torsion** while increased blood flow can be seen in **epididymitis.**

Ultrasound

- Hypoechoic areas with distinct borders may suggest a testicular seminoma.
- Calcifications and cystic areas with indistinct borders occur in non-seminomatous neoplasms.

DISPOSITION

- Initiate antibiotics for the treatment of epididymitis.
- A suspected testicular torsion may not allow time for diagnostic procedures and immediate surgical intervention may be needed to save testicular function.
  - If an ultrasound was done and indicates testicular torsion, patients should be referred to urology for immediate surgical intervention (detorsion).
  - Orchidopexy should also be considered for the contralateral testicle.
- An incarcerated hernia that cannot be easily reduced must also be referred to surgery for urgent intervention.
- Varicoceles may be non-urgently referred to urology depending on their grading.
- Counsel patients that "blue balls" may be relieved by masturbation with ejaculation.

Scrotal Masses

BACKGROUND

Scrotal "lumps" can be caused by varicoceles, spermatoceles, hydroceles, testicular tumors, hernias, and calcification of the appendix testes.

ASSESSMENT

HISTORY

History of Present Illness

- Determine when the testicular mass was first noted. **Congenital hydroceles** can be a lifelong phenomenon.
- Is there pain associated with the scrotal mass? Dull pain suggests a **varicocele or tumor** while sharper pain suggests an **inguinal hernia.**
- Is the mass constant or intermittent **(hernia)?**
- Does the patient describe a hard mass that is fixed to the testicle (**testicular tumor**) or a mass that is fluctuant and separate from the testicle (as occurs with **varicoceles, spermatoceles, hydroceles or hernias**)?
- Has the patient had any recent infection such as epididymitis or orchitis which would suggest a **reactive hydrocele**?
- Is there a history of trauma to the scrotum? Hematomas inside the scrotum can calcify.
- Is there a sudden increase in size of the scrotum following trauma (**reactive hydrocele**)?

Past Medical History

- Does the patient have medical problems causing hypoproteinemia (i.e. protein-losing enteropathy or nephritic syndrome) that could lead to extravasation of fluid into the scrotum?
- Has the patient been immunized against mumps?
- Is there a history of sexually transmitted infections (STIs)?

Review of Systems

- Are there any accompanying systemic symptoms such as back pain or shortness of breath which suggest **testicular cancer metastases**?

PHYSICAL

Genital

- Should be done with patient in a standing position.
- Visually inspect the scrotum for signs of swelling, trauma and varices.
- **Testicular tumors** are detected as hard lumps (as small as 0.5 mm) that are fixed and attached to the testicles.
- The epididymis is localized posterolaterally to each testicle. A hard swelling or out-pocket off of the epididymis suggests a **spermatocele.**
- **Hydroceles** are often noticed anterior to the testicle. Holding a light source to this swelling can cause the light to disperse within the scrotum and will illuminate the entire scrotal sack.
- A "bag of worms" may be appreciated superior to the testicle. This represents dilation of the pampiniform plexus of veins and indicates a **varicocele.**
  - Varicoceles may be left-sided (more common) or bilateral.
  - An isolated right-sided varicocele should raise suspicion of an abdominal or retroperitoneal process restricting blood return to the vena cava.
  - Varicoceles may enlarge in size during a Valsalva maneuver.
- Examine the inguinal canal by placing your fifth finger through the external ring of the canal. Have the patient perform a Valsalva to increase his intra-abdominal pressure. If present, a hernia may push the finger out of the canal. Following this maneuver one may see swelling protrude from the canal.
  - If intestinal contents protrude through the inguinal canal, the clinician may be able to auscultate bowel sounds by placing the stethoscope on the mass.

STUDIES

Urinalysis

- The presence of white blood cells may suggest **epididymitis** or a **reactive hydrocele.** This should be followed-up with testing for Gonorrhea and Chlamydia.

Human Chorionic Gonadotropin

- Is useful as a tumor marker: the beta subunit component is elevated with seminomas and choriocarcinomas.

Ultrasound

- **Testicular seminomas** are seen as hypoechoic areas with distinct borders in the testicle.
- Intra-testicular calcifications and cystic areas with indistinct borders can be seen with **non-seminomatous neoplasms**.
- A varicocele may be seen with ultrasound, but this diagnosis is usually made clinically.
  - Dilated pampiniform plexus of veins suggests a **varicocele.**
- **Spermatoceles** may be seen as a cystic outgrowth off of the epididymis.
- A **hydrocele** will be seen anterior to the testicle.

DISPOSITION

- A classic spermatocele does not require any further work up or consult unless painful.
- Urology consultation is usually required for treatment of all other testicular masses.
  - Testicular neoplasms found on ultrasound require urgent referral for orchiectomy and tumor staging.
  - Small, asymptomatic spermatoceles do not require any treatment; however, painful spermatoceles can be referred for removal.
  - Reducible hernias should be referred to general surgery for repair.
  - Congenital communicating hydroceles may require surgical repair as they are frequently associated with inguinal hernias.
  - Small varicoceles can often be monitored over time for changes and do not require further intervention. A varcicocelectomy should be considered if there is:
    - Pain in the scrotum.
    - A decrease in testicular growth on the affected side.
    - A large varicocele visible without valsalva maneuver.

- Abnormalities on semen analysis (this study is not recommended in teens).

- When a reactive hydrocele is present, it is important to determine the hydrocele's etiology. They will generally resolve once the underlying condition (e.g. trauma or infection) is treated.

What is unique about scrotal pain and masses in adolescents?

- Adolescents may deny or refuse to discuss sexual activity if they think that their parents may find out. The provider must excuse the parents from the room when taking a sexual history.
- Teens may minimize or even try to ignore symptoms out of fear that they might have cancer or will lose a testicle. This often translates in delay in seeking care and makes urgent evaluation more likely.
- If testicular torsion is suspected, the clinician may have to forgo diagnostic testing for urgent surgical evaluation and intervention.
- Large varicoceles (with or without testicular atrophy), noted early in puberty, require close follow-up for decreased testicular growth and possible referral to urology for evaluation.
- When assessing for varicoceles, adolescent males will likely be unwilling or unable to provide a semen sample to assess for sperm formation.

TEST YOUR KNOWLEDGE ANSWERS

85. A. The "bag of worms" along with the clinical presentation suggest that this teen has a varicocele. Because he has a Grade 3 varicocele (large and visible on inspection) that is accompanied by pain and discomfort, he should be referred to urology for evaluation and possible surgical treatment. Grade 1 varicoceles (small) are not visible on exam and only palpated with valsalva maneuver while Grade 2 varicoceles (medium) are palpated at rest without valsalva. Varicoceles are chronic conditions which generally do not need emergency evaluation or intervention. Ultrasound may confirm the diagnosis but it is generally not performed because most varicoceles can be comfortably diagnosed based on physical examination. While semen

analysis may assist the urologist in determining whether the varicocele is affecting male fertility, an adolescent male will likely be extremely uncomfortable when asked to produce a sample. This evaluation should be reserved for young adults. In this vignette, the boy is complaining about scrotal discomfort and the clinician notes decreased growth in the left testicle. These are both indications for urologic referral rather than simple reassurance.

86. B. This young man most likely has epididymitis caused by infection with gonorrhea or chlamydia. This will need to be treated with antibiotics, scrotal support and bed rest. Testicular torsion tends to have a more acutely painful presentation. The cremasteric reflex disappears and redness or swelling are not commonly part of the presentation. Similarly, incarcerated hernias do not present with redness or swelling of the testicle. Rather, they appear as a protuberance from the inguinal canal and may have bowel sounds associated with them. While testicular seminomas may present with pain, onset is usually insidious and unaccompanied by signs of acute inflammation. Examination will more likely reveal a hard, fixed mass on the testicle rather than swelling or tenderness to the epididymis. Spermatoceles are usually painless masses palpated on the epididymis or the distal vas deferens.

WEB REFERENCES

- American Urologic Association, The Acute Scrotum: http://www.auanet.org/content/education-and-meetings/med-stu-curriculum/acute-scrotum.pdf
- Centers for Disease Control and Prevention: Epididymitis (updated January 28, 2011): http://www.cdc.gov/std/treatment/2010/epi didymitis.htm
- Koester MC. 'Initial Evaluation and Management of Acute Scrotal Pain', Journal of Athletic Training. 2000; 35(l): 76–79, retrieved from http://www.ncbi.nlm.nih.gov/pmc/articles/PMC1323443/pdf/jathtrain00001-0078.pdf
- Taskinen S, *et al.* 'Testicular tumors in children and adolescents', Journal of Pediatric Urology. 2008; 4: 134–137, retrieved from http://www.sepeap.org/archivos/pdf/10892.pdf
- Tiemstra JD, Kapoor S. 'Evaluation of Scrotal Masses', American Family Physician. 2008 Nov 15:78(10): 1165–1170, retrieved from http://www.aafp.org/afp/2008/1115/pll65.html
- Trojian TH, Lishnak TS, Heiman D. 'Epididymitis and Orchitis: An Overview', American Family Physician. 2009 Apr l; 79(7): 583–587, retrieved from http://www.aafp.org/afp/2009/0401/p583.html

Additional Clinician and Patient Resources:

- American Urologic Association: Boys, Sports & Testicular Injury: When to Wear a Cup (July 7, 2009): http://www.auanet.org/content/press/press_releases/article.cfm?articleNo=148
- Medline Plus, Testicular Disorders: http://www.nlm.nih.gov/medlineplus/testicular disorders.html
- Men's Health Forum, Physical Health Penis and Testicles: http://www.malehealth.co.uk/topic/physical-health/penis-and-testicles
- Urologyhealth.org: The Official Website of the American Urological Association Foundation: http://www.urologyhealth.org/adult/
- Young Men's Health, Testicular Torsion: http://www.youngmenshealthsite.org/testicular_torsion.html

58

HIP PAIN AND LIMPING

Elizabeth G. Cius

TEST YOUR KNOWLEDGE

87. Which one of the following descriptions is most consistent with a diagnosis of slipped capital femoral epiphysis (SCFE)?
    A. 15 year old female long distance cross country runner who presents with groin pain that worsens with activity and improves with rest.
    B. 14 year old male with acute onset of hip pain in the setting of fever and chills.
    C. Obese 12 year old female with gradual onset of pain in her thigh that radiates to her knee associated with limping.
    D. Healthy 13 year old female that presents with vague nighttime hip pain that significantly improves with ibuprofen.
    E. All the above.

Refer to end of chapter for answer on page 646.

An obese 13 year old male presents to clinic with his mother with complaints of knee and thigh pain that started about 2–3 weeks ago. He cannot recall a specific injury to the hip but is a football player and may have gotten "roughed up" in practice. He is now limping and wants to know what he can do to make it better so he can return to play.

BACKGROUND

- Increased sports participation and obesity prevalence have made hip problems a common complaint of teens in the outpatient setting.
- Most causes of hip pain can be determined by a careful history and physical exam (Table 1).
- Slipped capital femoral epiphysis (SCFE) is a serious cause of hip pain in adolescence and is a frequently missed diagnosis requiring a high level of suspicion.
- SCFE occurs when the proximal femoral epiphysis is displaced from the femoral neck through the growth plate.
- The mean age of presentation is 12 years in females (premenarche) and 13.5 years in males (not yet reached Tanner stage IV).
- In many patients with SCFE, the presentation is knee pain rather than hip pain.
- SCFE is a surgical emergency; treatment delay may result in permanent disability.

RISK FACTORS

- Overweight/Obesity: Most teens who develop SCFE are at or above the 90th percentile of weight for age and sex.
- Growth Spurt and unfused growth plates place teens at higher risk.
- At presentation, if the patient is younger than 8 or older than 16 years, or has a weight below the 50th percentile for age or height below the 10th percentile for age, consider the following:
  - Endocrine disorders such as hypothyroidism and growth hormone deficiency.
  - Renal failure.
  - History of radiation therapy.
  - Genetic disorders such as Down syndrome.

ASSESSMENT

HISTORY

History of Present Illness

- Determine pain characteristics (Table 2):
  - Location? Hip lesions can manifest as referred pain to the knees, anterior thigh or groin.
  - Injury? Did the pain start after **trauma** to the area or occur without injury?
  - Duration? Acute onset usually accompanies **trauma** or **infection.** An insidious onset is associated with an **overuse injury, SCFE, Legg-Calves-Perthes disease** (**LCPD**) which occurs in prepubertal children, or chronic diseases such as **rheumatoid arthritis** or a **tumor**.
  - Quality? Is the pain severe, constant, intermittent, worse or better with activity? Does it wake the teen from sleep?
  - Are there alleviating (i.e. medications, ice, rest or compression) or aggravating factors (i.e. weight bearing, exercise or direct pressure to the area)?
- Has the patient ever injured this area before or sought care for this pain in the past?
- Is the pain associated with other concerning symptoms? Acute hip pain in the setting of fever, chills and a swollen warm joint suggests **septic arthritis.**
- **Appendicitis** can present as hip pain if the psoas muscle is inflamed.
- Is the patient sexually active? While not commonly seen in the hips, **gonococcal septic arthritis** should be considered, especially if the patient has concomitant embolic lesions (arthritis-dermatitis syndrome).

Past Medical History

- Does the patient have a medical condition that explains or contributes to current hip pain?
  - Overweight or obese.
  - Endocrinopathies such as **hypothyroidism, hypogonadism, growth hormone deficiency** or **panhypopituitarism.**
  - Genetic disorders such as **Down syndrome** or **Rubenstein-Taybi syndrome.**

- Rheumatologic disorders such as **juvenile rheumatoid arthritis (JRA)**, **systemic lupus erythematosus (SLE)** or **psoriatic arthritis.**
- Musculoskeletal disorders such as **osteoarthritis** of the hip or knee.
- A malignancy such as **Ewing's sarcoma** or **leukemia.**
- Hematologic condition such as **sickle cell disease (SCD)** are associated with avascular necrosis of the femoral head.

Past Surgical History

- Has the patient ever had a surgical procedure?
  - For 30–60% of patients diagnosed with unilateral SCFE, there is an increased risk that the contralateral hip will slip in the future.

Review of Systems

- Constitutional symptoms such as weight change, fatigue, weakness, fever, chills or night sweats suggest an **infectious** or **oncologic etiology**.
- Skin, hair or nail changes may indicate underlying **psoriasis, JRA** or **thyroid disease.**
- Muscle weakness, joint pain, swelling or stiffness suggest **rheumatologic disorder.**
- Numbness or tingling in the lower extremities, sensory changes, or bowel/bladder incontinence suggests **lumbar spine pathology**.
- Cold intolerance and constipation are consistent with **hypothyroidism.**

PHYSICAL

First: Observe without touching.

- Observe the position of the feet while the patient lies supine. Asymmetric positioning, with one foot in external rotation, suggests hip pathology.
- Expose the patient's legs and compare the affected hip to the unaffected side for deformity, overlying ecchymosis, erythema or swelling.
- Observe the patient's gait.
- Evaluate the patient's range of motion and compare to the unaffected side.
- Check for Trendelenburg's Sign:

  - As the patient stands on one leg (the affected side), pelvic tilting towards the unaffected side is considered a positive test indicating weakness of the hip abductor.
  - A positive test can be associated with **SCFE, developmental dysplasia, LCPD,** or weakness/paralysis of the hip abductor muscles.

- Assess for leg length discrepancy.
  - While lying supine, have the patient bring their heels towards their buttocks with feet together.
  - Any difference in the height of knees is associated with leg length discrepancy (Galeazzi Test). One can also measure the leg length from the anterior superior iliac spine to the lateral malleoli bilaterally.

Second: Perform the exam.

- In limping patients with knee pain, a normal knee exam points toward the need to examine the hip!
- Always examine the joint above and below the site of pain or injury.
- Palpate the affected hip (note that palpation of the hip joint may not always be helpful given joint depth).
  - Is there effusion or increased warmth over the joint?
  - Pain over the greater trochanter suggests **greater trochanter bursitis.**
- Strength testing should be preformed and compared to contralateral side.
- Log roll the affected hip and compare with unaffected side. Pain with this maneuver is seen in traumatic, infectious and inflammatory processes.
- Evaluate the hip for internal rotation. Place the patient in a prone position, knees flexed, ankles and feet rotated laterally. Limited internal rotation may indicate **SCFE, transient synovitis** or **septic arthritis**.

STUDIES

Laboratory studies are of limited value.

- If septic arthritis is suspected, a CBC with differential, ESR, CRP and blood cultures should be obtained.

- If symptoms (i.e. myxedema, constipation or cold intolerance) suggest an endocrinopathy (i.e. thyroid disease), corresponding tests should be considered (i.e. TSH).

X-Ray

- New onset hip pain or limp should be evaluated radiologically.
- Obtain at least 2 views of the affected and unaffected (for comparison) sides: the anteroposterior (AP) and lateral views.
- A lateral view can be obtained by frog leg positioning or by cross-table views. In cases of significantly decreased range of motion, the cross-table view is preferred.
- Most cases of SCFE are diagnosed by the following radiologic findings:
  - Steel sign: A double density seen at the metaphysis on AP film.
  - Widening of the growth plate when compared to the unaffected side.
  - Decreased epiphyseal height compared to the unaffected side.
  - Klein's line: A line is drawn along the superior edge of femoral neck on AP film. This line should cross the growth plate but if the growth plate falls below the line, findings are consistent with SCFE.

CT Scan with or without Contrast

- Details bone and soft tissue anatomy.
- May rule out appendicitis, deep soft tissue infection or tumor.
- Helps standardize severity of the slip in patient's with chronic SCFE.

MRI with or without Contrast

- Detects radiologically occult "preslips" in SCFE.
- Osteonecrosis of the femoral head may be more obvious by MRI (versus x-ray) to identify LCPD or SCD.
- Osteomyelitis is more easily identified by MRI.

Bone Scan

- Evaluates blood flow and metabolic activity to the area and can identify an underlying infection or neoplasm.

Ultrasound

- Evaluates the soft tissue surrounding the joint and is often used to guide joint effusion aspiration in cases of septic arthritis.

TREATMENT

- Therapy will depend on the etiology of hip pain or limping. For example, SCFE is considered an orthopedic surgical emergency.
- Once the diagnosis of SCFE is made, the goals of care are to prevent further slippage and associated complications including osteonecrosis.
- Following diagnosis, immediately have patient non-weight bearing with use of crutches or wheelchair.
- Patients should be referred to orthopedic surgery for definitive treatment. SCFE is typically repaired by a single cannulated screw in the center of the epiphysis.
- Delays in treatment may result in permanent disability. Surgery is indicated as soon as the diagnosis is confirmed.

DISPOSITION

- Outcome of SCFE is based on slip severity (e.g. mild, moderate or severe) and whether the slip is stable or unstable.
- Stable slip: The patient is able to walk and bear weight with or without crutches.
  - After repair, the teen will have a period of limited weight bearing for 6–8 weeks after which regular activities can be resumed.
  - Return to sports is dependent on the range of motion preserved.
  - Typically carries an excellent prognosis.
- Unstable slip: The patient is unable to bear weight even with crutches.
  - Associated with a higher rate of complications.
  - 20–50% will develop osteonecrosis with an increased risk for osteoarthritis.
- Between 1/3 to 2/3 of patients with unilateral SCFE may develop SCFE in the contralateral hip joint. There is ongoing debate over whether

prophylactic pinning of the unaffected hip should be preformed at the time of SCFE repair.

What is unique about hip pain and limping in adolescents?

- SCFE and apophyseal avulsion fractures are conditions unique to adolescents, because their growth plates have not yet fused, placing them at higher risk.
- When obtaining x-rays, contralateral views of the unaffected hip are essential to compare the extent of fusion of the growth plates.

TEST YOUR KNOWLEDGE ANSWER

87. C. SCFE typically occurs before epiphyseal plate closure and during maximal growth with a mean age of onset of 12 years in females and 13.5 years in males. Being overweight or obese is a major risk factor for the development of SCFE with most patients in the 90th percentile for weight for age or greater. Pain in SCFE may either be acute (duration less than 4 weeks) or chronic, and is located in the hip, thigh, knee or groin region. The case scenario in choice A most accurately describes a femoral stress fracture. The case scenario in choice B should raise a clinician's suspicion for septic arthritis. Finally, the case described in choice D most likely describes a patient with an osteoid osteoma.

Table 1. Common Causes of Hip Pain/Limping.

Condition	Clinical Features	Studies	Treatment
Slipped Capital Femoral Epiphysis 10–15 Years	• Acute (<4 weeks) or chronic presentation of painful limp • Non-specific hip, knee, groin or thigh pain • Overweight/obese • Uni- or bilateral • More common in African Americans and Pacific Islanders	• Positive Trendelenberg sign or leg length discrepancy • Painful, limited internal rotation on exam • X-ray diagnostic in most cases	• Make immediately non-weight bearing • Refer to orthopedic surgery for definitive management
Femoral Stress Fracture 12–18 Years	• Runners or endurance athletes • Insidious onset of anterior thigh pain that is initially worse with activity and progresses to pain at rest • Consider female athlete triad (amenorrhea, disordered eating and osteoporosis)	• Positive Hop Test (pain when hopping on affected leg) • Hip X-rays may not be helpful in early stage • If strongly suspected, MRI or bone scan can be more reliable	• Non-weight bearing until evidence of healing (2–4 weeks) with gradual return to play
Apophyseal Avulsion Fracture 12–25 Years	• Acute onset of pain after sudden, forceful muscle contraction • A "pop" is commonly reported	• Pain with passive stretch and active contraction of involved muscle • Pain to palpation over involved apophysis	Rehab program to gradually increase ROM and strength
Osteoid Osteoma 10–20 Years	• Pain is initially mild and intermittent but progresses to severe and constant • Pain at night is common • May have swelling or deformity of hip	• Decreased range of motion and atrophy of quadriceps • X-ray may be sufficient to make diagnosis; however, if negative and with a high index of suspicion can have MRI/bone scan	• Benign condition • Typically has excellent response to NSAIDs or ASA • May need surgery to remove if pain persists

(Continued)

Table 1. *(Continued)*

Condition	Clinical Features	Studies	Treatment

Septic Arthritis Any Age	• Acute onset of pain and limp in an ill and febrile patient
	• Refusal to bear weight
		• ESR > 40
		• WBC > 12,000
		• Blood culture
		• Lyme testing if in prevalent region
		• U/S will show effusion
		• U/S guided aspiration of joint fluid is gold standard for diagnosis
			• Hospital admission:
			  • Drain effusion
			  • IV antibiotics
			  • Immobilize joint and control pain

Tumor or Neoplastic Condition Any Age	• Insidious onset of pain in hip, groin or thigh • Associated night pain and "B symptoms" (Weight loss, night sweats, fever)	• CBC with differential • MRI • Bone marrow aspirate	Refer to Oncologist
Greater Trochanteric Burstitis Older Adults but Can be Seen in Teens	• Chronic intermittent lateral hip pain • Common in obese teens or those who run or climb	• Painful to direct palpation over the greater trochanter • A clinical diagnosis	• Rest, ice and NSAIDs • Stretching exercises for iliotibial band • May consider steroid injection

Table 2. Pain Characteristics and Associated Conditions.

Pain Characteristic	Associated Conditions
Constant and severe pain	Fracture Septic arthritis Osteomyelitis Sickle cell disease complication
Intermittent and less severe pain	SCFE Juvenile idiopathic arthritis Legg-Calves-Perthes disease (pre-pubertal) Transient synovitis (prepubertal)
Pain increases with activity	Overuse injuries Stress fractures
Pain decreases with activity	Rheumatologic conditions
Night pain	Tumor (Ewing's sarcoma) Leukemia Osteoid osteoma (benign)
Knee pain	SCFE (*referred pain seen in 15% of SCFE cases*)
Lateral thigh pain	Lumbar spine pathology: Herniated disc Vertebral osteomyelitis Greater trochanteric bursitis Ilotibial band syndrome (associated with snapping sound)

WEB REFERENCES

- Houghton KM. 'Review for the generalist: evaluation of pediatric hip pain', Pediatri Rheumatol Online J. 2009; 7: 10, retrieved from http://www.ncbi.nlm.nih.gov/pmc/articles/PMC2686695/
- Johanns J, Knopp W. 'What's causing your young patient's hip pain?', The Journal of Family Practice. 2010 October; 59(10): 555–561, retrieved from http://www.jfponline.com/Pages.asp?AID=8993
- Sawyer JR. Kapoor M. The Limping Child: A Systematic Approach to Diagnosis', American Family Physician. 2009 Feb l; 79(3): 215–224, retrieved from http://www.aafp.org/afp/2009/0201/p215.html

- Solduk L, Sogut O, Kaya H, Gokdemir MT, Ozkanli U. 'An Adolescent Patient With Hip Pain: Slipped Capital Femoral Epiphysis', J Clin Med Res 2011; 3(2): 99–100, retrieved from http://www.jocmr.org/index.php/JOCMR/article/view/503/315

Additional Clinician and Patient Resources:

- American Academy of Family Physicians (AAFP), General Sports Information: http://www.aafp.org/online/en/home.html
- American Academy of Pediatrics (AAP) Council on Sports Medicine and Fitness: http://www.aap.org/sections/sportsmedicine/SportsShorts.cfm
- American College of Sports Medicine: http://www.acsm.org
- American Medical Society of Sports Medicine: http://www.amssm.org
- Livestrong.com, Hip Pain in Adolescents (Sept 12, 2011), http://www.livestrong.com/article/542289-hip-pain-in-adolescents/
- TeensHealth from Nemours, Slipped Capital Femoral Epiphysis (SCFE), http://kidshealth.org/teen/diseases_conditions/bones/SCFE.html

59

NEUROLOGICAL EMERGENCIES: SEVERE HEADACHES, WEAKNESS, INCOORDINATION AND ALTERED MENTAL STATUS

Rick Place

TEST YOUR KNOWLEDGE

88. A CT scan is acutely indicated in each of the following conditions *EXCEPT*:

    A. Pseudotumor cerebri
    B. Intracranial bleeding
    C. Guillain-Barré syndrome
    D. Cerebellitis
    E. Acute ischemic stroke

Refer to end of chapter for answer on page 660.

A 14 year old female presents with complaints of lower extremity weakness and difficulty urinating. She had been taking cold medicines and today she feels as though she can barely walk.

BACKGROUND

- Neurologic emergencies comprise a wide array of pathologies that involve the central and peripheral nervous system.
- Adolescents may consult for sudden acute and severe headaches, sensory changes or paresthesias, focal motor weakness, acute incoordination and altered mental status.
- Etiologies include infectious, vascular, connective tissue and immune disorders.
- The goal of patient evaluation is to identify the location of a possible lesion and make a definitive diagnosis.

ASSESSMENT

HISTORY

History of Present Illness

Acute and severe headaches

- A common reason for consultation and the biggest question for the sufferer is often: "Is this a brain tumor?"
- While headaches do occur with **brain tumors**, brain tumors are not common causes of headaches.
- Increased intracranial pressure may result in a headache. Classically, this is a headache that awakens the patient from sleep and may be associated with vomiting; however, the sensitivity of these findings is low.
- A sudden onset, severe headache suggests an intracerebral vascular accident (i.e. **intravascular hemorrhage, subarachnoid hemorrhage**) and must be evaluated as such. These patients will look ill.
- A headache preceded by an aura may be a teen's first **migraine**. Auras typically involve the occipital lobe and are described as visual disturbances and occasionally brief periods of blindness. They often resolve before the onset

of the headache. Confusion may be an aura equivalent noted in **complex migraines**.

- Subacute, persistent, severe global headaches with or without vision changes in an obese teen should raise the suspicion of **pseudotumor cerebri**: a classic neurologic finding is papilledema from increased intracranial pressure which can lead to optic atrophy and blindness.
- **Meningitis** *MUST* be a consideration for headaches in the context of fever and neck stiffness.
    - **Viral** and **bacterial meningitis** can only be differentiated by the results of a lumbar puncture and CSF cultures.
    - Several days of persistent headache *without fever* is not uncommon in **viral** and **Lyme meningitis**.
    - Acute headaches in a patient with HIV is a high risk complaint requiring further investigation to rule out **pansinusitis** or **cryptococcal meningitis**.
- Other systemic illnesses such as pyelonephritis, influenza, and strep pharyngitis may produce moderately severe headache as part of a constitutional syndrome.

Acute sensory changes or parasthesias

- Common complaints in adolescents that are frequently difficult to prove or disprove. The key to the evaluation is that the neurologic distribution makes sense.
- **Transient ischemic attacks** (TIA) may produce transient sensory changes in a characteristic neurologic distribution. TIAs can occur in teens.
- Sensory changes that precede or are concurrent with a headache may be part of a **complicated migraine**.
- The exception to the rule that sensory (and motor) changes following a neurologic distribution are disorders with lesions that "differ in time and place" such as **multiple sclerosis** (MS) or **acute disseminated encephalomyelitis** (**ADEM**).

Acute focal motor weakness

- **Ischemic stroke** is of immediate concern when there is sudden onset motor weakness.

- **Sickle cell disease, thrombophilias (hypercoagulable states)** and **neoplasm** all predispose to ischemic stroke, while other conditions such as **Moyamoya disease** (chronic occlusive intravascular vasculopathy) or **vascular malformations** contribute to a hemorrhagic stroke.
- **Bell's palsy** is an idiopathic paresis of cranial nerve VII. Teens may complain of a concomitant headache, which can confuse the clinical picture.
- The onset of unilateral weakness, visual changes and severe headache may herald the presence of a **cerebral venous sinus thrombosis** in predisposed individuals (e.g. those with diabetic ketoacidosis or thrombophilia).
- **ADEM**, a post-infectious, demyelinating disorder can affect the entire central nervous system (including the spine) and may present with focal weakness anywhere.
- **Guillain-Barré syndrome** is also a post-infectious acute inflammatory demyelinating process that presents with ascending paralysis from the legs up.

Acute incoordination (cerebellar dysfunction)

- May present acutely with **cerebellar stroke** or may develop insidiously with **cerebral neoplasm** or **cerebellitis**.
- Cerebellar ataxia from **cerebellitis** is generally a post-infectious disorder that is most commonly associated with **mycoplasma**, **varicella**, and other viral etiologies.
- **Vertigo** (vestibular dysfunction) may present as ataxia (versus "spinning").

Acute altered mental status

- Rarely a primary neurologic abnormality, and is usually secondary to some other cause; diagnosis will depend on the associated symptoms.
- Occasionally, **partial complex seizures** will present with periods of confusion in the absence of other signs and symptoms.
- Other causes of acute altered mental status are **drug ingestion**, **meningitis**, **intracranial bleeding** and **confusional migraine**.
- Associated symptoms can focus the diagnostic evaluation:
  - Back pain in the presence of lower extremity symptoms suggests the possibility of a **spinal cord lesion**; this is a very time-dependent diagnosis.
  - Fever suggests an infectious etiology.

- History of depressive symptoms may raise suspicion of an intentional suicidal overdose.
- Assessing rectal and urinary function/incontinence is important, particularly when there is a question of a spinal process (back pain and associated weakness).

Past Medical History

- Can provide context for any acute neurologic condition (e.g. a known history of sickle cell disease can focus the differential).

Family History

- May be important for several conditions including: **migraine headaches** and **stroke (thrombophilia)**.

Medications

- May produce or contribute to neurologic conditions.
- **Pseudotumor cerebri** is more common in obese patients, those who rapidly gain weight and/or those on medications such as tetracycline, steroids, and oral contraceptives.
- Oral contraceptives may also be associated with migraine and strokes.

PHYSICAL

Comprehensive Neurologic Exam

- Mental status assessment: Determine if the teen is able to demonstrate that they are alert and oriented to person, place and time.
- Cranial nerve exam: The phrase "cranial nerves 2-12 intact" implies a formal and complete cranial nerve exam, including formal hearing test of *each* ear.
  - Cranial nerve 2: Anisocoria (unilateral dilated pupil) is concerning but can be a variant. If the patient does not appear acutely ill, an impending herniation is unlikely.
  - Visual field defects may be present in **acute migraines** or **occipital lesions**.
  - Abnormal extraocular movements (EOM), controlled by cranial nerves 3,4 and 6, must be evaluated.

- **Abducens palsy** (cranial nerve 6) with lateral gaze paralysis, may be a sign of increased intracranial pressure.
- General weakness of the EOM may herald the onset of **Miller-Fischer variant of Guillain-Barré Syndrome.**
- The trigeminal nerve (cranial nerve 5) is examined by testing sensation on each cheek.
- Facial weakness (cranial nerve 7) is almost universally due to **Bell's palsy**.
- In endemic areas, facial nerve palsy is often secondary to **Lyme disease** (often, there is an associated headache).
- **Peripheral Bell's paresis** may be distinguished from a central lesion: the patient with a peripheral lesion is unable to raise the unilateral eyebrow, whereas the patient with the central lesion can lift both eyebrows because of fibers that cross before creation of the peripheral nerve.
- The glossopharyngeal and vagus nerves (cranial nerves 9 and 10) are responsible for swallowing and can be tested by assessing strength and symmetry of palatal rise and quality of the voice.
- Patients with late stage **Guillain-Barré syndrome** may experience bulbar weakness, including difficulty handling secretions and guttural speech.

- Motor exam: may be performed by testing both upper and lower extremities for strength and symmetry. Additionally, testing each extremity for proximal and distal strength is critical, as some disorders will selectively affect different muscle groups.
  - **Guillain-Barré syndrome** will typically present with distal motor weakness (lower preceding upper extremity) and includes loss of reflexes as well as proprioception.
  - Focal motor weakness (paresis = partial; paralysis = complete) is notable with focal CNS lesions caused by **stroke**, **ADEM**, **neoplasm** or other insult.
  - Focal weakness that resolves is characteristic of a **TIA** (from embolic or ischemic occlusion); however, brief episodes of weakness may also be seen with migraines (**complicated migraine**) or after a generalized seizure (**Todd's paralysis**).
  - Generalized weakness is a more subjective finding but may be noted with early **Guillain-Barré syndrome**.

  - Generalized weakness is often a manifestation of more systemic issues, such as profound **hypokalemia, Addison's disease, botulism,** or even as a presenting complaint in **acute renal failure**.
- Reflex exam: Reflexes may become diminished early with peripheral motor weakness, particularly **Guillain-Barré syndrome**.
- Cerebellar function: Test by finger to nose (or ankle over shin) testing. Abnormalities identify dysmetria.
  - Ataxic gait may be the only sign of cerebellar deficit and is the most frequently omitted part of the neurologic exam. A patient may appear perfectly normal in bed or sitting, but be unable to stand or walk normally.
  - Romberg, standing while placing one foot in front of the other, is a test of proprioception and assesses the dorsal column of the spinal cord.

Digital Rectal

- It is critical to assess for rectal tone whenever a spinal process is suspected. These are extremely time dependent processes that require a rapid diagnosis.

STUDIES

- Laboratory tests may be important to advance the diagnostic process, establish diagnosis or provide clarification.
- The most important test for aiding the diagnosis of an unspecified neurologic condition is diagnostic imaging.

Complete Blood Count (CBC)

- Will identify anemia or leukocytosis.

Basic Metabolic Panel

- Will identify hypokalemia and assess renal function.

C-Reactive Protein

- Elevation could be useful to identify an infectious condition such as **spinal epidural abscess** but is otherwise nonspecific.

Cerebrospinal Fluid Studies

- Elevated white counts can be seen with **meningitis, encephalitis** and **cerebellitis.**
- Isolated increases in CSF protein may be noted in **Guillain-Barré syndrome.**
- Elevated RBCs in the CSF that do not clear between tubes 1 and 4 are concerning for the possibility of subarachnoid blood (which may not be noted on the CT scan).
- Elevated opening pressure indicates increased intercranial pressure, which can be seen with brain tumors and meningitis.
- In the absence of tumor, infection or obstruction, elevated opening pressure is diagnostic for pseudotumor cerebri.

Comprehensive Toxicology Screen

- A simple **drug screen** is rarely useful due to the limited number of agents identified.
- May identify the etiology of altered mental status; however, the episode is usually resolved by the time results are available. Hence, a good history often best identifies the exposure.

Computerized Tomography

- Offers an immediate diagnosis or exclusion of **intraventricular** or **intracranial hemorrhage** or **neoplasm.**
- In addition, it is frequently helpful to evaluate for **subarachnoid hemorrhage, brainstem neoplasm, ischemic stroke, cerebral venous sinus thrombosis, increased intracranial hemorrhage** and **hydrocephalus.**

Magnetic Resonance Imaging (Brain and/or Spinal Cord)

- May be necessary to diagnose **MS, ADEM, cerebral venous sinus thrombosis** and **brainstem neoplasm.**
- May show anatomic evidence of injury attributable to **TIA.**
- Can diagnose **spinal cord compression** from vertebral pathology or spinal epidural abscess.

SPECIAL TESTS

EEG (Electroencephalography)

- Is useful to identify the possibility of **partial complex seizures** and is essential if subclinical **status epilepticus** is considered.

Electromyography and Nerve Conduction Studies

- Helps to diagnose **Guillain-Barré syndrome** and **botulism**.

DISPOSITION

- Many of the conditions listed above will result in hospital admission, either because of the severity of the acute condition or the potential for progression.
- Some of these conditions are self limited but others will require consultation with a neurologist, such as complicated migraines or partial complex seizures.
- Other specialists may also be needed:
  - Hematology should be involved if thrombophilia is suspected.
  - Ophthalmology can make important contributions in cases of pseudotumor cerebri.
  - Psychiatric consult if an intentional overdose is suspected or confirmed.

What is unique about neurologic emergencies in adolescents?

- Some serious, time-dependent neurologic conditions initially present with relatively subtle manifestations: i.e. mild weakness with Guillan-Barré syndrome, strange combinations with ADEM, persistent headache with pseudotumor cerebri.
- It is easy for teens to get lost in the ocean of "psychosomatic noise" that is typical of the adolescent resulting in a delayed diagnosis.
- As with many adolescent disorders, teens are frequently at the cusp of more adult conditions. Few people would question a story of transient, but

resolved, right arm weakness in a 70 year old male; many would entertain skepticism in a 14 year old female. Nevertheless, all complaints must be addressed on their own merits through a complete neurologic assessment.

TEST YOUR KNOWLEDGE ANSWER

88. C. A CT scan is frequently helpful to evaluate pseudotumor cerebri, intracranial bleeding, acute ischemic stroke and cerebellitis. Guillain-Barré Syndrome is a post-infectious, acute inflammatory demyelinating process that presents with ascending paralysis (leg up). For this condition, collecting cerebrospinal fluid is indicated, as it may show increases in CSF protein with typical albumino-cytologic dissociation.

WEB REFERENCES

- Abu-Arafeh I and Macleod S. 'Serious neurological disorders in children with chronic headache', Arch Dis Child. 2005; 90: 937–040, retrieved from http://www.ncbi.nlm.nih.gov/pmc/articles/PMC1720577/pdf/v090p00937.pdf
- Arce D, Sass P, and Abul-Khoudoud H. 'Recognizing Spinal Cord Emergencies', American Family Physician. 2001 August 15; 64(4): 631–639, retrieved from http://www.aafp.org/afp/2001/0815/p631.html
- Haydel MJ, *et al.* 'Indications for Computed Tomography in Patients with Minor Head Injury', The New England Journal of Medicine. 2000 July 13; 343(2): 100–105, retrieved from https://secure.muhealth.org/~ed/students/articles/NEJM_343_pQ100.pdf
- Honda H and Warren DK. 'Central Nervous System Infections: Meningitis and Brain Abscess', Infect Dis Clin N Am. 2009; 23: 609–623, retrieved from http://xa.yimg.com/kq/groups/16749867/2098091879/name/Central+Nervous+System+Infections-+Meningitis+and+Brain+Abscess.pdf
- Lewis DW. 'Headaches in Children and Adolescents', American Family Physician. 2002 February 15; 65(4): 625–633, retrieved from http://www.aafp.org/afp/2002/0215/p625.html
- Macleod S and Appleton RE. 'Neurological disorders presenting mainly in adolescence', Arch Dis Child. 2007 February; 92(2): 170–175, retrieved from http://www.ncbi.nlm.nih.gov/pmc/articles/PMC2083313/

Additional Clinician and Patient Resources:

- DiagnosisPro: http://diagnosispro.com
- PediatricStrokeNetwork: www.pediatricstrokenetwork.com

60

SEIZURES

Robyn Miller

TEST YOUR KNOWLEDGE

89. A mother complains that her 16 year old son has been "jumpy" for the past few months. He drops something every morning (i.e. his tooth brush, book bag or cup of milk) and she is worried that he is using drugs. He is aware of the problem but blames it on the stress of football and the upcoming championships. Which one of the following is the *MOST* likely explanation?

    A. Post-Concussive Syndrome
    B. Juvenile Myoclonic Epilepsy
    C. Absence Seizures
    D. Startle Epilepsy
    E. Myoclonic Stress Reaction

90. Jackie is a 15 year old girl who was found having a seizure in her room. She has no known history of epilepsy and is otherwise healthy. Of note, her parents are going through a divorce and were arguing when her mother walked past and found Jackie on the bed shaking, grunting and crying. She was taken to the emergency department where she had an event similar to the first but was able to squeeze the physician's hand on command. What is the *MOST* appropriate treatment?

    A. Support with oxygen and administer IV ativan stat.
    B. Support with oxygen and load with phenobarbital.
    C. Support with oxygen and load with dilantin.
    D. Support with oxygen, administer IV ativan stat, and obtain a head CT.
    E. None of the above.

Refer to end of chapter for answers on page 668.

Daniel is a 15 year old male who was skateboarding at a local park when his younger brother found him on the ground confused and sleepy.

BACKGROUND

- Seizures are the physical findings or changes in behavior that occur during an episode of abnormal electrical activity in the brain.
- Based on whether consciousness is preserved, seizures can be divided into two categories: complex and partial (Table 1).
- Seizures are primarily caused by either neurologic or metabolic disease.
- Most seizures last less than 5 minutes and stop without intervention.
- A seizure that lasts longer than 30 minutes without return to baseline mental status is known as status epilepticus.
- Sudden unexplained death in epilepsy (SUDEP) is a rare cause of death in pediatrics (1-2.1 death per 10,000 patient years).

ASSESSMENT

HISTORY

History of Present Illness

- The first step in the evaluation of a seizure is to determine if one occurred: many events can mimic seizures. Seizures are often unwitnessed but if observed, assess for the following:
  - Loss of consciousness or change in mental status
  - Falling or loss of muscle control
  - Shaking movement of the entire body
  - Muscle twitching spreading up or down a limb
  - Loss of bowel or bladder function
  - Memory of the event
  - Fatigue or increased sleepiness following loss of consciousness (post-ictal state)
  - Bitten tongue or other injuries.

- Seizures can be triggered by many causes. Determine if the teen has:
  - Been sleep deprived
  - Used alcohol or drugs
  - Had a recent fever
  - Complained of neck pain or stiffness
  - Experienced head trauma within the past few hours to days

Past Medical History

- Cardiac problems, such as arrhythmias, may present similarly to seizures.
- Teens diagnosed with **thrombocytopenia** (platelets less than 10,000/ml) can have intracranial bleeding from minor trauma, with resultant seizure activity.
- A history of developmental delay suggests a genetic syndrome such as **tuberous sclerosis.**
- **Systemic lupus erythematosus** (SLE) can present with seizures from vasculitis in the brain.
- Seizures can result from **hypoglycemia.**
- Water intoxication causing seizures secondary to hyponatremia occurs with **syndrome of inappropriate antidiuretic hormone secretion** (SIADH), **psychogenic polydipsia,** or water loading in patients with anorexia nervosa prior to a "weigh in."

Family History

- Determine if there is a family history of genetic disorders, seizures or brain tumors.

Medications

- Has the teen been diagnosed with epilepsy and are they on antiepileptic drugs (AEDs)?
  - Childhood medication doses may be rendered ineffective if not adjusted as a teen grows.
  - AEDs raise the seizure threshold and cessation of AEDs can lead to an increase in seizure activity.

Social History

- Has there been a decline in school performance? **Absence seizures** often manifest as starring spells of which the patient is unaware and can cause lapses in memory.
- Screen for depression, anxiety and problems at home or school. Stress may manifest as a **pseudoseizure.**
- Assess for alcohol or drug use or abuse.
    - If the teen reports alcohol use, determine quantity, frequency and last drink. Seizures may be triggered by **alcohol withdrawal.**
    - **Heroin use** can lower the seizure threshold by decreasing GABA, the main inhibitory neurotransmitter in the brain.
    - Stimulant abuse can trigger seizures.

Sexual History

- **Pregnancy** can be complicated with **eclampsia**, defined by protein in the urine, elevated blood pressure, and seizures.
- **HIV** can lead to opportunistic infections that may cause seizures.
- Untreated **syphilis,** rare in today's society, may lead to neurosyphilis and associated seizures.

Review of Systems

- Headaches that wake a teen from sleep suggests an **intracranial mass.**
- Blurry or double vision may also indicate an **intracranial mass.**
- Complaints of syncope, lightheadedness, dizziness and nausea suggest a neurocardiogenic cause.

PHYSICAL

Vital Signs

- Elevated blood pressure or tachycardia suggests **drug intoxication** (i.e. stimulants).
- Fever suggests an infectious etiology.
- Bradycardia can be associated with increased intracranial pressure.

General Appearance

- The post-ictal state often follows a seizure, during which the teen may be tired or sleepy, or report feeling groggy.
- Soiled underwear or the smell of urine is a sign of lost bowel or bladder function, respectively.

HEENT

- Observe for signs of head trauma such as lacerations or edema.
- Examine the tongue and mouth for signs of injury or bleeding: loss of motor control can accompany seizure activity and may lead to uncontrolled and sustained contractions of masseter muscles.
- Observe pupils. They may be dilated with stimulant (i.e. cocaine or amphetamine) ingestion, or constricted with heroin ingestion.
- Papilledema is a sign of increased intracranial pressure.

Neck

- Nuchal stiffness or rigidity is a sign of meningitis/meningismus.

Cardiovascular

- An abnormal rhythm warrants an investigation for cardiac etiologies.

Neurologic

- Abnormal speech, asymmetric faces, hemiplegia and sensation deficits are all worrisome signs of a mass effect on the brain, either caused by blood or a tumor.
- Hemiplegia may be secondary to Todd's Paralysis, a transient state of paralysis following a seizure that resolves without intervention.
- Brisk reflexes and/or a positive Babinski, are upper motor neuron signs.

Skin

- Port-wine stain, facial angiofibromas, hypopigmented macules or shagreen patches are signs of a neurocutaneous disorder.
- Petechia may indicate infectious etiology such as meningitis.

STUDIES

Laboratory studies are not routinely recommended by the American Academy of Neurology for the evaluation of seizures and work up should instead be guided by clinical findings.

Complete Blood Count

- Elevated white blood cell count, neutrophils or bands may be present with infection.
- Neutropenia may indicate HIV or other viral infection.
- Thrombocytopenia increases the risk for brain bleeds after minor trauma.

Comprehensive Metabolic Panel

- Hypoglycemia and hyponatremia can cause seizures.
- Hypocalcemia may lead to tetany, which can be confused with seizures.

Antiepileptic Drug levels

- Subtherapeutic levels can trigger seizures.

SPECIAL TESTS

Electroencephalogram (EEG)

- All patients presenting with a first time seizure without an identifiable cause should have an EEG performed.
- If the patient is stable, the EEG can be scheduled as an outpatient.
- A seizure is a clinical diagnosis and cannot be diagnosed by an EEG; however, an EEG may provide evidence to define seizure type or epilepsy syndrome.

Urine Toxicology Screen

- Opioid, cocaine, amphetamine, and ecstasy/MNDA intoxication may cause seizures and should be considered in the work up.

Alcohol Level

- Alcohol withdrawal may present as seizures.

Prolactin Level

- If a psychogenic seizure is suspected, an abnormal serum prolactin level obtained within 10–20 minutes of the seizure may dispel the diagnosis.
  - A serum prolactin level greater than or equal to twice its baseline is consistent with a complex seizure.
  - Partial seizures may have a modest elevation in prolactin.
  - Normal levels do neither exclude a tonic clonic seizure nor support a diagnosis of psychogenic one.

Lumbar Puncture (LP)

- If there is a suspicion for intracranial infection an LP must be done.
- Depending on the level of clinical suspicion, studies should be sent for HSV, cryptococcus and other infectious etiologies.

CT Scan

- A CT scan should be performed before an LP in any patient suspected of having an intracranial mass.
- The MRI is superior to CT in evaluating for intracranial masses; however, in an emergency a CT is preferred.

TREATMENT

- Treatment is targeted at the underlying cause: if there are electrolyte abnormalities they should be corrected. If there is head trauma with a resultant bleed, then treatment of the bleed will treat the seizure.
- Seizures with no identifiable cause are considered idiopathic.
- Continued seizure episodes with no other underlying cause can be classified as epilepsy and require consultation with neurology, as some may require lifelong management with AEDs.
- Patients that present in status epilepticus in an outpatient setting require treatment with a rectal suppository of diastat and a repeat dose may be necessary. These patients will require further evaluation in the emergency department. If there is IV access, an initial dose of ativan is preferred, followed by fosphenytoin if the seizure continues longer than 5 minutes.

What is unique about seizures in adolescents?

- Most adolescents with chronic disease strive to "just be normal." An illness requiring daily medications, increases the risk of noncompliance and may result in poor control of the disease.
- Juvenile myoclonic epilepsy is a specific epileptic disorder that presents between the ages of 12 and 18 years. This condition does not remit spontaneously and will need lifelong treatment with AEDs, most commonly valproic acid.
- The most challenging aspect of treating adolescents with seizures are the limitations this disorder can place on driving. Most states require between a 3 and 18 month seizure free period before reinstating the driver's license and clinicians should become aware of their state specific requirements.
- Adolescence is a time of increased stress and developing but often poor coping skills. This can lead to psychogenic seizures, with greater prevalence in females.
- Coping with stigma and accepting and adapting to a recurring condition needs to become part of the developmental tasks of epileptic adolescents (Chapter 63).

TEST YOUR KNOWLEDGE ANSWERS

89. B. Juvenile Myoclonic Epilepsy (JME) is a seizure type that is characterized by sudden, brief, bilaterally synchronous and simultaneous muscle contractions. The contractions mainly affect the shoulders and upper muscles, but can involve the lower extremities or the entire body in a generalized tonic clonic seizure. The myoclonic or generalized tonic clonic seizures most commonly occur right after wakening either from a nap or night sleep. Absence seizures are characterized by starring spells and not muscle jerks. Post concussive syndrome is characterized by poor concentration, headaches, problems with memory, fatigue, irritability and insomnia following a head injury. Startle epilepsy is characterized by seizures triggered by unexpected sensory stimuli, usually loud noises. They usually develop in children that have some type of brain pathology from an injury that occurred early by the second year of life.

90. E. Psychogenic seizures are a manifestation of psychological distress. They often present in adolescence and have a co-morbid diagnosis of depression, PTSD, or dissociative and personality disorders (most commonly borderline personality disorder). Video imaging capturing an episode with a concomitant normal EEG is a classic finding.

Table 1. Seizure Classification.

Complex	**Partial**
Electrical discharge in both hemispheres	Electrical discharge is focal
Absence	Simple partial
Myoclonic	Complex partial
Tonic-clonic	Secondary generalized

WEB REFERENCES

- Adams SM and Knowles PD. 'Evaluation of a First Seizure', American Family Physician. 2007 May 1; 75(9): 1342–1347, retrieved from http://www.aafp.org/afp/2007/0501/p1342.html
- Baker GA, Spector S, McGrath Y, Soteriou H. 'Impact of epilepsy in adolescence: AUK controlled study', Epilepsy & Behavior. 2005; 6: 556–562, retrieved from http://www.epilepsyfoundation.org/livingwithepilepsy/parentsandcaregivers/parents/upload/YEBEH200510a.pdf
- Kanner AM and Shafer PO. 'Seizures and Teens: When Seizures Aren't the Only Problem', EP Magazine. 2006 November; 50–55, retrieved from http://www.epilepsy.com/pdfs/Except_parent_art5 .pdf
- Macleod S and Appleton RE. 'Neurological disorders presenting mainly in adolescence', Arch Dis Child. 2007 February; 92(2): 170–175, retrieved from http://www.ncbi.nlm.nih.gov/pmc/articles/PMC2083313/
- Mcabee GN, Wark JE. 'A Practical Approach to Uncomplicated Seizures in Children', American Family Physician. 2000 September 1;62(5): 1109-1116, retrieved from http://www.aafp.org/afp/2000/0901/pll09.html
- Riviello JJ, *et al.* 'Practice Parameter: Diagnostic assessment of the child with status epilepticus (an evidence-based review): Report of the Quality Standards Subcommittee of the

American Academy of Neurology and the Practice Committee of the Child Neurology Society', Neurology. 2006; 67: 1542–1550, retrieved from http://www.childneurologysociety.org/docs/default-source/default-document-library/dasfasa.pdf?sfvrsn=O

Additional Clinician and Patient Resources:

- Centers for Disease Control and Prevention, Parent Resource Guide: http://www.cdc.gov/epilepsy/pdfs/resource_guide.pdf
- Child Neurology Society: www.childneurologysociety.org
- Epilepsy Foundation®, Children and Teens with Epilepsy: http://www.efepa.org/living-with-epilepsy/children-and-teens-with-epilepsy/
- Epilepsy Therapy Project: www.epilepsy.com
- International League Against Epilepsy: www.ilae-epilepsy.org

61

ADOLESCENT SEXUAL ASSAULT/RAPE

Kathy Woodward

TEST YOUR KNOWLEDGE

A teen you have cared for since infancy presents for a camp physical exam. You know her family well and provide care to her siblings. During the review of systems of genitourinary symptoms, your quiet and withdrawn 14 year old female patient timidly admits that she has been having some vaginal discharge and intermittent dysuria for about a year. She then breaks into tears and reports that her uncle has been "messing with her" for the past 2 years. The contact has progressed to vaginal intercourse once or twice a month for one year. The last sexual contact was last night.

91. Which one of the following statements is most likely to be true?
    - A. Since you know the family well, your only obligation is to tell her mother so that the family can handle the situation.
    - B. You are not surprised that she is still a cheerleader and on the honor roll at school.
    - C. You can handle this entire situation in your office, without involving any other professionals.
    - D. All the above are true.
    - E. None of the above statements is true.
92. An appropriate response to this disclosure would be:
    - A. To finish the physical exam, complete the camp form and arrange for a return appointment with more time.
    - B. Ask her if she dislikes her uncle and just wants to get him in trouble.
    - C. Inform her that you are going to have to report this situation to the authorities, who have a special team of professionals who will help her and her family.
    - D. Ask her if she is also having sex with a boyfriend.

Refer to end of chapter for answers on page 676.

BACKGROUND

- Adolescents represent 10-25% of cases investigated for child maltreatment cases in the U.S., and are also victims of dating violence, sexual harassment, rape, sexual assault and human trafficking (Table 1).
- Both adolescent females and males can be victims of sexual assault and rape.
- Normal adolescent development tasks of autonomy and independence can place teens at higher risk as they may lack cognitive and social skills needed to develop healthy relationships or defend themselves from adult or peer predators/offenders.
- All health care providers are mandatory reporters if they suspect sexual abuse or rape. Most jurisdictions have assembled multi-disciplinary teams to handle the legal, medical and psychological aspects of sexual victimization.
- It is important to understand and become familiar with local reporting procedures and resources.

ASSESSMENT

HISTORY

- Document enough history to report the case to authorities.
- Spare the youth from recounting the story multiple times; this can be traumatic and risks impeaching the witness if the same account is not given each time.
- Focus on Who, What, When and Where:
  - **Who?** If the perpetrator is a stranger, peer or acquaintance over 16 years, in some states, it is up to the older teen (and the age, 16 to 18 years, varies by jurisdiction) to report a rape or sexual assault. Reporting is mandatory if the victim is under 16 years of age and there is a 7 year statute of limitation. However, if the perpetrator is a family member, teacher or coach, there is mandatory reporting with no statute of limitation.
  - **What** happened? Within the first 72 hours of sexual assault, it is preferable that a specially trained provider such as a Sexual Assault Nurse Examiner (SANE), Sexual Assault Response Team (SART) or Sexual

Assault Forensics Examiner (SAFE), take the history from the patient (Table 2). If more than 72 hours have elapsed since the rape or sexual assault, either the clinical provider or sexual assault center can obtain this information.

- **When?** If less than 72 hours, patient should be evaluated at a sexual assault center. If greater than 72 hours, may refer the patient to a sexual assault center or evaluate in your office.
- **Where?** Must use a sexual assault center in the jurisdiction where the crime was alleged to have occurred. Teens and families can seek assistance for sexual assault at their local centers but if the crime/abuse did not occur there, access for forensic rape kits may not be possible.

PHYSICAL

Genital Exam

- An examination of the external genitalia can reassure the teen that despite the abuse, there is no physical damage to their body.
- It also allows for documentation that sexually transmitted infections (STIs) with cutaneous lesions are not present such as human papillomavirus (HPV), herpes simplex virus (HSV) and syphilis.
- Exam should be performed even if the teen discloses rape or assault well after the first 72 hours, to ensure that there is no residual trauma.

STUDIES

Forensic Rape Kits

- The local police department is responsible for purchasing and processing forensic rape kits.
- Local counties that have their own sexual assault centers *will not bring rape kits into other jurisdictions.*
- The forensic rape kit and colposcopic examination is best performed in a SANE/SART/SAFE program (Table 2).
- Rape kits allow forensic DNA evidence to be collected if the sexual assault occurred in the last *72–96 hours.* DNA evidence can be found for longer duration in fatal cases.

Colposcopy

- Colposcopic documentation of genital trauma has become an important forensic tool in criminal cases. Genital findings may still be present after the 72 hour window.

Screening for STIs, HIV and Pregnancy

- Can be performed in the clinician's office but should be processed with a "chain of custody" in case there are any legal options pending.
- All laboratory services or hospitals have procedures for documenting "chain of custody" for laboratory tests and specimens.
- In **late disclosures of sexual assault,** there will not be any DNA evidence to collect; however, the health care provider should screen for STIs, HIV and unintended pregnancy.

Hepatitis B and C are also Recommended screening by some centers.

TREATMENT

- Goals of treatment include prevention of medical complications of rape or sexual assault including unintended pregnancy and/or STIs.
  - Unintended pregnancy can be prevented with the use of Plan B (150 mcg of levonogestrel) as a single oral dose within 72–120 hours after unprotected intercourse.
  - Prophylaxis for gonorrhea and chlamydia with Ceftriaxone 250 mg given IM and Azithromycin 1 gram given orally, should be given if STIs are suspected and before test results return. Treatment with antibiotics decreases the need to retest the patient in 2 weeks.
  - Other STIs have longer incubation periods and prophylaxis treatment is not recommended by the CDC. Vaginal infections such as trichomoniasis, bacterial vaginosis (BV), or post-antibiotic candidal infections, may not be found until 6–8 weeks after the sexual assault.
  - Viral STIs can have a much longer incubation period before detection. Regardless of HPV vaccine status of the adolescent victim, an external genital exam should be repeated in 6–12 weeks to assess for HPV, HSV, trichomoniasis and bacterial vaginosis.

- The adolescent should also return for repeat HIV testing at 6–12 weeks post rape or assault.
- HIV prophylaxis should be considered in cases of assault and rape.

- Victims of rape or sexual assault should be carefully screened for signs of PTSD, anxiety or depression and consider a mental health referral for further evaluation and possible therapy (Table 3).

What is unique about rape or sexual assault in adolescents?

- Younger teens do not often realize the magnitude of coercive relationships or that these relationships constitute sexual abuse.
- Some adolescents may experience shame or guilt following sexual assault or rape and decide not to disclose the experience. This is especially true for adolescent males.
- For this reason, many instances of rape or sexual assault may be reported months or years after the fact (e.g. incest), if at all.
- Teens can exhibit varied and far ranging responses to rape:
  - What appears to be a cavalier attitude may be avoidance;
  - An eating disorder may be the reaction to an intrusive thought (e.g. in response to forced fellatio);
  - Promiscuous behavior may be a conditioned response for seeking love and affection;
  - Substance abuse may be a teen's attempt to self-medicate;
  - Oppositional behavior may be an attempt to exert control for the first time;
  - School refusal may have more to do with gossip, the perpetrator, bullying and/or harassment, safety issues, and other generalized fears as a result of the trauma.
  - Depression, anxiety and suicidal attempts may follow sexual abuse.
  - Somatization, especially chronic pelvic pain, may indicate prior sexual abuse.

- The short term result of sexual abuse disclosure may include the teen's removal from home for safety (if the perpetrator lives with them). This removal, and/or the refusal of family member's to believe the victim, might be perceived as punishment and corroboration of the perpetrator's threats that "no one will believe you."

- While many adult victims of sexual assault experience years of sexual and relationship dysfunction, these post trauma effects may be exacerbated in young victims whose *only* sexual experiences have been abusive.
- When these victims become adult parents, they may become hyper-vigilant about protecting their children from abuse. Some may develop an unhealthy anxiety about their children's genital appearance or their behaviors.

TEST YOUR KNOWLEDGE ANSWERS

91. B. A sexual assault team is the best team (most experienced and skilled) to evaluate victims of sexual assault, in most jurisdictions. Health care providers are mandatory reporters and must report rape/sexual assault to the appropriate authorities. If the assault occurred less than 72 hours prior to patient presentation, the patient and his/her family can be referred to a sexual assault center or the emergency department for further work-up and evaluation. If it is more than 72 hours since the assault occurred, the patient can be evaluated by the primary care clinician or referred to a sexual assault center if appropriate. While some teens will have symptoms related to the assault including PTSD with sleep disturbance, fatigue, anxiety and depression that can affect school grades, activities and behaviors, it is also true that some teens may have the strength and resiliency to maintain their grades, activities and normal behaviors despite the traumatic experience of rape or sexual assault.
92. C. If a teen discloses a rape or sexual assault during a routine visit, the focus of the visit should shift to providing compassionate care to the teen victim of rape or sexual assault. Physical exams can be rescheduled for a later date.The teen ought to be commended for her bravery in disclosing her terrible experience.

Table 1. Rape and Sexual Assault.

- Rape, or "first-degree sexual assault," refers to non-consensual sexual intercourse that is committed by physical force, threat of injury or under duress.
- Lack of consent can include the victim's inability to say "no" to intercourse, due to the effects of drugs or alcohol.
- Rape can occur when the perpetrator and victim have a pre-existing relationship ("date rape"), or even when the offender is the victim's spouse.
- "Statutory rape" occurs when adults (18 years or older) engage in sexual intercourse with a person who has not reached the age of consent and usually, there has to be a minimum 4 year age difference (jurisdiction dependent).
- Rape, like other crimes, has to be reported and investigated in the jurisdiction where the rape occurred.

Table 2. SANE, SART and SAFE.

SANE: Sexual Assault Nurse Examiners	• A program that seeks to treat the emotional, physical, and legal needs of rape victims with greater consideration and sensitivity. • Female nurses are trained to handle the physical examination of the victim and to obtain physical evidence using a sexual offense collection kit. • Nurses are also taught how to interview the victim about the assault and keep good records, which are critical to a successful criminal prosecution of the suspect.
SART: Sexual Assault Response Team	• Community professionals who work jointly to minimize the trauma to victims of sexual assault when they seek medical or legal advice. • SART coordinate their efforts to reduce the number of questions a victim must answer when law enforcement personnel and prosecutors collect evidence. • Members of a SART unit consist of personnel from emergency departments and law enforcement offices. • Wider scale than SANE programs; SANE and SART often work in conjunction.
SAFE: Sexual Assault Forensic Examiners	• Developed in some communities and serve the same function as SANE programs.

Table 3. Recommendations for Therapy.

Consider referring for therapy when the teen:

- shows worse/negative/regressed level of functioning.
- loses interest in activities.
- becomes withdrawn or aggressive.
- becomes self-injurious.
- is suicidal or homicidal.
- exhibits low frustration tolerance.
- has low self-esteem or self-worth.

WEB REFERENCES

- Centers for Disease Control and Prevention. 'Sexually Transmitted Diseases Treatment Guidelines', 2010. MMWR2010; 59(No. RR-12): l–110, retrieved from http://www.cdc.gov/std/treatment/2010/STD-Treatment-2010-RR5912.pdf
- Child Welfare Information Gateway. Mandatory Reporters of Child Abuse and Neglect: Summary of State Statutes (current through August 2012): https://www.childwelfare.gov/systemwide/laws_policies/statutes/manda.pdf
- National Institute of Justice: Responses to Sexual Violence: Effectiveness of SANE/SART Programs (Modified May 30, 2012): http://www.nij.gov/topics/crime/rape-sexual-violence/response.htm#effectiveness

Additional Clinician and Patient Resources:

- American Academy of Child & Adolescent Psychiatry: Child Sexual Abuse and How to Respond (2011 Press Releases): http://www.aacap.org/cs/2011_press_releases/child_sexual_abuse_and_how_to_respond
- Avert. Averting HIV and AIDS: Worldwide Ages of Consent: http://www.avert.org/age-of-consent.htm
- Child and Family Services Agency. Mandated Reporter Training: http://dc.mandatedreporter.org/pages/Welcome.action
- Most jurisdications operate rape crisis centers that can be found with an online search, such as: DC Rape Crisis Center: http://www.dcrcc.org/
- National Insitute of Justice: Laws to Make Campuses Safer (October 1, 2008): http://www.nij.gov/nij/topics/crime/rape-sexual-violence/campus/laws.htm
- Rape, Abuse, & Incest National Network, patient information and access to a national sexual assault hotline: http://www.rainn.org/

- Rape, Abuse & Incest National Network: What is a SANE/SART?, retrieved from https://rainn.org/get-information/sexual-assault-recovery/medical-information/SANE-SART
- Rape crisis information, online resources and hotlines: http://www.ibiblio.org/rcip/crisiscenters.html
- U.S. Department of Health and Human Services, Child Welfare Information. General Information on Child Abuse and Neglect: http://www.childwelfare.gov

62

THE SUICIDAL ADOLESCENT

Maureen E. Lyon

TEST YOUR KNOWLEDGE

93. Which one of the following statements is true?
    A. Suicide attempts are used by teens to get attention and are not related to actual completed suicides.
    B. Medication side effects can be associated with suicidal behavior.
    C. Adolescent boys with high grade point averages are at high risk for suicide attempts.
    D. All the above are true.
    E. None of the above are true.
94. Which one of the following statements is true?
    A. Depression is the most common mental illness in adolescents who make a suicide attempt.
    B. The best predictor of a completed suicide in a teen is a past injurious suicide attempt.
    C. Adolescent girls are more likely to make suicide attempts, but adolescent boys are more likely to complete suicide, because the means they use are more lethal.
    D. All the above are true.
    E. None of the above are true.

Refer to end of chapter for answers on page 686.

"My daughter says that she just doesn't want to live — she just broke up with her boyfriend of 9 months and is really depressed. She once overdosed on Tylenol and I'm worried!"

BACKGROUND

- Suicide is the third leading cause of death in the U.S. for youth between 10 to 24 years.
- The top three methods used in suicides of young people include firearms (46%), suffocation (37%) and poisoning (8%).
- Each year 149,000 youth between the ages of 10 and 24 receive medical care for self-inflicted injuries at Emergency Departments throughout the U.S.
- Cultural variations in suicide rates also exist with Native Americans, Alaskan Natives and Hispanic youth having the highest rates of suicide related fatalities.
- Perceived parent and family connectedness, emotional well-being for girls and high grade point average for boys, are protective against suicide attempts.
- There are many possible antecedents of adolescent suicide attempts (Table 1).

ASSESSMENT

HISTORY

History of Present Illness

- Determine if there is suicidal intent, a plan and/or means of self-harm.
- Determine if self-harm has occurred (patient overdosed but told no one).
- Assess for means of self harm such as a gun or potentially harmful medications at home.
- Depressed or irritable mood of at least two weeks duration, difficulty concentrating or paying attention, decreased ability to make decisions, increased insomnia, changes in appetite, withdrawal from friends or social isolation, alcohol or illicit drug use and/or suicidal ideation suggests **major depressive disorder.**

Past Medical History

- Does the teen report past suicidal ideation?
- A teen who has threatened to harm or has harmed someone may have a **conduct disorder** and has a higher risk of completed suicide with access to lethal means.
- Has the teen ever been or recently been diagnosed with pregnancy?

Family History

- Has a family member or friend attempted or completed suicide?
- Is there any family discord or evidence of poor parental support systems?
- Is there a family history of depression or substance abuse?

Medications

- Has the patient recently started or discontinued an SSRI (associated with agitation and suicidal behavior in some adolescents), suggestive of **medication side effect**?
- Is the patient taking propanolol or anticonvulsant medications? These can worsen suicidality.
- Some antiretrovirals taken by HIV positive teens have been associated with increased risk of suicidal ideation as a **medication side effect.**

Social History

- Determine if the teen has experienced any academic problems.
- Does the patient report any sleep problems or insomnia?
- Has the teen been the subject of bullying at school, home or cyberspace?
- Has the teen experienced abuse or neglect (e.g. no food to eat or clothes to wear or referral to child protective services in the past)?
- Has the teen had a history of fighting or injury from fighting? Any related suspensions or expulsions from school?
- Does the teen have access to firearms or other lethal weapons?
- Has the teen experienced a threat of separation from a parental figure? In fights, have parental figures threatened to send a teen to military school or to live with another relative? If so, these teens are more likely to attempt suicide.
- Is the teen actively questioning his or her sexual orientation?

- Has the teen ever abused drugs or alcohol?
- Has the teen ever been incarcerated or in youth rehabilitative services?

PHYSICAL

Vital Signs

- May be altered in a patient who does not acknowledge overdose.

Neurologic Exam

- Is the patient lucid? Exhibiting unusual behaviors raises suspicion for recent drug use or drug overdose.

Skin

- Examine for any signs of self-injurious behaviors, such as scars from self-cutting or burning on arms or other parts of the body.

STUDIES

Drug Screen

- Consider testing if the teen reports prior or recent history of drug use, presents acting unusually or if there is a report of progressive decline.

Pregnancy Test

- Should be considered in all sexually active teens.

HIV Antibody Screen and Screening for Other STIs

- Consider testing in a teen who is sexually active or engages in other risky behaviors such as IV drug use.

TREATMENT

- Teens presenting to the clinician's office with suicidal ideation should be urgently referred to the emergency department for psychiatric evaluation and to determine if inpatient treatment is warranted. To do this effectively, a parent or responsible adult needs to be contacted.
- Confidentiality should be waved and this should be explained to the patient.

- The general clinician can:
  - Create a clinic environment that supports all teens including suicide survivors and work to eliminate the stigma associated with behavioral health care.
  - Refer suicide attempters to the emergency room with a request for a psychiatry evaluation for treatment.
  - Become familiar with appropriate support services in the community:
    - Facilitate access to affordable behavioral health care by using community mental health centers.
    - Refer teens to mental health services to be screened and tested for depression, anxiety disorder, psychotic disorder not otherwise specified, bipolar disorder or schizophreniform disorder.
    - Refer teens with substance abuse issues to adolescent addiction counseling programs.
    - Learn about school counseling programs and local hotlines.
    - Consider referral to a family-based, multi-system therapy which uses a three pronged approach:
      - Educate parents about appropriate parenting skills, decrease negative parenting interactions and decrease coercive styles of interacting that promote aggression and later delinquency.
      - Strengthen family relationships, connectedness and emotional cohesion.
      - Enhance family problem-solving skills.
  - Maintain regular communication with the teen's psychiatrist or therapist to ensure appropriate follow up.

SUICIDE PREVENTION

- Inquiry about emotional health, family interactions, school achievement and general sense of connectedness. Create an atmosphere that facilitates detection of suicidality.
- Ask depression and suicide screening questions at routine visits.
- Educate parents and other caretakers about means restriction:
  - Limit access to firearms and other weapons in the home. Guns and ammunition should always be stored in separate locked boxes.

  - Lock up medications. In cases where a teen has made a suicide attempt or has expressed suicidal ideation and is on medication, consider directly observed treatment with parental handling of medication.

- "No Suicide" contracts have not been found to be effective prevention strategies.
- Educate parents about the importance of nurturing their teens. This starts well before adolescence:

  - Praise for positive behavior.
  - Spend time with children.
  - Read to children starting in infancy.
  - Teach and model positive social skills.
  - Role model nonviolent conflict resolution for children.

What is unique about suicide attempts in adolescents?

- Most teens who commit suicide have a history of prior suicide attempt. It is estimated that 10% of adolescent suicide attempters will eventually commit suicide.
- Suicide rates are increasing for African-American and other minority youth who have had historically low rates of suicide in the past.
- Injurious suicide attempts by teens are over 100 times more frequent than completed suicides.
- Parents and/or friends are usually the ones to raise the alarm that something is wrong.

TEST YOUR KNOWLEDGE ANSWERS

93. B. Some antidepressants, anticonvulsants, HIV associated anti-retroviral medications and beta blockers are associated with increased agitation and suicide attempts among adolescents. Changing to a different medication may be necessary and sufficient to eliminate suicidal ideation. The U.S. Food and Drug Administration (FDA) recently proposed that makers of all antidepressant medications update the existing black box warning on their products' labeling to include warnings about increased risks of

suicidality in young adults ages 18 to 24 during initial treatment (generally the first one to two months).

94. D. Although bipolar disorder and psychosis are strongly associated with adolescent suicide attempts, a previous diagnosis of depression is the most common diagnosis in a teen who makes a suicide attempt. While girls may be more likely than boys to attempt suicide, boys are more likely to successfully complete suicide as they choose more lethal means in their attempts. In 2006, the suicide death rate among males 15–24 years of age was 6 times higher than females in the same age group — a trend that generally continues throughout life. Serious attempts (e.g. told no one, lethal means or only found by accident) should result in hospitalization so that a comprehensive assessment of the psychosocial conditions leading to the attempt can be assessed and preventive measures be put in place to support the teen's return to home and school.

Table 1. Antecedents of Adolescent Suicide Attempts.

History of mental health treatment especially for depression
History of previous suicide attempt
Friend suicide attempt or completion
Alcohol or marijuana use
School problems including bullying
Weapon-carrying at school
Violence victimization
Violence perpetration
Same-sex romantic attraction
Threat of abandonment (by family member, boyfriend or girlfriend)

WEB REFERENCES

- Borowsky IW, Ireland M and ResnickMD. 'Adolescent Suicide Attempts: Risks and Protectors', Pediatrics. 2001 March l; 107(3): 485–493, retrieved from http://pediatrics.aappublications.org/content/107/3/485.abstract
- Centers for Disease Control and Prevention. 'Programs for the Prevention of Suicide Among Adolescents and Young Adults', MMWR. 43(RR-6): 1–7, retrieved from http://wonder.cdc.gov/wonder/Prevguid/m0031525/m0031525.asp#head001000000000000

- Greydanus DE and Shek D. 'Deliberate Self-harm and Suicide in Adolescents', Keio J Med. 2009 September; 58(3): 144–151, retrieved from https://www.jstage.jst.go.jp/article/kjm/58/3/58_3_144/_pdf
- Hatzenbuehler ML. 'The Social Environment and Suicide Attempts in Lesbian, Gay, and Bisexual Youth', Pediatrics. 2011 May 1; 127(5): 896–903, retrieved from http://pediatrics.aappublications.org/content/127/5/896.full.pdf+html?sid=ae4bcfce-8747-488f-a28b-832520a0b!5f
- Johnson GR, Krug EG and Potter LB. 'Suicide Among Adolescents and Young Adults: A Cross-National Comparison of 34 Countries', Suicide and Life-Threatening Behavior. 2000 Spring; 30(1): 74–82, retrieved from http://thefamilysite.info/demo/files/2011/08/Suicide-Among-Adolescents-and-Young-Adults-A-Cross-National-Comparison-of-34-Countries.pdf
- 'Practice Parameter for the Assessment and Treatment of Children and Adolescents With Suicidal Behavior', Journal American Academy of Child Adolescent Psychiatry. 2001 July; 40 (7 Supplement): 24S–51S, retrieved from http://download.journals.elsevierhealth.com/pdfs/journals/0890-8567/PIIS0890856709603555.pdf
- Shain BN, and the Committee on Adolescence. 'Suicide and Suicide Attempts in Adolescents', Pediatrics. 2007 September 1; 120(3): 669–676, retrieved from http://pediatrics.aappublications.org/content/120/3/669.full.pdf+html?sid=ae4bcfce-8747-488f-a28b-832520a0b!5f

Additional Clinician and Patient Resources:

- National Suicide Prevention Lifeline: http://www.suicidepreventionlifeline.org/
- American Academy of Child and Adolescent Psychiatry. Facts for Families: No. 10: Teen Suicide and \ Suicide attempts, suicide prevention and support for suicide survivors: http://www.aacap.org/cs/2010_press_releases/aacaps_facts_for_families_informs_public_about_teen_suicide
- American Association of Suicidology: Warning Signs: http://www.suicidology.org/c/document_library/get_file?folderId=232&name=DLFE-31.pdf
- Centers for Disease Control and Prevention. Suicide Prevention (last updated October 17, 2012): http://www.cdc.gov/ViolencePrevention/suicide/
- KidsHealth from Nemours, About Teen Suicide: http://kidshealth.org/parent/emotions/behavior/suicide.html

SECTION V

SPECIAL CARE

63

CHRONIC ILLNESS AND ADHERENCE TO TREATMENT

Daniel N. Davidow

TEST YOUR KNOWLEDGE

95. Which of the following statements is true?
    - A. An adolescent who has had a chronic condition since early childhood has mastered it and is not expected to have problems during the teen years.
    - B. While it is important for teens to become independent, family monitoring is essential to ensure treatment adherence.
    - C. Fear of long term consequences due to non-adherence usually persuades teens to take medication consistently.
    - D. All the above.
    - E. None of the above.

Refer to end of chapter for answer on page 699.

A 14 year old star baseball player and straight-A student presented with hematuria. Within a year, he was diagnosed with focal sclerosing glomerulonephritis requiring renal transplant. No longer able to play baseball, his grades deteriorated AND he became angry and sullen. He began to skip his medications, risking rejection of the kidney that his mother had donated.

BACKGROUND

- Caretakers and healthcare providers can understandably become frustrated when teens are non-adherent to their treatment regimen. They need to learn about this phenomenon to better deal with it.
- Different factors contribute to non-adherence to treatment:
  - Difficulty coming to terms with the condition.
  - Normal adolescent development and experimentation.
  - Feeling overwhelmed or confused.
  - Interfering life stressors or the impact of the condition on the teen's daily life.
  - Having a reason to be ill, or not having a reason to be well.

ASSESSMENT

Acceptance of the Diagnosis

- Most adolescents coming to terms with a chronic illness or disability pass through stages of **shock, denial, anger, depression**, and/or **bargaining**, in no particular order, before reaching the resolution of **acceptance.**
- Each stage can be brief, recurrent or prolonged depending upon the teen.

Resilience versus Vulnerability

- Some people have natural resilience to handle challenges effectively and there is an ongoing effort to better understand these traits.
- An emotionally fragile teen may become stuck in a certain phase of grief.
- An **anxious or phobic** person could become mired in **shock or denial**, while an **oppositional or defiant** patient can become stuck in the **anger or bargaining** phase.

- Teens have very active fantasies and can easily live in denial.
- Resilient characteristics can be helpful and protective:
  - A competitive or obsessive teen may focus on being the best patient or on proving that they will not be held back by illness.

Prior Life Experiences

- Traumatic life experiences, especially those causing shame or guilt, can predispose a patient toward anger or depression, e.g. the teen may believe that they deserve the illness as punishment.

Onset of Illness

- A teen diagnosed with a chronic illness at birth, such as cystic fibrosis, has had more time to come to accept their diagnosis than a teen who suddenly develops an illness, such as diabetes, in his mid-teen years.
- Nevertheless, childhood adjustment does not necessarily preclude problems from occurring during adolescence.

Support Network

Family members and peers play a significant role in a teen's ability to accept their medical condition, either helping or hindering the process.

- Family members also process the diagnosis and progress through stages of grief.
  - A parent may become depressed and emotionally unavailable over the loss of his child's valued future potential.
  - An anxious parent may become over-controlling and thereby cause a power struggle over treatment with their child.
- Families may show enmeshed or disengaged dynamics, open or closed communication styles, hyper or hypo-reactive patterns, a tendency to overprotect the ill child or a tendency to scapegoat, all of which will affect the patient's adaptation.
  - Siblings may be supportive or jealous of the patient.
  - Parents may model positive or negative behaviors.
  - Religious or cultural values may be helpful or counterproductive.

Treatment Expectations

- Whether an adolescent feels overwhelmed by the diagnosis of a chronic illness depends on the factors discussed above and the impact of potential treatment strategies on the teen's life and daily function.
- Caretakers may not realize how difficult or complex a treatment regimen is for a particular teen, or how much discomfort is caused by the treatment.
- Each teen's and family's resources must be considered in developing a treatment plan.
  - An "inconvenience" for one teen may feel like a significant lifestyle restriction for another, or an impossible task by yet another.
  - Teens may hesitate to disclose that they don't understand or parents can't afford prescribed treatments.
  - Teens may also be embarrassed by the stigma associated with taking medications.
- Medication side effects are a common reason that teens stop treatment adherence without notifying their provider.
  - Medications can have physical side effects and emotional consequences such as irritability, somnolence, exaggerated gag reflex or fear of needles, leading to a negative association with the treatment.
- Illness symptoms may sometimes be preferred to treatment side effects. For example, a teen diagnosed with hyperthyroidism may feel more energetic and powerful when medications are not taken. Adolescent girls may even welcome the weight loss of the hyperthyroid state.
  - Fear of long term consequences of non-adherence do not usually persuade teens to take medications consistently:
    - Young teens may not have developed the ability to project themselves into the future and older teens may have a sense of **omnipotence** which allows them to ignore potential adverse consequences of their actions.
    - The threat of adverse consequences can backfire and cause teens to prove "it won't happen to me."
- Some teens with chronic illness or disability feel no motivation to take care of themselves because of a pessimistic or fatalistic outlook.
  - These teens may lack direction or goals, or feel that their life choices are limited.

    - They may believe there are no reasons to pursue goals if their lifespan is going to be shortened by their condition.

- There are some patients who do not follow prescribed treatment regimens because, for reasons which are not usually obvious, they have a need to be ill or do not have enough reason to be healthy.

Psychosocial Maintenance of Illness

- Teens may find it useful to maintain their illness status for secondary gain, they may suffer from a conversion reaction or sadly, be victims of being made ill or disabled.
- Of these reasons, **secondary gain** is usually the easiest to uncover.
    - For example, an entire family can subsist on a patient's disability income, placing the patient in an emotional bind.
- A **conversion reaction** is caused by an emotional conflict being "converted" into a physical symptom. Patients will resist giving up the symptom until the emotional conflict is resolved.
    - Sexual abuse is a common cause of conversion symptoms, but these symptoms can be provoked by other emotional conflicts as well.
- **Symbiotic dependency** can occur when a teen enjoys being dependent on parents while simultaneously the parents' emotional needs are met caring for their teen.
    - If the dynamic becomes exaggerated and pathologic, the patient or parent may create or exaggerate an illness, as in **Munchausen's Syndrome** or **Munchausen's by Proxy**.

TREATMENT

- Caring for teens with chronic illness or disability requires helping teens surmount or circumvent the obstacles which impede their path toward optimal functioning and independence.
- Healthcare providers must help teens uncover the reasons for their non-adherence to formulate effective solutions. This may require special appointment times, such as the end of the day because:

    - Non-adherence to treatment is dangerous and can worsen complications of a medical condition or be life threatening.
    - Reasons for non-adherence may not be obvious or may be deliberately obscured.
- Success in addressing those challenging situations is possible if the four "R's" are practiced:
    - **Relate** to the patient:
        - In a comfortable setting, take time to find out about the patient, the family dynamics and to investigate the situation.
        - The provider must develop a rapport by being warm, caring, genuine and open minded. Teens will not open up to adults who are judgmental.
    - **Respect** the thoughts and opinions of teen patients.
        - Rather than dictate a treatment strategy, it is usually more advantageous to negotiate a treatment strategy which may allow teens to "buy-in" to the plan over time.
    - **Review** information about the disease and/or treatment with the patient and family to dispel misconceptions and educate about treatment options.
        - Sometimes lack of adherence is due to a simple misunderstanding.
        - The treatment regimen should be simplified whenever possible.
        - Look for problems with medication side effects or interactions.
    - Explore **reasons** for the conflict or refusal of care.
        - A reason can anticipate a solution, but finding it won't immediately solve the problem.
        - There may be more than one concern.
        - The patient's difficulties must be valued and not discounted.

DISPOSITION

- A multidisciplinary team approach is often necessary to treat teens living with chronic illness.
    - This team may include:
        - The Physician or Nurse Practitioner primary provider
        - The **patient and family members**
        - Specialist providers

- Nurse Educators
- Psychotherapists
- Rehabilitation therapists
- Social Workers or Case Managers
- Nutritionists
- Teachers

- The primary care provider should know about treatments prescribed by specialists to closely monitor medication interactions.
- The electronic medical record (EMR) can facilitate communication.
  - For those without access to EMR, networking via an email list-serve can keep providers up-do-date when the patient is seen by the other team members.
- Specialized treatment approaches may be necessary to address more complex situations:

Counseling

- Provides an opportunity to discuss ways in which normal development can be misinterpreted as pathologic.
  - As examples, a teen who asserts his independence through a power struggle with his parents does not have "Oppositional Defiant Disorder" and a teen who adapts different personae as she establishes her identity does not have "Borderline Personality Disorder."
- Teens may not be developmentally ready to accept responsibility to manage their illness.
- A teen may request a "responsibility holiday," when parents take over care for a short duration, so the teen can avoid becoming burned out.

Psychotherapy

- Used to address more serious situations, often related to sexual, physical or emotional trauma complicating the illness or disability.
- Individual, family, group therapy, or some combination of these may be needed.
- Specialized therapies may be needed, such as
  - Motivational interviewing techniques for patients with very little motivation or energy for change.

  - Hypnotherapy or cognitive behavioral therapy for chronic pain or conversion reaction.
  - Groups to address substance abuse, eating disorders or learn relaxation techniques.
  - Community clubs or activities which provide social interaction and opportunities for independence, such as a church youth group, Boy Scouts, other clubs or sports.
  - Mentors, or Big Brother/Big Sister programs.

- Psychotropic medication is needed if depressive or anxious symptoms interfere with counseling or psychotherapeutic efforts.
- Goal setting and positive reinforcement can be helpful in moving the patient or family past a habitual negative pattern of behavior.
- Consider specific rehabilitative therapy, such as speech, physical, occupational, pet therapy or therapeutic horseback riding.
- Confinement in a hospital or residential facility is indicated if the behaviors are dangerous, self-destructive or if it becomes necessary to separate the patient from family when there is severe symbiotic dependency.

What is unique about chronic illness in adolescents?

- Being a teen is difficult enough. Teens negotiate the process of becoming an adult; juggle the demands of family, academics, and extracurricular interests; all while trying to develop an identity and future goals. It becomes even harder to address these issues while also dealing with a chronic illness.
- The diagnosis of a chronic illness or disability can be overwhelming and can interfere with normal adolescent development.
- Efforts to assert independence can result in power struggles with caretakers over treatment decisions.
- A chronic illness can make a teen feel different from his or her peers and can interfere with being accepted, leading to prolonged parental dependency, anger or resentment.
- The teen may deny or hide their condition to better 'fit in,' which could involve neglecting needed treatments or medications.
- A teen living with chronic illness may gravitate to a fringe peer group and become involved in risk taking behaviors to fit in.

- An accepting peer group allows teens to safely separate from their family, to establish an identity and set of core values.
- When an illness or disability affects a teen's body image or self-esteem, the normal development of *ego identity* or *sexual identity* can be affected, leading to problems with personality integration and emotional connectedness.
- Meeting the challenges of treating adolescents with chronic illness or disability can be a rewarding endeavor that can help patients transition to adulthood with an optimal level of functional independence and self sufficiency.

TEST YOUR KNOWLEDGE ANSWER

95. B. It is important for teens to exercise their capacity for managing their chronic illness so they can transition to becoming adults with competent self-care skills. Nevertheless, throughout this process, the family needs to provide guidance and protection, including monitoring of adherence to treatment. Consequences of non-adherence are "too distant" and hence do not significantly impact adolescent adherence to treatment. A child with a chronic condition to which he/she has adapted well, may face new difficulties and develop new problems and distress upon entering adolescence.

WEB REFERENCES

- Neinstein LS. 'The treatment of adolescents with a chronic illness', West J Med. 2001 November; 175(5): 293–295, retrieved from http://www.ncbi.nlm.nih.gov/pmc/articles/PMC1071594/
- Sawyer SM, Drew S, Yeo MS and Britto MT. 'Adolescents with a chronic condition: challenges living, challenges treating', Lancet. 2007 Apring 28;369:1481-89, pdf from researchgate.net
- Suris JC, Michaud PA & Viner R. 'The adolescent with a chronic condition. Part I: developmental issues' Arch Dis Child. 2004; 89: 938–942, retrieved from http://adc.bmj.com/content/89/10/938.full
- Suris J-C, Michaud P-A, Akre C and Sawyer SM. 'Health Risk Behaviors in Adolescents With Chronic Conditions', Pediatrics. 2008 November; 122(5); elll3–elll8, retrieved from http://www.pediatricsdigest.mobi/content/122/5/elll3.full
- Yeo, M. 'Chronic Illness and disability', BMJ. 2005 March 26; 330(7439): 721–723, retrieved from http://www.ncbi.nlm.nih.gov/pmc/articles/PMC555640/

Additional Clinician and Patient Resources:

- The C. Everett Koop Institute at Dartmouth, Chronic Illness Resources for Teens: http://geiselmed.dartmouth.edu/koop/resources/chronic_illness/
- Child and Family Web Guide Tufts University, Chronic Illness Support: http://www.cfw.tufts.edu/?/category/resources-%20recreation/5/topic/chronic-illness-support/124/
- Healing Well.com: http://www.healingwell.com/
- Medline Plus: http://www.nlm.nih.gov/medlineplus/copingwithchronicillness.html
- PBS, Who Cares: Chronic Illness in America: http://www.pbs.org/inthebalance/archives/whocares/
- TeensHealth from Nemours, Dealing with a Health Condition: http://kidshealth.org/teen/yourmind/problems/dealchroni c_illness.html

64

DIFFICULT CONVERSATIONS: BAD NEWS, DISCLOSURE AND ADVANCE DIRECTIVES

Donna Marschall

TEST YOUR KNOWLEDGE

96. When communicating difficult information to teens, which of the following is *NOT* recommended?
    - A. Present straightforward information about the diagnosis.
    - B. "Chunk" information into brief segments.
    - C. Provide extensive diagnostic information.
    - D. Allow patients time to absorb and sit with potentially distressing information.
    - E. None of the above are recommended.
97. Which of the following statements are true?
    - A. Adolescents need to be asked for assent before initiating treatment of a serious illness.
    - B. Seeking advance directives is unlikely to cause distress in mature adolescents.
    - C. Physicians should refer their patients to professionals trained in communication to communicate "bad news."
    - D. All the above.
    - E. None of the above.

Refer to end of chapter for answers on page 706.

At 13 years old, Janet is unaware of her perinatally acquired HIV diagnosis. Over the years, her parents have told her that she needs to take special "vitamins" to treat a "blood condition" and have asked her doctors to not disclose her diagnosis. She has started to ask more direct questions about her medical status.

BACKGROUND

- Discussing certain topics with adolescents can be difficult, and particularly so when the clinician has to reveal "bad news."
- Discussions between clinicians and adolescents in medical settings may involve complex, emotionally intense information, such as the possibility of dying from an illness or requiring an amputation. This can be difficult for patients and clinicians to tolerate and manage.
- Appropriate and successful handling of these discussions is an important step in conveying genuine concern that increases the likelihood that patients will engage in the medical process.
- Prior experience, support or stress at home or at school, and individual characteristics can all affect an adolescent's ability to hear, understand and process the information given by their providers. Certain topics can be particularly difficult:
  - **Diagnosis disclosure:** Perceptions of diagnoses can elicit negative feelings that are shaped by societal attitudes, beliefs and misinformation. Serious chronic illnesses such as HIV, cancer and end stage renal disease can be particularly stressful.
  - **Prognosis:** Even potential "positive" outcomes may still entail loss of, or disruption in, daily functioning such as exercise restrictions or treatment side effects.
  - **Treatment:** Protocols that are complex can impose a significant burden on patients (e.g., taking multiple daily medications or painful physical therapy regimens).
  - **Advance Directives:** Proposed in case the patient becomes incapacitated (Table 1).
  - **Breaking confidentiality:** *As required by law* when reporting abuse or neglect to Child Protective Services or reporting suicidal or homicidal intent.

SPECIAL CONSIDERATIONS

- Difficult discussions can elicit strong feelings in clinicians. It is not uncommon to feel nervous and anxious, uncomfortable, sad and even angry when discussing these tough topics. As such, it is important for care providers to understand their own feelings while interacting with their patients. Clinicians should:
  - Be aware of their own emotional "hot spots" (known areas of discomfort and anxiety, such as death or disfigurement) and be aware of one's physical and emotional response when faced with those issues (e.g., feeling agitated/anxious/irritable or a strong desire to avoid the difficult conversation).
  - Seek out mentoring support from supervisors when these issues arise. Physicians should be honest and clear with their supervisors. For example: "I'm having difficulty figuring out how to tell my patient he has HIV. I'm nervous and I'm not sure how to continue."
  - Appropriately acknowledge these feelings with patients; avoid appearing aloof or detached: "It's hard for me to share this news with you but it is important."
  - Seek out assistance from non-physician colleagues who are trained communicators (e.g., psychologists, child life specialists, social workers or chaplains) for mentoring/suggestions.
  - Physicians should take care to *NOT* "pass the buck" and rely solely on colleagues to communicate bad news. There are recommended techniques to convey difficult information (Table 2).

ASSESSMENT

- Assess patient and caregiver ability to understand what they are being told. Patients and caregivers may be emotionally overwhelmed or have trouble processing complex information.
  - Be cautious not to interpret limited verbal response and nodding as true comprehension of the information being shared.
  - Present information in small segments, "chunking," and check in with the patient to ascertain level of understanding: "That was hard to hear. What are you thinking now?"

- Avoid asking yes or no questions to get a better sense of what the patient understands.
- Assess the patient's comprehension and ability to intellectually and emotionally manage information: "Your results show that you are HIV positive. What does that mean to you?"
- Determine, to the extent possible, the patient's ability to handle potentially distressing feelings and be prepared to respond to those feelings.
- Assess cultural issues such as norms and communication etiquette for each family.
    - Ask adult caregivers, "How should I give information to your son?"
    - Be respectful and compassionate to build rapport at difficult times, despite cultural differences.
    - Use trained translators as necessary. Do not rely on other family members to translate sensitive information.
    - Maintain appropriate eye contact. If possible, be on the same physical level with patients. Don't "hide" behind barriers like a desk.
    - Find a private setting to talk. If possible, do *NOT* disclose bad news over the telephone.

DISPOSITION

- Communicating bad news with adolescent patients and their caregivers is an involved process. Providers need to:
    - Convey potentially difficult information in ways that are clear, calm, and responsive to the anxieties of both patients and caregivers.
    - Determine whether adult caregivers should be present with the teen during discussion or if the physician should meet with each separately. Keep in mind the teen's legal rights within your jurisdiction. Some medical results (e.g., pregnancy, HIV) may need the teen's consent before being shared with a caregiver.
    - Allow the patient time to absorb information conveyed before continuing.
    - If the patient indicates s/he wants to leave immediately, ask if you can have just a few minutes with him or her and use this time to help the patient enlist support: "Can I call someone for you to meet you here?

What are you planning to do today after you leave here? I'd like to give you my office phone number should you have questions later."

- Some patient responses require immediate action by the provider. If a patient is extremely distressed and at-risk for self-harm: "I should just go walk in front of a bus," the provider should contact an emergency mental health provider to assess the patient.
- Physicians may also provide 24 hour emergency contact numbers such as a teen hotline number or a psychiatrist on-call service.

What is unique about communicating "bad news" with adolescents?

- Adolescence is a period of striking physical, cognitive and emotional development, and adolescent patients can vary significantly in their capacity to handle difficult information. Carefully assess each patient's level of understanding and development on an individual basis.
- Adolescence is a time when teens trend towards becoming autonomous and independent. Efforts should be made to provide as much detail as is appropriate and to seek assent for procedures and treatment plans.
- Cognitive or emotional age may not be consistent with chronological age. A 17 year old who appears mature may have low tolerance for stress and present much younger than his age.
- Some adult caregivers may seek to "protect" adolescents from receiving "bad news" and request that physicians avoid or soften any communications with their patient. However, adolescents are often much more aware of the circumstances of their medical situation than their caregivers know, and they can play an important role in their own care.
- Caregivers should be cautioned that avoiding frank and open medical discussions with their teens can confound the teen's ability to cope with difficult medical news. They may perceive that their caregiver (and/or physician) is withholding important information or deceiving them.
- Building a working alliance with the adolescent is paramount to treatment adherence.

TEST YOUR KNOWLEDGE ANSWERS

96. C. Providing extensive diagnostic information with medical terminology may result in confusion and LESS understanding. It is better to present clear and straightforward information that can enhance trust and future communication. Patients also benefit from receiving information in brief and distinct statements, also known as "chunking." In addition, they need to be allowed time to absorb new and distressing information.
97. A. Adolescents need to be asked for assent to treatment. While this is not a legal prerequisite, respecting the adolescent's need for autonomy is both ethical and important for engaging them in the medical process. Physicians need to assume the responsibility of communicating bad news. Some conversations, such as eliciting advance directives, cause distress and anxiety even in the most mature adolescent. Rather than referring, seeking guidance from professionals with specialized training including experienced colleagues, chaplains, social workers and psychologists, can aid physicians as they contemplate difficult conversations.

Table 1. Advance Directives (ADs).

- Also known as living wills, these are instructions given by a patient and their family specifying health decisions, should the patient become incapacitated due to their illness.
- A useful tool to guide treatment decisions at times when patients and families are most uncertain and overwhelmed, and intended to ensure that a patient's wishes for their care are ultimately honored.
- The discussion of ADs are legally mandated for adult patients, but this is not so for adolescents. Some providers and families may feel that discussing an AD would cause anxiety in teens.
- Adolescent patients' decision-making capacity for their health care should be assessed on a case-by-case basis.
- The potential risk for distress can be mediated by clear communication with adolescents. Failure to consider this option may lead to increased distress and anxiety at a later point during the patient's illness.
- Consultation can be sought with supervisors, mental health and/or palliative care teams to determine the appropriateness of and most judicious approach to developing an AD with a patient.

Table 2. Recommendations for Conducting Difficult Interviews with Adolescents.

Recommendation	Examples of What to Say
Ask teens who they would like to have present with them when meeting.	"Is there someone here with you today whom you would like to be part of this meeting?" "How can we include your parents in this discussion?"
Talk *with* teens, not *at* them. Avoid talking "over" patients by focusing communication only with caregivers.	*While making eye contact with the patient:* "Thank you for coming in today. We have important things to discuss about your health. What do you already know about why you're here?"
Use clear, concise and accurate language. If disclosing a diagnosis, write it down.	"Your lab results came back, and they show that you have Hodgkins Disease — a form of cancer. Let me write this down for you so you know exactly what your diagnosis is called."
Try to determine the patient's level of understanding and knowledge. Don't overload with information. Avoid using medical jargon.	"Have you ever known anybody with cancer? What have you heard about it?" "You have Type 1 Diabetes. This means you will need to take medicine every day to manage this disease and stay healthy. I will explain every step of the treatment for you."
Avoid rote speech. Personalize information by using patients' names.	"I have told you a lot of information today, Mary. I know you and your mom have been very worried since I first saw you last week. Do you have any questions about what I've told you?"
Pay attention for signs of emotional distress, and acknowledge and ask about these feelings. Avoid trying to "rescue" your patient and make them "feel better." Have tissues available.	*You observe that your patient's head is down, quiet and tearful*: "I can tell that this is hitting you hard. What are you thinking right now?"
Solicit questions and answer what has been asked.	"What would you like to know that I haven't already said? What more would you like to know about your diagnosis?"
Ask patients and family members to repeat back information in their own words.	"I've told you a lot of information. Sometimes I don't explain things as well as I would like and I want to make sure that today I explain it well. What is your understanding of what I've said?"

(*Continued*)

Table 2. (*Continued*)

Recommendation	Examples of What to Say
Don't mislead adolescents. Don't tell them it "will be fine" if it won't. Everyone's perception of what is "fine" is different.	"This treatment will improve your chances of surviving this illness but it will have side effects such as hair loss."
Provide a plan of action and arrange follow-up meetings.	"We have a good team and will all work together to treat your illness. Here are the things that you and I need to do next [...]. We will meet in two weeks to go over what we've done."
Seek assent from adolescents for any medical decisions. Treat the assent process with the same level of respect as when seeking consent from caregivers.	"We have gone over what we feel is the best plan. Before we start, it is very important that you are on board with the plan as you are the key player in your treatment. Do you agree with this plan? Do you have any concerns?"

WEB REFERENCES

- Aitken PV. 'Incorporating Advance Care Planning into Family Practice', American Family Physician. 1999 Feb l; 59(3): 605–612, retrieved from http://www.aafp.org/afp/1999/0201/p605.html
- Lyon ME, *et al.* 'Who Will Speak for Me? Improving End-of-Life Decision-Making for Adolescents with HIV and Their Families', Pediatrics. 2009 Feb l; 123(2): el99–e206, retrieved from http://pediatrics.aappublications.org/content/123/2/el99.long
- National Institutes of Health State-of-the-Science Conference Statement, 'National Institutes of Health State-of-the-Science Conference Statement on Improving End-of-Life Care (December 6–8, 2004): http://consensus.nih.gov/2004/2004EndOfLifeCareSOS024html.htm
- Wiener L, *et al.* 'How I Wish to be Remembered: The Use of an Advance Care Planning Document in Adolescent and Young Adult Populations', Journal of Palliative Medicine. 2008 December; 11(10): 1309–1313, retrieved from http://www.ncbi.nlm.nih.gov/pmc/articles/PMC2650081/

Additional Clinician and Patient Resources:

- American Academy on Communication in Healthcare: http://www.aachonline.org
- Initiative for Pediatric Palliative Care: http://www.ippcweb.org
- WebMD, Understanding Your Health Choices: Conversations Before the Crisis (2005): http://www.webmd.com/balance/understanding-health-choices-conversations-before-crisis

65

SCREENING FOR VIOLENCE AND ABUSE

Anisha Abraham

TEST YOUR KNOWLEDGE

98. The second leading cause of mortality in adolescence is?
    - A. Motor vehicle accidents
    - B. AIDS
    - C. Homicide
    - D. Suicide
    - E. Other accidents
99. Regarding bullying and teens, which one of the following statements is true?
    - A. 5% of teens are estimated to be involved in bullying or being bullied.
    - B. Bullying occurs more frequently among females than males.
    - C. School-associated deaths are quite common and the most common cause is revenge for bullying.
    - D. Bullies are generally physically aggressive and have a strong need to dominate others.
    - E. Teens who bully are unlikely to have any long-term difficulties or consequences.

Refer to end of chapter for answers on page 716.

"My son was recently in another fight and hurt his hand. He has had several fights in the past and has been suspended from school. What can we do to help him?"

BACKGROUND

- Violence is defined as the threatened or actual use of force against an individual or group.
- Violent behavior among teens results from multiple factors including genetics, family, culture and environmental influences.
- Health providers can play an important role in the identification and prevention of violence through careful screening for bullying, partner violence, fighting and abuse.

RISK FACTORS

Perpetrators

- **Individual:** Being male, history of early aggressive behavior, ADHD, oppositional defiant disorder, intense emotional response to threats, poor academic performance and/or history of physical or sexual abuse.
- **Family:** Antisocial parents or siblings, parents who use harsh physical punishment, poor parental supervision, parental alcohol or drug abuse and/or parental separation or divorce.
- **Environment:** Living in an urban area, rejection by prosocial peers, association with peers engaged in problem behaviors and/or lack of experience with nonviolent alternatives for resolving conflict.
- **Other factors:** Exposure to media violence (television, computer, music, and videogames), access to firearms, gang involvement and substance use.

Victims

- Prior exposure to violence or family history of violence.
- History of physical abuse, forced sexual contact or feeling controlled or worthless.
- Occasionally, victims can become perpetrators of violence.

ASSESSMENT

HISTORY:

- Ask a detailed psychosocial history.
- Ascertain specific violence risks by using the **FISTS** Questionnaire (Table 1).
- Assess for somatic complaints such as fatigue, headaches, sleep or eating disturbances, as well as irritability, anger outbursts, difficulty concentrating, depression, feelings of detachment, and a sense of foreshortened future.
- Determine if there has been a change in academic or social function.
- Be aware of special considerations: history of abuse, bullying, partner violence or fighting.

Abuse (Physical, Psychological and Sexual)

- Physical abuse includes punching, beating, kicking, shaking or otherwise inflicting physical harm.
- Psychological abuse (verbal or emotional abuse) includes acts that cause serious behavioral, cognitive, or mental problems such as repeated intimidation and insults.
- Sexual abuse involves fondling genitals, intercourse, rape, sodomy, and exploitation through prostitution or pornography.
- Victims can develop low self-esteem and feelings of worthlessness that may manifest as abrupt behavioral changes, such as self-destructive and/or sexualized behaviors.

Bullying

- Almost 30% of teens are estimated to be involved in bullying, as victim or perpetrator.
- Bullying can involve direct (i.e. hitting, threatening or intimidating) or indirect attacks (i.e. spreading rumors).
- Bullying is more frequent among males than females. Males are more likely to be hit, slapped or pushed, while females are more often targets of rumors and sexual comments.

- Bullying can lead to anxiety, poor concentration, school avoidance, and low self-esteem.
- Bullies are physically aggressive and impulsive with a strong need to dominate others.
- Teens (particularly males) who bully are more likely to participate in other delinquent behavior like shoplifting.
- Prevention is linked to raising awareness, increasing teacher/parent involvement, creating strict rules against bullying, and providing support to youth.
- School-associated deaths are rare, but when it occurs, the most common cause is retaliation for bullying.
- Encourage teen victims to report bullying to authorities and parents.

Partner/Dating Violence

- Violence perpetrated by male partners is usually related to beliefs of entitlement while violence by female partners is usually related to emotional reactions such as jealousy.
- Risk factors include a dominating negotiation style and anger management problems.
- Can occur regardless of sexual orientation.
- Victims are at high risk of experiencing mental health problems and subsequent abuse.
- Create strategies that promote healthy relationships.

Fighting

- Fighting is more common among teens who are: male, younger, use alcohol and drugs and carry weapons.
- Teens who are involved in frequent fights often do not know how to control their anger or avoid conflicts, and generally believe that fighting is the only solution.
- Ask specifically about weapon use, access to a weapon or knife, involvement in a gang or crew and means of responding to difficult situations.
- Advise parents and guardians to limit firearm access at home and store weapons safely (guns and ammunition stored separately in lock boxes out of reach of children).

- Counsel teens on conflict negotiation techniques such as trying to understand the other's point of view and considering alternative options for addressing the problem (i.e. avoid the problem by staying away, or diffuse the problem by taking it less seriously).
- Discuss consequences of actions such as benefits of violence versus benefits of walking away from a dispute.
- Consider counseling and referral for anger management.

PHYSICAL

General

- Look for signs of abuse including bruises on the skin, abrasions to the wrists and/or ankles, or bruises or lacerations to torso, face, mucosa or genitals.
- In cases of sexual abuse, examine for oral palatal, hymenal or rectal bruising as well as any evidence of sexually transmitted infections such as vaginal or penile discharge, genital warts, chancre or herpes lesions.
- Examine for fractures, burns, and patterns of recurrent injury over time.
- Observe for injuries inconsistent with the explained mechanism of action.

STUDIES

- In the case of sexual abuse, screen for sexually transmitted infections including gonorrhea, chlamydia, syphilis and HIV.
- Consider x-rays if fractures are suspected or CT/MRI if internal organ injury is suspected based on physical exam findings.

DISPOSITION

- Effective violence prevention strategies focus on: strengthening family relationships, teaching teens about the consequences of high-risk behaviors and encouraging them to stay in school.
- Teach alternative methods of handling anger and frustration and focus on individual strengths and positive coping skills.
- Help foster resilience factors that protect teens from violence such as a sense of purpose.
- For high risk youth, consider follow-up in the primary care setting or referral to mental health professionals. Physicians can also help identify

additional resources in the community such as homes for abused teens or other protective shelters in the community.

- Comply with state-specific mandatory reporting laws for teens: report abuse to legal authorities and social work services when appropriate.
- In cases where abuse may be ongoing, assess safety of victim, offer information on resources, encourage counseling, promote planning for specific situations and offer follow up.

What is unique about violence in adolescents?

- Homicide is the second leading cause of death among young people in the U.S., and the leading cause of death for African-American and Hispanic youth.
- Protective factors against interpersonal and self-inflicted violence include: zero tolerance for bullying, positive social orientation, school commitment and involvement in social activities.
- Adolescents aged 16–24 years experience the highest per capita rates of intimate violence, nearly 20 per 1000 females. About one in three high school students have been or will be involved in an abusive relationship.
- Early intervention, mentoring and positive youth development have shown efficacy in preventing youth violence.

TEST YOUR KNOWLEDGE ANSWERS

98. C. Motor vehicle accidents are the leading cause of death of teens in the U.S. followed by homicide and suicide as the second and third leading causes.
99. D. Bullies are generally physically aggressive and have a strong need to dominate others. Almost 30% of teens are estimated to bully or be bullied. Bullying occurs more commonly among males than females. Males tend to use direct means (i.e. hit) while females tend to be more indirect (i.e. spread rumors). School-associated deaths are rare although the most common cause is revenge for bullying. Teens who bully are more likely to be involved in anti-social behaviors as adults (i.e. stealing). Teens who are bullied may suffer behavioral problems including anxiety and low self-esteem.

Table 1. FISTS Questionnaire.

Fighting	In how many Fights have you been involved?
Injuries	Have you ever been Injured in a fight?
Sexual Violence	Has anyone forced you to have Sex against your will?
Threats	Has anyone ever Threatened you before?
Self-Defense Strategies	Do you carry a weapon? Do you have access to a weapon? How do you handle conflict? Are you part of a gang?

WEB REFERENCES

- Centers for Disease Control and Prevention, 'Youth Violence' (last updated October 18, 2012), retrieved from http://www.cdc.gov/violenceprevention/youthviolence/
- Finkelhor D, Turner H, Ormrod R, Hamby SL. 'Violence, Abuse, and Crime Exposure in a National Sample of Children and Youth', Pediatrics. 2009; 124(5): 1411–1423, retrieved from http://www.pediatricsdigest.mobi/content/124/5/1411.full.pdf%20
- Nansel TR, *et al.* 'Bullying Behaviors Among US Youth: Prevalence and Association With Psychosocial Adustment', JAMA. 2001; 285(16): 2094–2100, retrieved from http://jama.jamanetwork.com/article.aspx?articleid=193774
- Office of the Surgeon General (US); National Center for Injury Prevention and Control (US); National Institute of Mental Health (US); Center for Mental Health Services (US). Youth Violence: A Report of the Surgeon General. Rockville (MD): Office of the Surgeon General (US); 2001. Available from: http://www.ncbi.nlm.nih.gov/books/NBK44294/
- Ybarra ML, *et al.* 'Linkages Between Internet and Other Media Violence With Seriously Violent Behavior by Youth', Pediatrics. 2008 November; 122(5): 929–937, retrieved from http://www.pediatricsdigest.mobi/content/122/5/929.full

Additional Clinician and Patient Resources:

- AAP-Connected Kids: http://www.aap.org/ConnectedKids
- Centers for Disease Control and Prevention:
- Injury and Violence Prevention: www.cdc.gov/injury
- Understanding Bullying FactSheet (2011): http://www.cdc.gov/violenceprevention/pdf/bullying_factsheet-a.pdf
- Division of Violence Prevention: www.cdc.gov/ncipc/dvp/dvp.htm
- Love is not Abuse: www.loveisnotabuse.com
- National Sexual Violence Resource Center: http://www.nsvrc.org/

- National Youth Violence Prevention Resource Center: www.safeyouth.org
- Partner Violence: www.cdc.gov/violenceprevention
- Stop Bullying Now Campaign: www.stopbullyingnow.hrsa.gov
- Violence Policy Center: Research, Investigation, Analysis, & Advocacy for a Safer America: http://www.vpc.org/studyndx.htm

66

CYBERBULLYING AND SEXTING

Sadhana Dharmapuri

TEST YOUR KNOWLEDGE

100. The parents of a cyberbullying victim can sue the parents of the bully in civil court for:

    A. Defamation of character
    B. Intentional infliction of emotional harm
    C. Invasion of privacy
    D. All the above
    E. None of the above

Refer to end of chapter for answer on page 723.

"I can't go to school anymore! I sent this guy a sexy picture of me because he said he would go out with me. He sent it to all of his friends. Now everyone is calling me a slut. I want to die!"

BACKGROUND

- **Cyberbullying** is bullying which uses electronic technology (i.e., email, chat rooms, instant messaging, web pages and text messaging) as a means of harassing, embarrassing and threatening others.
  - There are no geographical limitations to cyberbullying.
  - All teens are at risk of being cyberbullied, but girls are more likely to be victims.
  - Traditional schoolyard bullies are 2.5 times more likely to be online bullies.
  - Perpetrators are more likely to be known to the victim.
  - Cyberbullying can lead to despair and suicide.
  - 20–40% of victims have also admitted to being cyberbullies.
- **Sexting** is the act of sending sexually explicit messages or photos electronically, primarily between mobile phones.
  - Images are usually sent to romantic partners or interests, but can be distributed to others.
  - Males and females are equally likely to send naked images, although males are more likely to be the recipient of these pictures.
  - Older teens and those who pay their own phone bills are much more likely to send and receive "sexts."
- Cyberbullying and sexting have been identified as more problematic than traditional bullying because of accessibility to technology, anonymity and lack of supervision or regulation.

ASSESSMENT

HISTORY

- Establishing a trusting relationship with a teen by active listening and asking appropriate questions can often confirm a history of cyberbullying or sexting.

Victims

- Determine technology use.
  - Does the teen have access to computers and/or cell phones and which applications are used (i.e., twitter, chat rooms and/or social networking sites)?
  - How many hours are spent on each electronic device?
- Determine the teen's developmental stage as well as level of understanding of cyberbullying and sexting.
  - Does the teen understand consequences of posting inappropriate messages or pictures online or on a cell phone?
- Is there parental monitoring (i.e., computer located in shared family space and/or use of filters and applications to block programs)?
- Ask if the teen has ever been bullied or noticed someone else being bullied online.
- Has the teen ever posted or been sent a "sexy" or nude image online or on their cell phone?
- Ask parents if they have noticed changes in behavior such as increased anxiety when reading emails or instant messages or feelings of anger, depression and/or frustration after using the computer or cell phone. Has the teen started to avoid the computer or cell phone?
- Complete a thorough HEEADSSS assessment to ascertain any other risk factors.
- Assess how upset the teen is about cyberbullying? Does the HEEADSSS assessment reveal any suicidal or homicidal ideations?
- Assess for somatic complaints: stomach pain, fatigue, headache, weight loss, sleep disturbance and/or changes in eating habits.

Perpetrators

- Ask the teen if they have ever bullied someone online or sent inappropriate texts or pictures on their cell phone?
- Ask parents if they have noticed changes in their teen's behavior including: quickly switching screens or closing programs when parents come into the room, getting unusually upset if phone or computer privileges are restricted

or avoiding discussions about what they are doing on computers and cell phones.

- Determine if the teen has multiple online accounts.

PHYSICAL

Vital Signs

- Tachycardia or elevated blood pressure may indicate anxiety.

General Appearance

- Observe for signs of depression such as loss of interest in appearance with poor grooming or hygiene or unexplained weight loss?
- Is the patient tearful or upset by questions related to cyberbullying or technology use?

DISPOSITION

- Encourage teens and their families to talk about cyberbullying and sexting and what it means in the context of the teen's life.
- Counsel teens to delete hurtful texts or sexts that they receive and not to forward these messages.
- Discuss the repercussions of sending and posting inappropriate texts or pictures with teen patients.
- The internet is far reaching and many colleges and employers now have access to social networking media. Inappropriate texts and photos may be seen by potential college recruits and employers which could affect college application hiring status.
- Encourage adolescents to report cyberbullying or sexting to their parent or guardian, school officials, physician or even a police officer.
- Clinicians should become informed about state anti-bullying laws which vary by jurisdiction.
- Cyberbullying or sexting may be punishable by law: Teens who send explicit texts may also be punishable for violating child pornography laws.
- Schools may have anti-bullying policies in place that parents and clinicians can learn more about by speaking to appropriate school officials including the school principal and/or guidance counselors.

- If there are no policies in place, encourage schools to develop official anti-cyberbullying and anti-sexting policies.
- Inform educators and schools about the harmful effects of cyberbullying and sexting.
- Educate school officials about the benefits of confiscating any devices on which they find cyberbullying messages or sexts, and encourage subsequent notification of local law enforcement.
- Ultimately, schools, parents and community members need to work together to educate teens about guidelines for appropriate texting and posting (Table 1).

What is unique about cyberbullying and adolescents?

- Teens may or may not confide in their parents or others if they are victims of cyberbullying or sexting out of fears of punishment or embarrassment; therefore, any complaints should be taken seriously by parents and clinicians.
- Teens may not understand the full repercussions of their online or cell phone actions, including the permanence of such posts.
- Teens place a high value on the opinions of their peers and this makes them more susceptible to cyberbullying.
- Adolescence marks a time of self-expression and the discovery of eroticism. Increased anxiety and impulsivity may lead to sexting.
- The excitement of the moment, lack of self-reflection and inability to process long term consequences may also lead to cyberbullying and sexting.
- Many adolescents are more savvy about the internet and texting than their parents. This imbalance creates the perfect set up for decreased parental monitoring, especially when compared to the degree of monitoring and control parents assume in other aspects of teen lives.

TEST YOUR KNOWLEDGE ANSWER

100. D. Each of these civil actions or remedies is available to victims of cyberbullying. There have been reports where the family of a victim sues the family of the bully when neither teen is of legal age. Such cases can lead to significant monetary payouts to the victim.

Table 1. Online and Text Messaging Guidelines for Adolescents.

When posting online or texting messages, ask yourself the following questions:

Who is the intended audience?

- Assume that *everyone* (including family members) will see what you post online or text.
- Your may intend to have a targeted audience (i.e. your best friend), but you really have little control over who will see what you post or text (e.g. best friend may share with others).

How will your post or text be used?

- People, including so called friends, may use what you post or text to make fun of you or cause you harm.
- If your worst enemy had access to your post or text, could they use it to make life miserable for you?

What does your post or text say about you?

- Colleges, sports recruiters and/or potential employers may judge you negatively by your posts or texts, especially if you use inappropriate language and/or images.

What are potential consequences?

- Embarrassment.
- Rejection by peers.
- Loss of parental trust.
- Rejection from colleges, scholarship or employment opportunities.

How can I stay safe?

- Assume that all posts and/or texts are permanent.
  - How would you feel about a message posted or texted tomorrow? One week from now? One month from now?
  - If you're not sure, better to be safe and not post or text the message.
- Communicate only with people you know. Never share private or personal information with strangers.
- Involve your parents. Show them what you are creating, publishing and posting online to establish trust and show that you have good judgment.

WEB REFERENCES

- Committee on Injury, Violence, and Poison Prevention. 'Role of the Pediatrician in Youth Violence Prevention', Pediatrics. 2009 July l; 124(l): 393–402, retrieved from http://pediatrics.aappublications.org/content/124/1/393.full
- Eisenberg ME and Aalsma MC. 'Bullying and peer victimization: Position paper of the Society for Adolescent Medicine', Journal of Adolescnet Health. 2005 January; 36(l): 88–91, retrieved from http://www.jahonline.org/article/Sl054-139X(04)00212-5/fulltext
- Lenhart A. 'Cyberbullying' Pew Research Center (Jun 27, 2007), retrieved from http://pewinternet.org/Reports/2007/Cyberbullying.aspx
- O'Keefe GS, Clarke-Pearson K, Council on Communications and Media. 'The Impact of Social Media on Children, Adolescents, and Families', Pediatrics. 2011 April 1; 127(4): 800–804, retrieved from http://www.pediatricsdigest.mobi/content/127/4/800.full
- Tokunaga RS. 'Following you home from school: A critical review and synthesis of research on cyberbullying victimization', Computers in Human Behavior. 2010; 26: 277–287, retrieved from http://icbtt.arizona.edu/sites/default/files/tokunaga._r_cyberbullying.pdf

Additional Clinician and Patient Resources:

- Break the Cycle: Empowering Youth to End Domestic Violence: www.breakthecycle.org
- Cyberbullying Research Center: www.Cyberbullying.us
- Institute of Medicine, The Role of Information Communications Technologies In Violence Prevention: www.IOM.edu
- Love is respect.org: http://www.loveisrespect.org/
- Project Anti-Bully, Cyberbullying: http://projectbully.com/cyberbullying.html
- SafeKids.com: Online safety & civility: www.safekids.com
- Stop Bullying Now: http://projectbully.com/cyberbullying.html
- Young Women's Health:, Cyberbullying: http://www.youngwomenshealth.org/
- cyberbullying.html

67

TOBACCO USE AND CESSATION COUNSELING

Brooke Bokor

TEST YOUR KNOWLEDGE

101. Which one of the following statements is true?

   A. Most of the benefits from quitting occur within 5 years of smoking cessation.
   B. Adolescents must quit tobacco use before they can start the oral contraceptive pill (OCP) because of high thromboembolic risk.
   C. An expected trade-off of tobacco cessation is an unhealthy weight gain, about 20 pounds on average.
   D. All the above are true.
   E. None of the above is true.

102. After two years of brief smoking cessation counseling at each clinic visit, your 16 year old patient with moderate tobacco dependence finally asks for aid in cessation. Which one of the following statements is true?

   A. FDA product limitations prevent use of prescription or over-the-counter (OTC) smoking cessation aids in patients who are 16 years old.
   B. There is clear evidence of tobacco dependence medication effectiveness with adolescents, smokeless tobacco users, and light smokers.

Refer to end of chapter for answers on page 737.

C. Abstinence rates quoted in the FDA medication guides for buproprion and varenicline, are based on studies in which patients were provided a patient support program and weekly counseling, respectively, in addition to pharmacotherapy.
D. All the above are true.
E. None of the above is true.

"I know, Doc ... I've tried quitting before but I get stressed sometimes and smoking cigarettes helps me relax. And anyway, I'd probably gain a lot of weight if I quit."

BACKGROUND

- Among the 20% of U.S. teens who currently smoke cigarettes, 50.8% tried to quit during the 12 months before the 2009 YRBS survey.
- 8.9% of U.S. teens had used smokeless tobacco on at least 1 day during the 30 days before the survey, with increased prevalence among males.
- Adolescents are more likely to be concerned with the short term rather than long term consequences of smoking (Table 1).
- Influences to start, continue and become dependent upon nicotine are multi-factorial and go beyond peer pressure.
  - Tobacco marketing targets youth and new users with flavored products and disproportionate advertising in predominantly African-American neighborhoods.
  - There is a genetic variant of the nicotine receptor that increases the risk of nicotine dependence and heavy smoker status for people who do smoke.
  - Tobacco smoke has ingredients, other than nicotine, that have been found to reduce the enzyme monoamine oxidase throughout the body, resulting in higher dopamine levels in the brain that leads to the desire for repeated tobacco use.
  - Adolescent females may initiate smoking for weight reduction purposes.

ASSESSMENT

HISTORY

- The 5 A's: Ask, Assess, Advise, Assist and Arrange is a model for evaluating and treating patients who use tobacco.

ASK about Tobacco Use

- Ask teens when they are alone.
- Ask at every possible visit during the HEEADDSSS exam.
  - Is the teen a current or former user, have they never used, or are they exposed to second-hand smoke (may provide temptation at home when trying to cut down)?
    - Identify type of tobacco use: smokeless tobacco (e.g., chew), cigarillos (e.g., black'n milds), cigarettes, etc. (Table 2).
    - Clarify patterns of use. Some teens use intermittently, on weekends only, with friends, when they have enough money to buy tobacco, or off-season from sports.
- Determine cut down or quit attempts: how many attempts and duration of abstinence?
- Evaluate for anxiety and/or depression which may precede tobacco use or be present co-morbidly.

ASSESS level of Tobacco Dependence and Risk of Withdrawal Symptoms

- Use the modified Fagerstrom nicotine tolerance questionnaire to assess risk of withdrawal symptoms and need for cessation assistance medications (Table 3). Higher levels of dependence correlate with a greater need for quit assistance.
- Ask questions for smokeless tobacco and cigar users. Nicotine exposure increases the longer that tobacco is kept in the mouth and if juices are swallowed versus spit out.

ASSESS Readiness to Cut Down

- This is best done assessing readiness for change (Table 4).
- If the teen is *not* willing to cut down, the treatment goal is to promote *readiness* to stop tobacco use, rather than quitting tobacco use.
- Future quit attempts are enhanced by using the "5 R's" in a brief intervention designed to take 3 minutes or less: Relevance, Risks, Rewards, Roadblocks and Repetition (Table 5).
- This intervention, as brief as 3 minutes, has been shown to significantly increase cessation rates in those interested.

PHYSICAL

Vital Signs

- Assess for tachycardia or elevations in blood pressure.

General

- Note odor of tobacco on patient or parent, or presence of "smoker's cough."

HEENT

- Assess oral mucosa for ulceration.
- Assess teeth for discoloration.

Lung

- Examine for evidence of respiratory compromise such as prolonged expiration and/or wheezing.

Skin

- Assess nails for discoloration and note any yellow coloration of cigarette holding fingers.

STUDIES

Laboratory studies are of limited value and not routinely necessary when assessing tobacco use.

Lipid Levels

- Long-term use of tobacco can increase lipid levels.

Cotinine Level

- Salivary and urine cotinine levels (enduring nicotine metabolites) can be used to detect primary and secondary tobacco exposure. Sensitivity and specificity is high, even with intermittent smokers. This test is currently impractical outside of research settings.

TREATMENT

ADVISE Tobacco Users with a Clear, Strong, Personalized Message about Cessation

- **Clear:** "I strongly advise you to cut down and quit using tobacco and I can help you."
- **Strong:** "Cutting out tobacco use is one of the most important things you can do to protect your health now and in the future." Or "Occasional social smoking is still dangerous."
- **Personalized:** "Continuing to use tobacco makes you ..." Tie this statement to current symptoms or relevant short-term health concerns, such as social and/or economic costs. It may be useful to incorporate the teen's response to the "Risks" of tobacco use question.
- Advise tobacco using parents or other family members living with the teen to stop.

ASSIST Those Ready to Cut Down on Use

- Help set a quit or cut down date and develop a plan.
- Engage social support (i.e. parents or friends).
- Warn patients about nicotine withdrawal symptoms: expect peak symptoms within 24–48 hours of quitting abruptly and recession within 1 month (Table 6).
- Clarify patient's estimate of the length of each craving, often much longer than the average length of 5–10 minutes.
  - Ask teens to time their cravings to convince themselves that they can wait it out.
  - Coping strategies to deal with cravings and withdrawal symptoms include deep breathing, drinking water through a straw and distracting through activity.
- Practice problem-solving and refusal skills.
  - Develop strategies to address triggers (internal and external) and exposure to other tobacco users.
  - Encourage participation in activities incompatible with tobacco use (e.g., sports).

- Anticipate obstacles.
  - Lack of self-confidence or treatment access may be hidden challenges.
  - Co-payments for counseling sessions or pharmacotherapy are common barriers.
  - Post-cessation weight gain averages less than 10 pounds and is more common in females.
- Refer to a local quitline.
  - Quitline counseling by trained cessation experts has been shown to increase cessation among dependent adolescent tobacco users, is free, nationally available by phone or internet and often has an easy fax referral system for providers.
  - Pharmacotherapy aids, e.g., patches and gum, are provided for free to those >18 years in many states.
  - 1-800-QUIT-NOW (toll-free call)
- Refer to counseling.
  - Counseling plus pharmacotherapy is more effective than either treatment alone.
  - Adolescent counseling that incorporates sensitivity to readiness for change and uses motivational enhancement and cognitive behavioral therapy (CBT) remains first-line, with almost double the odds of abstinence at one year than no intervention.
- Pharmacotherapy
  - There are single and combination medication regimens for tobacco cessation, but consistent proof of their effectiveness in adolescents is lacking.
  - All methods are solely FDA approved for those >18 years age, but many are used off-label for those under age 18 years with moderate to severe tobacco dependence.
  - Factors to consider when starting pharmacotherapy: clinician familiarity with medications, contraindications, patient preference and age, previous patient experiences and patient characteristics (i.e., history of depression, pregnancy or weight gain).

Nicotine Replacement Therapies (NRT)

- Bind to nicotinic-cholinergic receptors, stimulating continued dopamine release (but at lower rates than with tobacco).
- Designed to wean patients off tobacco with controlled nicotine exposure treating cravings and withdrawal.
- Risk of additive nicotine adverse effects if also using tobacco.
- No known health risk from long-term use, but pregnancy category D.
  - Over the counter (OTC) products are available for sale to those >18 years.
    - The skin patch has the most continuous delivery of nicotine of all NRT, but doesn't allow titration during the day.
    - Chewing gum and nicotine lozenges allow for 30 minute cycles of relief as needed, alone or in combination therapy.
  - Prescription-only products are also available.
    - The oral inhaler is a cigarette-like shaped product that should be avoided if the teen has a history of severe bronchospasm.
    - A nasal spray is also available, but is the most addictive form of NRT.

Non-Nicotine Containing Products

- Buproprion SR and Varenicline are prescription-only tablets recommended for 3–6 month regimens.
  - Since 2009, both share the black-box warning with antidepressants regarding risk of activated mood (given shared mechanism of actions).
  - Buproprion has been associated with seizures in patients with bulimia.
  - These drugs are pregnancy category C.
  - No dosing adjustments are needed for lighter tobacco users.
- Buproprion SR
  - Inhibits neuronal uptake of norepinephrine, serotonin and dopamine.
  - Unclear mechanism for tobacco cessation.
  - Found to decrease cravings and is also an antidepressant.
  - Can be used in combination with NRT.

- Varenicline
  - Competitively inhibits the nicotinic-cholinergic receptors while providing partial stimulation at the receptors, thereby decreasing the reward from tobacco use and mediating withdrawal symptoms with lesser dopamine release.
  - Risk of additive nicotine adverse effects if also using tobacco or NRT.

Most Effective Regimens (in Combination with Counseling)

- Nicotine patch (> 14 weeks) + as needed NRT (gum or spray) or Varenicline 2 mg/day × 12 weeks triples the odds of abstinence at 6 months, with a 30–35% estimated abstinence rate, as compared to placebo (6%).
- Next best methods include the NRT patch + buproprion. Current studies in adolescents show only approximately 14% abstinence rates.
- In patients with co-morbid mental disorder, avoid buproprion in bipolar disorder and eating disorders; however, it may be a good choice for those with depression.
- The patch is safe in schizophrenia.
- Watch for mental illness relapse with "self-medication" tobacco use.
- If patients express concerns about weight gain, Buproprion SR or NRTs (especially the nicotine gum and lozenge) can delay weight gain. Sugarless gum and mints serve as low-calorie substitutes for oral fixation.

DISPOSITION

ARRANGE Follow-Up or Referral

- Contact the patient within 1–2 weeks of cessation attempt: in office, by phone, or through state quitline referral (1-800-QUIT-NOW).
- Make a second contact within 4 weeks, and then monthly for the first 3 months of cessation
- Frequent, brief contact will provide relapse prevention: discuss progress, difficulties, and encourage the next attempt if unsuccessful: "Most successful quitters have tried many times before."

RELAPSE PREVENTION

- Most relapse occurs within the first 2 weeks after the quit date and the risk decreases over time; however, the risk for relapse can persist for a long time for many tobacco users.
- Those who identify relaxation and stress control as a primary motivation for tobacco use will require new coping skills to respond to stressful situations, i.e., deep breathing techniques.
- Those who identify habit, handling, and routine as an integral part of their tobacco use will need to disrupt all normal behavioral routines of tobacco use and find other hand-to-mouth substitutes before the quit date to improve the transition to abstinence, i.e., keep lighters and tobacco out of finger's reach.
- Teach each user to delay their immediate response to cravings, e.g, choose to smoke only after their 5–10 minute craving subsides.

What is unique about tobacco use and cessation in adolescents?

- Current animal research through the National Institute on Drug Abuse (NIDA) suggests that adolescents have greater biochemical susceptibility to tobacco addiction.
- Adolescent tobacco use patterns are varied and often episodic, e.g., only on weekends. They may not self-identify as "tobacco users," nor make traditional commitments to "quitting" versus "stopping."
- Adolescents are developmentally tasked with experimentation and boundary testing: talk with them about non-destructive ways to express their individuality.
- Adolescents need to feel control over their own lives: create a sense of self-efficacy by framing quitting as control over the tobacco industry marketing efforts to influence adolescents.
- Adolescents may fear being rejected by peers when quitting: talk about actual prevalence of tobacco use among peers to combat "everyone else does it" comments.
- Of the scant trials with evidence about pharmacological interventions among adolescents (nicotine replacement and bupropion), none demonstrated effectiveness for adolescent smokers. Counseling remains first-line.

- Adolescents with attention deficit disorder (ADD) have a higher incidence of smoking then the general population, probably the result of "self-medication."
- Mental health issues (i.e., ADD, depression and eating disorders) may perpetuate tobacco use.

TEST YOUR KNOWLEDGE ANSWERS

101. A. Since the Framingham study publication, coronary artery disease (CAD) has been recognized as one of the most important consequences of smoking. As in cancer, the risk of myocardial infarction is increased with the number of cigarettes smoked per day, younger age at smoking onset, and the degree of inhalation. This study of women and men, also suggests that most of the benefit of quitting occurs within 5 years following cessation. Excess risk of developing CAD is reduced by 50% within 1 year of tobacco abstinence (Campaign for Tobacco-Free Kids, 2010).

The World Health Organization (WHO) guidelines state that an absolute contraindication for estrogen-containing contraception exists only for women age >35 years who smoke >15 cigarettes daily. For women under age 35, the benefits of contraception outweigh the risks despite tobacco use of any amount (as a singular risk factor for CAD). The risk of hemorrhagic stroke is increased in females that smoke and use OCP as compared to females that neither smoke nor use OCPs.

The average smoker weighs 4–10 pounds less than the average non-smoker due to transient rise in metabolism and appetite suppression with each use of tobacco. The weight gained by quitting smoking brings most ex-smokers up to what they would weigh if they had never smoked. The health benefits of smoking cessation far exceed any risks from the average 4–10 pound weight gain or any adverse psychological effects that may follow quitting. Because it can take weeks-months after cessation for metabolism to normalize, such weight gain is expected within and lasting for approximately 6 months of cessation (Tobacco Research and Intervention Program at the H. Lee Moffitt Cancer Center & Research

Institute at the University of South Florida, 2000; A Report of the Surgeon General, 1990).

102. C. Pharmacologic interventions alone are not as effective as when used in combination with a patient support program. In all studies with varenicline (Chantix®), patients (age >18 years) were provided with an educational booklet on smoking cessation and received up to 10 minutes of smoking cessation counseling at each weekly treatment visit according to Agency for Healthcare Research and Quality guidelines. Studies with buproprion (Zyban®) have shown that >30% of people quit smoking for at least 1 month while taking the drug and simultaneously participating in a patient support program. Nicotine nasal spray (Nicotrol®) trials utilized individual counseling or group support.

Off-label use of pharmacotherapy is legally permitted (but not regulated) for those under age 18, but should be determined on a case-by-case basis in those with at least moderate level tobacco dependence (American Cancer Society, 2010). However, there is insufficient evidence of effectiveness of medications for tobacco dependence in specific populations, i.e., pregnant women, smokeless tobacco users, light smokers, and adolescents (Fiore, 2008).

Table 1. Health Consequences of Tobacco Use.

Short-Term	• Wrinkles, yellow teeth and fingernails • Bad breath, smelly clothes, house or car • Reduced sex appeal • Excess phlegm and frequent upper respiratory illnesses • Reduced athletic stamina • Cost $$$ • Harm to pregnancy
Long-Term	• Cancers (lung, oral, cervical) • COPD • Dyslipidemia and atherosclerosis • Heart disease • Diabetes • Stroke • Erectile dysfunction
Other	• Poor role modeling for siblings, kids • Increased risk for low birth weight newborns • Increased rates of infections in exposed children • Higher health insurance premiums • Employment or housing disqualification

Table 2. Tobacco Products.

Product	AKA	Description
Chewing Tobacco	Chew Chaw Plugs Twists	Sweetened loose tobacco leaves in pouches. A wad is held between the cheek and gum and chewed to release flavor and nicotine. Juices are spit out, or swallowed if more addicted.
Snuff	Dipping	Ground or shredded tobacco leaves in tins or pouches, moist or dry. A pinch is held between the cheek and gum. Dry forms can be sniffed. Juices are spit out, or swallowed if more addicted.
Snus ("**snoos**")		Smokeless, spitless tobacco in pouches that are held between the upper lip and gum for $\leq$ 30 minutes then discarded. Promoted as an alternative product where smoking is prohibited. Lower than snuff in carcinogens due to steam curing.
Dissolvable Tobacco	Tobacco lozenges	Compressed powder tobacco that dissolves in the mouth, like small hard candies (marketed in candy-like packaging).
Cigarillos, Cigars	Black'n Milds Swisher Sweets	Any product with a tobacco wrapper is a cigar; thin ones are cigarillos. All include tobacco. Can be bought singly and over the counter, unlike cigarettes, due to differing regulations. "Blunts" are cigars with tobacco removed and replaced with marijuana.
Kreteks	Clove cigarettes	Contain about 30% clove spice, but contain higher content nicotine, tar, and carbon monoxide (CO) than conventional US cigarettes.
Bidis ("bee-dees")		Thin, leaf-rolled cigarettes from Southeast Asia +/− flavor. Taste, small size, easy access, and appearance similar to marijuana joints make them attractive to young smokers. Contain higher content nicotine, tar, and CO than conventional US cigarettes.
Hookah	Shisha Goza Narghile Water pipe	Flavored charcoal +/− tobacco smoked through water pipe over 30–60 minutes, often in a group. One session is associated with greater CO +/− similar nicotine intake as a single cigarette. Falsely thought to be filtered out by the water.

Table 3. Modified Version of the Fagerström Tolerance Questionnaire (mFTQ).

Score: Sum total of 0 − 2 = No Dependence; 3 − 5 = Moderate Dependence; 6 − 9 = High Dependence

1. How many cigarettes do you smoke per day? >26 cigarettes a day (2), 16–25 cigarettes a day (1), <15 cigarettes a day (0)
2. Do you inhale? Always (2), Quite often (1), Seldom (1), Never (0)
3. How soon after you wake up do you need tobacco? <30 minutes (1), >30 minutes after waking (0)
4. Which cigarette would you most hate to give up? First morning cigarette (1), Any other cigarette (0)
5. Is it hard not to use tobacco in places where it is forbidden (church, library, movies, etc.)? Yes (1), No (0)
6. Do you smoke if you are so ill that you are in bed most of the day? Yes (1), No or not usually (0)**
7. Do you smoke more during the first 2 hours than during the rest of the day? Yes (1) No (0)**

**"Yes" to either of the last 2 questions suggests the need for help in quitting.

Table 4. Stages of Change.

Precontemplative Stage	Not willing to quit
Contemplative Stage	Thinking about quitting
Preparation Stage	Ready to quit and getting ready to act
Action Stage	Quitting now
Maintenance Stage	Sticking to the plan

Table 5. The 5 R's: Enhancing Motivation to Quit Tobacco.

Relevance	*"Why would quitting tobacco be important to you?"* Motivation to quit is linked to perceived self-relevance.
Risks	*"What are the 'not-so-good' things about tobacco use in your life?"* Early adolescents are less likely to think about or respond to long-term consequences.
Rewards	*"What benefits of quitting tobacco might you notice?"* Have teens focus on immediate results and exhaust their list: e.g., food tastes better, they can save money, perform better in physical activities, their breath and clothes will smell better, etc.
Roadblocks	*"What situations or things might make it hard to quit tobacco?"* This may clarify treatment needs (e.g., withdrawal symptoms, weight gain, being around other tobacco users, inability to otherwise control stress or feelings).
	"What are the good things about tobacco use in your life?" Can be used as a reverse method of learning about roadblocks. Usual reasons include stress relief, stimulation, relaxation and pleasure. Adolescents benefit from concrete problem-solving counseling, e.g., role-playing.
Repetition	Repeat this motivational intervention each time an unmotivated teen visits the clinic. Remind those in the *relapse stage* that most people require 6–12 repeat quit attempts before succeeding.

Table 6. Tobacco Use Withdrawal Symptoms.

Symptoms	Frustration, irritability or anger Anxiety Insomnia and bad dreams Headaches Tiredness Dizziness (up to 2 days after quitting) Depressed mood Difficulty concentrating Restlessness Increased appetite Tobacco cravings
Signs	Decreased heart rate

WEB REFERENCES

- NIDA. Tobacco Addiction. Research Report Series. July 2009. NIH Publication #09-4342
- Milton MH, Maule CO, Yee SL, Backinger C, Maiarcher AM, Husten CG. Youth Tobacco Cessation: A Guide for Making Informed Decisions. Atlanta: U.S. Department of Health and Human Services, Centers for Disease Control and Prevention; 2004. www.cdc.gov/tobacco/quit_smoking/cessation/youth_tobacco_cessation/index.htm
- Masters NJ and Tutt C. 'Smoking Pack Years: Calculator (2010), http://smokingpackyears.com/faq.html
- Benefits from Quitting Tobacco Use Fact Sheet. Campaign for Tobacco-Free Kids, http://www.tobaccofreekids.org/research/factsheets/pdf/0246.pdf. accessed Oct 10, 2010
- Booklet 3: Smoking and Weight, Forever Free Series. Tobacco Research and Intervention Program at the H. Lee Moffitt Cancer Center & Research Institute at the University of South Florida. 2000. www.women.smokefree.gov/landing.aspx?rid=3
- The Health Benefits of Smoking Cessation: A Report of the Surgeon General, 1990. United States. Public Health Service. Office on Smoking and Health. http://profiles.nlm.nih.gov/NN/B/B/C/T
- American Cancer Society, Inc. 'Off-label Drug Use: What is off-label drug use?', http://www.cancer.org/Treatment/TreatmentsandSideEffects/TreatmentTypes/Chemotherapy/off-label-drug-use, accessed 11-22-10
- Fiore MC, Jaén CR, Baker TB, *et al.* Treating Tobacco Use and Dependence: 2008 Update. Clinical Practice Guideline. Rockville, MD: U.S. Department of Health and Human Services. Public Health Service. May 2008. www.tobaccoprc.org/download/file/ClinicalPracticeGuidelinesUpdate08.pdf
- Rosen IM and Maurer DM. 'Reducing Tobacco Use in Adolescents', American Family Physician. 2008 February 15; 77(4): 483–490, retrieved from http://www.aafp.org/afp/2008/0215Zp483.html

Patient Resources:

- www.teenquit.com: Free online teen-centered stop smoking tools, including calculator of tobacco costs, based on the Adolescent Smoking Cessation Escaping Nicotine and Tobacco (ASCENT) program
- www.ffsonline.org: Free basic or paid premium Freedom From Smoking® Online program uses ongoing email reminders, online modules, and chat rooms to teach quit techniques and offer personal quit support; through the American Lung Association
- www.mylastdip.com: Free online smokeless tobacco cessation site with age specific programs from Oregon Research Institute (requires enrollment by patient in online research study)
- www.Smokefree.gov: Free evidence-based information and professional assistance to help support the immediate and long-term needs of people trying to quit smoking. Also www.women.smokefree.gov

- www.goaskalice.colutnbia.edu: Go Ask Alice! is the free young adult-centered online bank of health questions and answers, including tobacco and drugs, produced by the Alice! Health Promotion Program at Columbia University.
- www.nosmokingroom.org: Free site for girls age 5–12 and their parents to participate in educational activities about tobacco prevention and cessation

Clinician Resources:

- http://www.ahrq.gov/clinic/tobacco/tobaqrg.htm: "Quick Reference Guide for Clinicians;" a summary of the Public Health Service-sponsored Clinical Practice Guideline, Treating Tobacco Use and Dependence: 2008 Update
- www.GlobalTobaccoControl.org: Free online training module, "Role of Healthcare Professionals in Tobacco Control," including lectures on adolescents and tobacco prevention and cessation, developed through the AAP
- www.aap.org/richmondcenter/resourcesChapters.html: Links to state-specific data, reports, advocacy information, and local contacts and coalitions
- http://rxforchange.ucsf.edu: Free training for providers and trainees, based on the U.S. Public Health Service Clinical Practice Guideline for Treating Tobacco Use and Dependence, including selected readings, lectures with animated PowerPoint slides, videotape of counseling sessions, and role playing with case scenarios.
- http://smokingpackyears.com: Free online calculator for conversion of tobacco use to pack years, including estimates for pipe, hookah, and smokeless tobacco.
- www.lungusa.org/stop-smoking: Facts, figures, and tobacco-product updates from the American Lung Association
- www.cdc.gov/tobacco: State-specific data and database of all tobacco-related articles from the Centers for Disease Control and Prevention
- http://www.surgeongeneral.gov/tobacco/tobaqrg.htm

68

SUBSTANCE USE AND ABUSE

David S. Reitman and
Gregg Joseph Montalto

TEST YOUR KNOWLEDGE

103. Benjamin, 16, admits to trying alcohol numerous times. He confides that he often drinks when he is by himself and that his friends have commented that his drinking is "out of control." He recently got into a significant fist fight while under the influence. After he sobered up he had no recollection of the event.

Which of the following statements is true?

A. Because most adolescents experiment with alcohol at some point, this situation can probably be viewed as a variant of normal teen behavior.
B. Benjamin scores a 3 on the CRAFFT questionnaire, indicating that he is at risk of significant substance abuse (Table 3).
C. Benjamin is probably psychotic and needs urgent admission to an inpatient substance abuse center.
D. Adolescents do not consider alcohol to be an illegal substance; therefore, his risk of drug abuse is low.
E. Alcohol is merely an exageration of normal behavior for this teen and other co-morbid disorders (such as depression, anxiety) are unlikely.

Refer to end of chapter for answers on page 753.

104. A 17 year old male presents to the ED with headache, malaise, nausea, and vomiting. He is tachycardic; diaphoretic and appears confused. His neurological exam is non-focal. Initial lab findings are normal including a comprehensive metabolic panel, complete blood count, and CSF protein, glucose and cell counts. On further inquiry, he admits to "robotripping" with his friends earlier in the day. Of the following, which is the *BEST* plan of care?

   A. After 4–6 hours of observation in the ED, discharge to home once his headache is controlled and the tachycardia resolves.
   B. After sending acetominophen levels, admit for observation.
   C. Call his parents to find out if he is taking any other medications.
   D. Obtain an EKG; if normal, discharge to home.
   E. B and C.
   F. None of the above.

105. A 15 year old female presents to the ED with agitation, tachycardia, hypertension, hyperthermia, and mydriasis. She is suspected of substance abuse but her drug screen is negative. Which of the following "legal highs" did she *MOST* likely use?

   A. *Salvia divinorum*
   B. Mephedrone
   C. Spice (JWH-018)
   D. Kratom
   E. None of the above

"I think that my son is doing drugs and I want to get a drug test to prove it."

BACKGROUND

- Adolescence is a time when teens may consider experimentation with drugs of abuse.
- The provider caring for teens has an important role in substance abuse screening, counseling and referring for treatment when necessary.
- Table 1 outlines drugs that could potentially be abused including commonly adulterated or misused household products, and "legal highs" that are widely available both over the counter and online. Table 2 details specific substances and their physiologic effects on the body.

ASSESSMENT

HISTORY

- As with most sensitive adolescent issues, parents and teens should be interviewed separately to facilitate an honest and accurate discussion of issues.
- A thorough HEEADSSS evaluation can raise red flags in suspected cases of substance abuse.

Home

- Determine whether the teen's friends are using any substances, as this can put the teen at increased risk of also trying them.
- Inquire about recent changes to mood and any changes in relationships with friends, family members, teachers/coaches, etc.
- Has there been any missing money?

Education

- Has there been any decline or failure in the teen's school performance? Does the patient or family report difficulty concentrating or completing tasks?

This might suggest **substance use** but also requires differentiation from a **mood disorder.**

- Has the family received reports of school truancy or problems with the law?

Eating

- Has there been any change in the teen's eating habits? Have the family or teen noted any recent weight gain or loss? Chronic use of stimulants such as cocaine or methamphetamine may be associated with weight loss while chronic use of alcohol or cannabis may be accompanied by weight gain.

Activities

- Have parents noticed any significant negative changes in the teen's social group or activities?

Depression

- Does the family or teen report changes in sleeping habits and patterns? Sleep alteration and fatigue may be a chronic feature of many substances (e.g. benzodiazepines, stimulants, alcohol, club drugs, etc.) but needs to be differentiated from other co-morbid causes such as **depression, anxiety** or **bipolar disorder.**

Drugs

- Have parents noticed any chemical soaked rags or clothes (products are "huffed" by soaking towels or rags and then pressing to the mouth), plastic or paper bags ("bagging" where chemicals are poured into bags and then inhaled) or found any unexplained abusable product such as aerosol sprays, lighters, whip cream containers, solvents, etc? This may suggest **inhalant abuse**.
- Have the parents noticed an inordinate number of credit card-type gift cards, which teens have been known to use to purchase online "legal high" substances?
- If a teen admits to substance use, the clinician must determine the severity or chronicity of drug dependence.

- Screening tools are available to determine the potential for substance dependence.
- The **CRAFFT** questionnaire is a validated tool which can aid clinicians in their assessment (Table 3).

Review of Systems

- Determine bowel regimen. Chronic constipation may be present with **opiate abuse.**

PHYSICAL

- By the time teens come to a medical provider, many of the immediate symptoms of substances may have resolved. It is important to alert parents to signs and symptoms of various substances as they may often see teens soon after use. These include:
  - Drunk or drowsy appearance lacking explanation.
  - Anxiety or irritability.
  - Chemical breath odor that would be characteristic of **inhalant abuse.**
- The physical examination may provide minimal benefit for the assessment. Nonetheless, the evaluating clinician should note the following:

Vital Signs and Anthropometric Measurements

- Including height and weight noting any significant changes to weight.

HEENT

- Hyperemic or eroded nasal mucosa may be associated with inhaled substances such as cocaine or stimulants.
- Bloodshot eyes may relate to frequent marijuana use.
- Myosis can be found with opiate use. Mydriasis can occur with stimulant and atropine-like compounds (Jimson's weed).
- Poor dentition caused by bruxism, hyposalivation and dental neglect are frequently seen with methamphetamine use ("meth mouth").

Abdomen

- Hepatomegaly may be present if the patient is an intravenous drug user and contracts Hepatitis B or C.

Genitourinary

- Exam of the genitalia, mouth and anus should be performed if the clinician suspects that the teen may be offering sexual services in exchange for money or drugs.

Skin

- Icterus
- Needle marks along any vein in the extremities with intravenous drug use.
- Cellulitis or abscesses may accompany injection sites.

Neurologic

- Tremors may be present with chronic use of alcohol, opiates or benzodiazepines.
- In adolescents with a known seizure disorder, alcohol or drug use may trigger a seizure.

Mental Status

- Acute psychosis has been seen with PCP, ketamine and a number of "legal highs," particularly the synthetic cannabinoids (e.g. Spice, K2), and bath salts (e.g. MDPV or mephedrone).
- Lonely and impulsive drug users are at higher risk for HIV and for depression so additional screening may be required.
- Note: Experienced marijuana smokers are able to "hide a high".

STUDIES

- Indications for drug testing an adolescent:
    - New onset psychiatric symptoms or worsening symptoms.
    - New onset physical symptoms (such as fatigue or appetite change) without other explanation.
    - Monitoring compliance during a drug rehabilitation program.

- Note: Routine urine drug screens do not test for "legal highs:" synthetic cannabinoids, MDPV, mephedrone, Salvia, inhalants, and others.

Toxicology Screens

- Urine Toxicology Immunoassay
  - Tests for drug metabolites in a standard panel that usually includes: opiates, alcohol, cocaine, marijuana, PCP and amphetamines.
  - Can be adulterated by the patient. A directly observed specimen is ideal and is required in forensic toxicology cases.
  - Cross-reactivity with other substances is possible (e.g. a positive PCP screen may be caused by dextromethorphan abuse).
  - Presence (or absence) of a positive immunoassay may depend on:
    - Quantity of abused substance
    - Time since last use
    - Frequency of use
- Mass Spectrometry and Gas Chromatography (MS/GC) can be used to confirm presence (or absence) of specific substances which may not be seen on the immunoassay (e.g. dextromethorphan).
- Other tests: Can sample buccal mucosa, blood or sweat for drug screening tests.

Liver Function Tests

- Elevated AST, ALT and GGT may indicate chronic liver disease.

STI Screening

If the clinician suspects a teen may be offering sexual services in exchange for money or drugs, consider screening for genital gonorrhea/chlamydia, anal gonorrhea/chlamydia, oral gonorrhea, and/or syphilis and HIV.

DISPOSITION

Outpatient Drug Treatment

- Individual cognitive behavioral therapy (CBT): Help the teen recognize situations or cues that lead to substance use and then teach them to either avoid the situation or use skills to subsitute the behavior when the cue is present.

- 12 step programs (e.g. Alcoholics Anonymous) and/or group therapy: many groups, specifically for adolescents can provide peer-based support.
- Outpatient drug treatment centers may provide multiple modalities (CBT, family therapy, group therapy and/or medication) for teens on a short or medium term basis.

Outdoor Behavioral Healthcare Programs (a.k.a. "Wilderness Programs")

- Removes the adolescent from the substance abusing environment for 1–2 months.
- Teens work with therapists in an intense group environment, sharing responsiblities in keeping themselves (and their colleagues) safe.
- Intensive group therapy and survival skills are integrated into programs.
- Teens frequently transition to a residential treatment program following the wilderness experience.
- Can be very expensive and generally not covered by private insurance programs.

Inpatient Treatment Programs

- Indications include:
  - Severe psychiatric co-morbidity
  - Psychosis
  - Severe depression or mania
  - Suicidality
- Detoxification
  - Required for physical dependence on alcohol, opiates or benzodiazepines.
  - Treatment and monitoring of withdrawal symptoms.
- Patients should expect at least a 1–2 week inpatient stay.
- May involve group therapy, family therapy, individual therapy, crisis intervention.
- Transition to residential treatment program or outpatient day programs.

Residential Treatment Programs

- Generally long-term treatment (1–12 months).
- Frequently treat dual-diagnosed patients (psychiatric illness with co-morbid substance abuse).
- Recommended as "step-down" treatment from the inpatient setting or as a longer term treatment for patients who have failed outpatient management.
- Frequently have an educational component designed to keep the teen on-track to complete their secondary education requirements.

What is unique about substance abuse in adolescents?

- Adolescents frequently present to the clinician because their parents suspect substance use. It is important to create a dynamic where both the teen and family feel safe and respected.
- If parents demand a drug screen, it is important to discuss the limitations of toxicology screening (i.e. may have negative results if the substance already "washed out" of system, or if testing for substances not in routine screening) as well as how the results will affect the family, with both the teen and parents.
- Confidentiality in adolescent substance abuse can be difficult to navigate.
  - Violating confidentiality may hinder the teen's trust in any provider with sensitive information regarding future substance use.
  - Conversely, unconditional confidentiality may allow a minor to continue to engage in substance using activities that could put their life in danger.
  - A clinician may need to tactfully break confidentiality if an adolescent engages in activities that could place their or another person's life in danger.
- Teens requiring substance abuse treatment should be enrolled in programs that are developmentally appropriate for adolescents.

TEST YOUR KNOWLEDGE ANSWERS

103. B. Benjamin's CRAFFT score of 3 suggests that he likely has some issues around alcohol use and this definitely requires further evaluation. This degree of substance use suggests pathology and is not indicative of normal teen behavior, even if alcohol is not considered an "illegal substance" by the patient. Benjamin does not exhibit symptoms of psychosis which

would warrant an urgent inpatient admission. Nevertheless, when a teen presents with a history of substance abuse, the clinician must evaluate whether or not a mood disorder or other mental health disorder may be contributing to the substance abuse.

104. E. Many OTC formulations that contain dextromethorphan also contain acetaminophen. Acetaminophen toxicity will often not clinically manifest itself in the first 24 hours; therefore, without knowing the exact formulation that was ingested, an acetaminophen level is critical. Calling his parents to find out if he is taking any other medications is important, particularly if he is taking any SSRI medications. The combination of dextromethorphan and SSRIs can lead to a serotonergic syndrome. An EKG in this clinical scenario, would be of low yield.
105. B. This patient presents primarily with adrenergic symptoms, which most closely matches the effects of mephedrone, a form of "bath salts."

Table 1. Common Drugs of Abuse.

Class	Substance	Street Names	Notes
Stimulants	Cocaine	Coke, Blow, Nose Candy, Crack (freebase)	Inhaled or smoked.
	Amphetamine Dextroam-phetamine	Dexies, Speed	Frequently diverted from prescription ADHD medication. Taken orally or intranasally.
	Methamphetamine	Crystal, Crystal Meth, Meth, Ice	Synthetic "club drug" that can be inhaled or smoked.
	MDMA	E, X, Ecstasy, XTC	Synthetic "club drug".
Cannabinoids	Marijuana Hashish	Weed, Ganja, Grass Brick	"Joint" = cigarette while a "blunt" = cigar. Can be laced with PCP, smoked/baked into cookies or brownies for consumption.
Synthetic cannabinoids	CP 47,497 and homologues HU-210 HU-211 JWH-018 JWH-073 JWH-200 Many others	Spice K2 Genie Zohai Smoke Sense Yucatan Fire	Available online and at many convenience stores.
Hallucinogens	Lysergic Acid Diethylamide	LSD, Acid, Sugar, White Lightening, Yellow Sunshine	Synthetic and usually eaten.
	Salvia	Diviner's Mint, Magjc Mint, Diviner's Sage, Sally-D, Mystic Sage, Herb-of-the Virgin	30:1 female to male use. Adverse events typically not drug-related; rather injury-related due to disinhibition. Smoked or absorbed via buccal mucosa. Available online and in convenience stores. Illegal in some states.

(*Continued*)

Table 1. (*Continued*)

Class	Substance	Street Names	Notes
Hallucinogens (Cont.)	Psilocybin	Mushrooms, 'shrooms	Mushrooms grown in ground.
	Phencyclidine	Angel Dust, PCP, Rocket Fuel, Whack	Can be laced with other drugs.
Opiates	Heroin	Smack, Junk, Horse, H	Can be smoked, eaten, injected, or inhaled nasally.
	Oxycodone	OCs, Oxys	
Kratom	Kratom	Thang, Kakuam, Thom, Ketum, Biak	Unique compound: induces stimulant-like euphoria at low doses, and opioid-like effects at higher doses. Used as far back as 19th century for opium detoxification. Chewed, smoked, brewed into tea. Plant native to swampy regions of Asia and Africa.
Bath Salts	MDPV (methylenedioxy-pyrovalerone)	Bath Salts, Plant Food	White or light tan powder.
	Mephedrone (4-methylmeth-cathinone)	Meow-meow, 4-MMC, m-CAT, Bounce, Bubbles, Mad Cow, Plant Food, Drone, Meph, Spice E, Charge, Rush, Ronzio, Fiskrens, MMC Hammer	Popular club drug in U.K. Insufflated (snorted), ingested or administered rectally. Water-soluble, can be injected. Easily addictive.

(*Continued*)

Table 1. (*Continued*)

Class	Substance	Street Names	Notes
Sedatives	Benzodiazepines	Benzos	
	Ketamine	K, Special K	
	Gamma-Hydroxybuterate	G	"Club drug" and "date rape drug".
	Flutrazepam	"Date Rape Drug," "Roofies"	Can cause anterograde amnesia.
Inhalants	Nitrous Oxide	Whippets, Laughing Gas	Found in whipped cream canisters.
	Volatile Fuels/Solvents	Air Blast, Bullet Bolt, Highball, Huff, Poor Man's Pot, White Out	More than 1000 household products including markers, spray paint, air freshener, hair spray, cleaners, etc.
	Alkyl Nitrates	Poppers, Locker Room, Rush	Combined with Viagra, can cause hypotension.
OTC drugs	Dextromethorphan	Triple C's, Robotripping, DXM, Skittles, Red Devils, Rojo	Cough syrup and OTC cold medications. Some DXM-containing products contain multiple ingredients (i.e. acetominophen), increasing risk for unintended adverse effects. Can induce serotonin syndrome, particularly in patients on SSRIs.

Table 2. Possible Acute and Chronic effects of Abused Substances.

Drug	Acute Effects	Chronic effects	Notes
Cocaine	Increased HR and BP Increased energy and alertness Decreased sleep Euphoria Decreased appetite Mydriasis Psychosis Agitation Sweating Nausea Pulmonary toxicity (if smoked) Rhabdomyolysis	Cognitive deficits Psychosis Nasal Septum ulceration Interstitial pneumonitis Angina pectoris Gastroduodenal ulcer Abruptio Placenta	Withdrawal with dysphoria, fatigue, increased sleep
Amphetamine Dextroamphetamine Methamphetamine	Increased HR and BP Increased energy and alertness Decreased sleep Euphoria Decreased appetite Psychosis Agitation Mydriasis Sweating Nausea Rhabdomyolysis	Cognitive deficits Psychosis Enamel erosion ("meth mouth") Erectile dysfunction	Withdrawal with dysphoria, fatigue, increased sleep Increased libido with ejaculatory dysfunction (Methamphetamine)
MDMA	Extroversion Euphoria Bruxism Mydriasis Dry mouth, increased thirst Hyperthermia Dizziness		Use can exacerbate underlying depression and anxiety. Hyponatremic seizures possible secondary to water intoxification.

(*Continued*)

Table 2. (*Continued*)

Drug	Acute Effects	Chronic Effects	Notes
	Concentration difficulties Intensified tactile sensations		
MDPV Mephedrone	Acute psychosis Intense alertness Euphoria Empathy, talkativeness Intense sensory input Sexual arousal Perceptual distortions Headache Tremors Blurred vision Seizures Anxiety/agitation/aggression Depression Tachycardia and hypertension Urinary retention		"Bath salts" and "plant food." Can't be certain of other potentially dangerous ingredients not listed on packaging.
Marijuana Hashish	Increased HR Orthostatic hypotension Conjunctival injection Gynecomastia Slowed reaction times Decreased cognition and memory Psychomotor slowing Appetite stimulation	Amotivational syndrome Long-lasting cognitive slowing Decreased pulmonary function Inhibition of growth hormone secretion	Withdrawal with insomnia, appetite loss, anxiety, irritability. Facilitates hepatic fibrosis in EtOH abusers.

(*Continued*)

Table 2. (*Continued*)

Drug	Acute Effects	Chronic Effects	Notes
Synthetic cannabinoids	Similar to marijuana	Similar to marijuana. Reports of imperative voices and recurrent paranoid hallucinations.	Withdrawal, with reports of internal unrest, tremor, palpitation, insomnia, headache, diarrhea, vomiting.
Lysergic Acid Diethylamide	Altered perceptions of shapes, colors and time sense Increased aural acuity Visual hallucinations Nausea Blurred vision Dizziness	Depression Psychosis	
Psilocybin	Euphoria Hallucinations (visual/aural) Synesthesias		
Phencyclidine	Vertical nystagmus Ataxia Confusion Delusions Hallucinations Hypertension Amnesia (anterograde) Dysphoria Seizures Respiratory suppression Coma Increased threshold for pain, violence and unusual strength		Vertical nystagmus is characteristic of PCP intoxication.

(*Continued*)

Table 2. (*Continued*)

Drug	Acute Effects	Chronic Effects	Notes
Heroin Oxycodone	Euphoria Analgesia Sedation Impaired judgement and cognition Hypotension Hypothermia Respiratory suppression Ataxia Coma	Constipation Abscesses (injected) Arteritis, thrombosis (if injected) Hepatitis Glomerulonephritis Aspiration pneumonia	Withdrawal symptoms include anxiety, irritability, diarrhea, vomiting, abdominal cramping, myalgias. Antidote: Narcan.
Kratom	At low doses, euphoria At high doses, similar to heroin and other opioids Nausea, vomiting, diarrhea Nystagmus and tremor	Anorexia, weight loss, hyperpigmentation, psychosis	Can cause opioid abstinence syndrome (see heroin above).
Salvia	Agitated delerium, confusion, decreased inhibition		In theory, symptoms can be reversed at the kappa opioid receptor with naloxone.
Benzodiazepines	Sedation Dizziness Weakness		
Ketamine	Dissociative state Catalepsy Nystagmus Respiratory depression	Cognitive deficits	
Gamma-Hydroxybuterate	Dizziness Ataxia Short-term amnesia Sedation		Can be used as a "date rape" drug

(*Continued*)

Table 2. (*Continued*)

Drug	Acute Effects	Chronic Effects	Notes
	Confusion Bradycardia Respiratory depression Vomiting		
Flutrazepam	CNS depression and sedation Anterograde amnesia		Clear liquid. Potentially lethal if combined with alcohol.
Nitrous oxide	Euphoria Intoxication Analgesia		
Volatile fuels/ solvents	Eye, nose and mouth inflammation Respiratory problems Arrhythmia CNS depression/death	Brain atrophy Cognitive defects Hepatotoxic esp. when combined with liver disease	
Alkyl nitrates	Headaches Dizziness Hypotension	Methemoglobinemia	
Dextrome-thorphan	Visual, tactile and aural hallucinations Excitability Dissociative experience Anxiety Lethargy Euphoria Disorientation/confusion Increased perceptions Blurred vision Ataxia Nausea Hypertension Respiratory distress Nystagmus Seizures Arrhythmia	Cognitive deficits	May show up as PCP on toxicology screen. Can cause serotonin syndrome, particularly in patients also taking an SSRI.

Table 3. CRAFFT Questionnaire.

Car	Have you ever ridden in a **Car** driven by someone (including yourself) who was "high" or had been using alcohol or drugs?
Relax	Do you ever use alcohol or drugs to **Relax**, feel better about yourself, or fit in?
Alone	Do you ever use alcohol or drugs when **Alone?**
Forget	Do you ever **Forget** things you did while using alcohol or drugs?
Friends	Have family or **Friends** ever told you that you to cut down on drinking or drug use?
Trouble	Have you ever gotten into **Trouble** while using alcohol or drugs?

- The teen who answers "Yes" to 1–2 questions should be given brief information regarding the dangers of substance dependence.
- A "Yes" answer to 2 or more questions requires further assessment and intervention as the teen may be at risk of significant substance dependence.

WEB REFERENCES

- Anderson CE and Loomis GA. 'Recognition and Prevention of Inhalant Abuse', American Family Physician. 2003 September; 68(5): 869–874, retrieved from http://www.aafp.org/afp/2003/0901/p869.html
- Calfee R and Fadele P. 'Popular Ergogenic Drugs and Supplements in Young Athletes', Pediatrics. 2006; 117(3): e577–e589, http://pediatrics.aappublications.org/content/117/3/e577.full?sid=9e55254b-d75c-435c-9796-18905cf75612
- The Endocrine Society Position Statement: Steroid Abuse (June 2008), http://www.endo-society.org/advocacy/policy/upload/Steroid-Abuse-Position-Statement-w-Header.pdf
- 'Practice Parameter for the Assessment and Treatment of Children and Adolescents With Substance Use Disorders', Journal American Academy Child Adolescent Psychiatry. 2005; 44(6): 609–621, retrieved from http://download.journals.elsevierhealth.com/pdfs/journals/0890-8567/PIIS0890856709616415.pdf

Additional Clinician and Patient Resources:

- ASK Adolescent Substane Abuse Knowledge Base: www.adolescent-substance-abuse.com
- The Center for Adolescent Substance Abuse Research: http://ceasar-boston.org/clinicians/crafft.php (for the CRAFFT questionnaire)
- Clubdrugs.gov, A Service of The National Institute on Drug Abuse: http://www.drugabuse.gov/drugs-abuse/club-drugs

- DEA Drugs and Chemicals of Concern: http://www.deadiversion.usdoj.gov/drugs_concern/index.html
- National Inhalant Prevention Coalition Website: http://www.inhalants.org
- National Institute on Drug Abuse: www.drugabuse.gov/
- Natural Medicines Comprehensive Database: www.naturaldatabase.com
- Office of National Drug Control Policy: http://www.ondcp.gov/streetterms
- Psychonaut Research Project: http://www.psychonautproject.eu/
- Teen Drug Abuse: http://www.teendrugabuse.us

69

JUDICIOUS USE OF PSYCHOPHARMACOLOGIC AGENTS

Daniel N. Davidow

TEST YOUR KNOWLEDGE

106. Which one of the following statements is *NOT* true?

A. Adolescents on neuroleptic medications have a lower risk of tardive dyskinesia than adults.

B. Beta blockers can help patients with PTSD remodel traumatic memories.

C. Lithium may be helpful to patients with recurrent and persistent suicidal ideation.

D. Neuroleptic malignant syndrome presents with high fever and muscular rigidity progressing to rhabdomyolysis, delirium and even death.

E. GABAergic anxiolytic medications may help with sleep and sensitivity to pain.

Refer to end of chapter for answer on page 775.

A 16 year old female is brought to clinic for consultation. Her mother reports that she is currently on multiple medications: Zoloft for "social anxiety," Ritalin for "ADD" and Depakote for emotional lability. When she started to show poor reality testing, Zyprexa was added as an antipsychotic to her medication regimen. She has now developed diabetes.

BACKGROUND

- The shortage of psychiatrists, specifically those specializing in child and adolescent care, is forcing clinicians to become familiar with and increasingly dispense psychotropic medications.
- Judicious use of psychopharmacologic agents implies that clinicians be *conservative, informed, cautious* and *responsive* when prescribing these medications.
  - *Conservative use*: Use when necessary and no more than necessary.
  - *Informed use*: Understand the patient's diagnosis and targeted symptoms. What is the reason for prescribing the medication and how will it help? Be aware of potential interactions and side effects of medications prescribed.
  - *Cautious use*: Weigh the risks versus benefits of medications, and recognize that there are risks which are not fully elucidated. Make attempts to balance the known risks, potential risks and unknown risks against the benefits of medication use.
  - *Responsive use*: Monitor teens closely to determine if treatment is effective and address questions, concerns or challenges to adherence to treatment. Monitor the effectiveness of the medication to ameliorate the target symptom, and address barriers and stumbling blocks impeding treatment adherence.
- Clinicians need to understand the different categories of medications, their actions and side effect profiles (Table 1).

ASSESSMENT

HISTORY

- Making the diagnosis of a psychiatric illness is a thoughtful and disciplined process of evaluation, *not* made by merely "meeting DSM criteria." DSM criteria are designed to describe a diagnosis but NOT to define that diagnosis (many conditions present with similar behavior patterns).
- Patients must be appropriately assessed, as many psychiatric symptoms overlap and proper treatment depends on a comprehensive evaluation, including:
  - An unhurried and thorough interview of the patient and family with questions about the patient's past and current experiences and level of functioning.
- Determine if target symptoms are debilitating or significantly restricting the teen's function.
  - Is anxiety or depression preventing the teen from socializing or participating in previously enjoyed or productive activities?
  - Is the symptom disrupting family life?
  - Is aggression, impulsivity or delusion putting the teen at risk in her current environment?
- Determine if the teen is at risk to harm self or others, or at risk to be harmed or victimized.
  - If so, hospitalization may be necessary for safety and close monitoring.
  - If not, learn about the teen's support network and environmental stressors which might complicate treatment (such as legal, financial or social problems).
- Determine if the teen is a good candidate for psychotherapy and if such therapy should be used either before prescribing medication, or concurrently with medicine.
  - Are psychotherapeutic resources available and accessible?
  - Is the teen cognitively capable of participating in a discussion with a therapist to learn to make positive changes?
  - Have previous psychotherapeutic efforts failed? If so, why?

- Determine if there are medical conditions which could be adversely affected by psychotropic medication side effects, or if other medications are being used which could have undesirable interactions with prescribed psychotropics.

STUDIES

- When indicated, send laboratory tests for medical conditions which can mimic or exacerbate psychiatric problems (i.e. Porphyria, Wilson's disease, hyperthyroidism or pheochromocytoma).

SPECIAL TESTS

- Psychological or educational testing may be necessary to derive a complete understanding of the challenges the teen faces. These tests inform about intelligence, learning disabilities, skills and other areas of weakness.
- Some medications require laboratory tests for clearance.
  - For example, before initiating lithium, thyroid function tests, BUN and creatinine should be ordered to establish normal baseline thyroid and renal function.
- Some medications can also be measured for adherence or toxicity such as lithium or valproate.

TREATMENT

Consider Risks when Initiating Psychopharmacologic Agents

Known risks

- Include documented side effects and the risks of not taking the medication. Some medications have higher or lower associated risk of known side effects (Table 1).
- Avoid polypharmacy. Multiple medications given simultaneously:
  - Interact and affect each other's blood levels or create additive side effects or risks.
  - Add more variables and make assessment of benefits difficult.
  - Make treatment compliance difficult or unlikely.

- Use one medication that treats most of the targeted symptoms with the fewest side effects possible.

Potential risks

- Teens may use medications inappropriately in overdose, or abuse the addiction potential of the medication by selling or sharing medicines.
- Be aware of this possibility and maintain a high index of suspicion, especially with high risk medications such as stimulants, benzodiazepines and quetiapine.

Unknown risks

- Medication effects on the developing brain are not fully known and the brain isn't considered fully developed until a person is in their mid-20's.
- There should be a valid reason for initiating medication such as the inability to function successfully without it, or inability to meaningfully participate in therapy.

Psychopharmacologic Agents

- Table 2 illustrates case scenarios and choice of medication.
- Some of these medications are unlikely to be prescribed by a generalist, but knowledge about them is important because patients will report their use and often ask for "a refill."

Antidepressants

Often categorized by neurotransmitter effect. Some have mixed effects and others are more specific.

- **Selective serotonin reuptake inhibitors** (SSRI's) treat depression, anxiety and obsessive/compulsive characteristics.
  - Some SSRI's are sedating (trazodone, mirtazapine, nefazodone), some are activity neutral (citalopram, sertraline) and some are activating (fluoxetine, paroxetine).
  - Watch for **serotonin syndrome** if introducing or withdrawing these medicines quickly.

    - Symptoms may include: tachycardia, hypertension, hyperthermia, flu-like symptoms, myoclonus, restlessness, agitation, anxiety, nausea or vomiting.
    - Treat serotonin syndrome with benzodiazepine or propranolol.

- **Noradrenergic** (atomoxetine) **or dopaminergic** (buproprion) medicines can improve cognitive function and attention but can lead to agitation or aggression in high doses.

- **Tricyclic and tetracyclic antidepressants** have serotonin and noradrenergic effects, are anxiolytic and help relieve OCD symptoms.
  - Most are activating, but imipramine and amitriptyline can be sedating.
  - Imipramine helps with cognitive organization and attention and has been used to treat **enuresis.**
  - The sedating medicines often improve sleep architecture.
  - Doxepin has H2 receptor blocking effects to control stomach acid injury.
  - Newer mixed serotonin and noradrenergic medications have specific use profiles (venlafaxine for depression in opiate addicts, and duloxetine in chronic pain syndromes).
- Some medications provide antianxiety benefits.
  - **GABAergic** anxiolytic medications (eszopiclone, pregabalin) may also help with sleep and sensitivity to pain.
  - **Benzodiazepines** (alprazolam, diazepam, lorazepam) are also GABAergic anxiolytics, but have much more addictive potential.
  - Neuroleptic medications (typical and atypical antipsychotics) have powerful anti-anxiety benefits.
    - Risks of dystonic movements or neuroleptic malignant syndrome may outweigh benefits.
  - **Beta blockers** (propranolol) interrupt the feedback loop for anxiety, which may help patients with PTSD remodel traumatic memories.
  - **Buspirone** is an anxiolytic medication that also has potential cognitive benefits for memory and learning.

Mood Stabilizing Medicines

- Improve mood fluctuations and anger symptoms. Most are anti-epileptic and work by reducing cortical irritability.

- Valproate, lamotrigine, carbamazepine, oxcarbazepine, gabapentin, and tiagabine are most commonly used as mood stabilizers.
- Lamotrigine is associated with **Steven's Johnson syndrome,** carbamazepine with **pancytopenia** and valproate with **hepatitis;** although rare, these are potentially fatal side effects usually preventable with close monitoring.
- Valproate can rarely cause **polycystic ovarian syndrome** or **pancreatitis.** Liver enzymes and amylase should be monitored, especially if the teen reports abdominal pain or nausea.
- Lithium and topiramate have more serious side effect profiles.
  - Lithium is a membrane stabilizer and excellent mood regulator but can cause **hypothyroidism, diabetes insipidis and nephritis.** Avoid use in patients with diabetes mellitus and be aware of **teratogenic risk.** It has been found effective to combat recurrent and persistent suicidality.
  - Topiramate has a specific and unique benefit for reduction of cravings and is used to help with binge eating or bulimia and in various types of addictions, but can cause cognitive blunting, confusion and irritability.
- Clonidine and guanfacine inhibit norepinephrine release and help improve impulse control and decrease anger.
  - Known to improve attention, concentration and are also known to help decrease tics.

Neuroleptic Medicines

- Used as anti-aggressive and mood stabilizing medications, especially the "atypicals" such as risperidone, olanzepine, quetiapine and ziprasidone.
- Risperidone and olanzepine tend to cause weight gain and can lead to diabetes while ziprasidone often decreases appetite.
- Quetiapine has mood stabilizing and antidepressive effects.
- Psychotic or delusional symptoms are best controlled by neuroleptic medications.
  - Newer antipsychotic agents have less risk of causing **tardive dyskinesia** than older medications but still present some risk.
  - Baclofen, clonidine, benzodiazepines, or tetrabenazine may be necessary to treat the serious movement disorders which can occur during use or withdrawal of neuroleptics, but tardive dyskinesia is sometimes irreversible.

  - Young adolescents have a higher risk of tardive dyskinesia compared to adults.
  - Extrapyramidal side effects (stiffness, shuffling gait) can be warning signs of risk for tardive dyskinesia.
  - Request an **Abnormal Involuntary Movement Scale (AIMS)** assessment at regular intervals on patients taking neuroleptics to document symptoms.

- **Propranolol** can also be used for anger control by blunting autonomic "flooding," especially in cognitively impaired or brain injured patients. It also helps control tremors.
- Ziprasidone and quetiapine are least likely to cause weight gain but ziprasidone is more likely to **prolong the QT interval** or cause akathisia (restlessness).

  - Monitor EKG recordings serially.
  - Effects on the QT interval by different medications (e.g. thioridazine or nefazodone, calcium channel blockers, -azoles and -mycins) are additive.
  - Benztropine or propranolol may be necessary to treat akathisia if this side effect occurs.

- Aripiprazole is less likely to cause cognitive blunting and can even improve attention or cognition but has a tendency to provoke irritability and agitation or worsen psychosis in higher doses. Start at a low dose and increase gradually.
- Chlorpromazine can be used in low doses as an adjunct antipsychotic, anxiolytic or for help controlling nausea or pain.
- Monitor for **Neuroleptic Malignant Syndrome** with characteristic high fever, muscle rigidity leading to rhabdomyolysis and delirium (unpredictable and potentially fatal).

  - Treat with aggressive hydration, cooling, dantrolene, bromocriptine or benzodiazepines.
  - Hotline: 888-667-8367

Stimulants or Anticholinergic Medicines

- Cognitive/attentional weaknesses are addressed by norepinephrine/dopamine stimulants or by anticholinergic medications.

- Methylphenidate, dextroamphetamine and methamphetamine, like cocaine, increase available dopamine and should be used in the lowest effective dosage.
  - Overdosing can cause over-focusing (slowing processing speed), skin or nail picking, irritability, agitation, aggression and psychosis.
  - Mood swings can be seen when the medication wears off and the patient feels tired or depressed.
  - Short acting forms of these medications can be crushed and snorted by patients who abuse them, resulting in addiction.
  - Close monitoring of prescription refills is necessary to prevent sale or misuse of these Schedule II Drugs.
  - A teen who keeps "losing" his prescriptions for methamphetamine, may be selling, abusing, or sharing the medication.
- Alternatives to stimulants for attention and focus include buproprion, atomoxetine, imipramine, clonidine, guanfacine and aripiprazole.
- Dopaminergic agents, such as bromocriptine, amantadine and memantine are often used to improve cognition following brain injury but have the same risk profile as the stimulants described above.
- Anticholinergic medications, such as donepezil, inhibit anticholinesterase, and are used to stimulate memory following brain injury or in dementia.
  - May cause nausea or restlessness.
- Most psychotropic medications are pregnancy category C or D for teratogenicity risk. If category B, there is probably "not enough data" to define risk.

DISPOSITION

- Diagnosis, while valuable, is not a precondition to determining treatment.
- Some diagnoses respond best to specific medications or classes of medicines.
  - Example: If a patient has anxiety or depression and not ADD, treatment of an attentional weakness with stimulants could make the condition worse.
- Symptom clusters with specific syndromes allow for more accurate communication.

  - Example: A patient with Tourette's Syndrome would be expected to show tics as well as obsessive-compulsive traits, impulse control and attentional focus problems.
- Diagnosis may provide an understanding of the origin or intensity of target symptoms and guide decisions about whether medication is necessary.
  - Example: Anxiety generated by a situational problem may be more amenable to psychotherapy alone than obsessive-compulsive disorder or paranoid delusional anxiety.
- Rather than treating the diagnosis, controlling the target symptom is often the objective in medication selection.
  - May target depressive, anxiety, obsessive, compulsive, anger, impulsive, psychotic or delusional symptoms; cognitive or attentional weaknesses or severe mood lability.
  - The response of target symptom(s) to the medication must be evaluated objectively by obtaining feedback from the teen and family members as well as direct observation over time.
  - If there is more than one target symptom, a single medication that treats multiple symptoms would be preferable to the use of multiple medications.
- Arrange for appropriate follow up to ascertain responsiveness to medication.
  - Try to collect information from the teen, family, school and/or other relevant settings to assess the extent of the teen's successes or challenges.
  - LISTEN to the teen and respond to concerns.
  - Help the teen to understand the rationale for medication use, and try to negotiate acceptance of the plan.
  - Even mild side effects, such as headache, insomnia or decreased libido can cause discontinuation of treatment.
  - Is the medication causing a financial burden on the family?
  - What environmental factors are influencing the symptoms?
  - Does the patient need an alternative placement for structure or safety or to decrease the intensity of emotional stimulation?
  - Is the patient struggling against inappropriate expectations?
- Is the patient making use of adjunctive treatment?

  - Consider individual, family, group, cognitive behavioral, interpersonal, dialectical behavior therapies, etc.
  - Maintain a list of community support resources or social services to use if needed.
- If appropriate (i.e. the problem was situational), attempt to wean medications when it appears that the symptom has been ameliorated and the teen is more functional.

What is unique about diagnosing psychiatric conditions and initiating psychopharmacologic agents in adolescents?

- When making a diagnosis, consider adolescent specific concerns:
  - Personality Disorders cannot be diagnosed until a person's personality (ego, identity) is fully formed in adulthood.
  - Teens experience situational problems differently than adults as they cope with and manage environmental stressors or traumatic experiences according to their developmental stage. They may not disclose these situations until trust is developed. Post Traumatic Stress Disorder (PTSD) or Adjustment Disorder symptoms can look like many other psychiatric diagnoses.
  - Sexual identity is forming during adolescence and sexual orientation confusion often causes anger, anxiety or depressive symptoms.

TEST YOUR KNOWLEDGE ANSWER

106. A. Young adolescents on neuroleptic medications have a higher risk of tardive dyskinesia than adults. All other statements are true. Beta blockers have been found to help patients with PTSD remodel traumatic memories. Lithium is the only medication that can treat recurrent and persistent suicidal ideation. Neuroleptic malignant syndrome is characterized by high fever, delerium, muscular rigidity, rhabdomyolysis and occasionally death. Gabaergic anxiolytic medications can help with sleep and pain syndromes.

Table 1. Medication Side Effects.

Medication Risk	Higher	Lower
Seizure	Tricyclics Buproprion Neuroleptics	Anti-epileptics Lithium
Prolonged QT	Ziprasodone Thioridazine Nefazodone	Olanzepine
Irritability/aggression	Stimulants Dopaminergics Tricyclics Fluoxetine Paroxetine	Sertraline Citalopram
Tics	Stimulants Dopaminergics Quetiapine	Clonidine Guanfacine
Movement disorder	Neuroleptics	Buspirone Propranolol
Cognitive blunting	Neuroleptics Topiramate	Aripiprazole
Sedation	Trazodone Mirtazepine Imipramine Amitriptyline Clomipramine Clonidine Doxepin Ziprasodone Quetiapine	SSRI's Aripirazole Guanfacine
Depression/suicidal thoughts	Propranolol SSRI's	Neuroleptics
Weight gain/diabetes	Risperidone Olanzepine Aripiprazole	Quetiapine Ziprasodone
Teratogenicity	Lithium	Doxepin
Potential for addiction	Benzodiazepines Stimulants	Buspirone Clonidine Imipramine

Table 2. Choosing the Right Medication: Case Scenarios.

Class	Medication	Case Scenario
Tricyclic antidepressant	Imipramine	Teen with learning disability and attentional weakness who is obsessively anxious, has difficulty sleeping and enuresis.
Anxiolytic	Buspirone	Teen with developmental disability and situational anxiety, to avoid cognitive blunting.
Beta blocker	Propranolol	If anxiety is trauma related such as a brain injured teen who has a coarse tremor and outbursts of disinhibited rage.
Mood stabilizing	Valproate or Lamotrigine	Teen with bipolar disorder, type I and a history of diabetes.
	Clonidine	Teen with Tourette's Syndrome to improve tics, impulse control and attention.

WEB REFERENCES

- Agency for Healthcare Research and Quality, National Guideline Clearinghouse. Practice parameter for the assessment and treatment of children and adolescents with anxiety disorders: http://www.guideline.gov/content.aspx?id=10549
- The Center for Health and Health Care in Schools, The School of Public Health and Health Services, The George Washington University. Psychotropic Drugs and Children. A 2007 Update: http://www.healthinschools.org/~/media/Files/psychotropic07.ashx
- U.S. National Library of Medicine, PubMed Health. Clinical Guidelines for the Management of Anxiety: http://www.ncbi.nlm.nih.gov/pubmedhealth/PMH0008474/> http://www.guideline.gov/content.aspx?id=15096
- U.S. National Library of Medicine, PubMed Health. Clinical Guidelines for the Management of Anxiety. Depression in Children and Young People: Identification and Management in Primary, Community and Secondary Care: http://www.ncbi.nlm.nih.gov/pubmedhealth/PMH0015779/

LIST OF QUESTIONS & ANSWERS